FOODS THAT HEAL

A practical A–Z guide to over 1,000 food remedies to prevent, cure and soothe

Dr C. Norman Shealy, MD, PhD
Founder of The American Holistic Medical Association

Thorsons

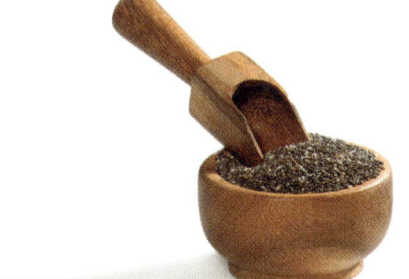

HarperCollins*Publishers*
HarperCollins*Publishers*
1 London Bridge Street
London SE1 9GF

www.harpercollins.co.uk

HarperCollins*Publishers*
Macken House, 39/40 Mayor Street Upper
Dublin 1, D01 C9W8, Ireland

First published by HarperCollins*Publishers* in 2014
This updated edition published in 2025

3 5 7 9 10 8 6 4 2

Copyright © HarperCollinsPublishers 2014, 2025

Norman Shealy asserts the moral right to be identified as the author of this work.

Cover designers: Peter Clayman and Louise Evans
Interior designer and picture researcher: Jacqui Caulton
Editorial Director: Caitlin Doyle
Senior Editor: Sarah Varrow
Proofreader: Lisa Eyre
Indexer: Ben Murphy

A catalogue record of this book is available from the British Library

ISBN 978-0-00-879737-9

Printed and bound in Malaysia

All rights reserved. No part of this publication may be reproduced, stored in a retrieval system or transmitted, in any form or by any means, electronic, mechanical, photocopying, recording or otherwise, without the prior permission of the publishers.

Without limiting the exclusive rights of any author, contributor or the publisher of this publication, any unauthorised use of this publication to train generative artificial intelligence (AI) technologies is expressly prohibited. HarperCollins also exercise their rights under Article 4(3) of the Digital Single Market Directive 2019/790 and expressly reserve this publication from the text and data mining exception.

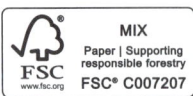

NOTE FROM THE PUBLISHER
Any information given in this book is not intended to be taken as a replacement for medical advice.
Any person with a condition requiring medical attention should consult a qualified
practitioner or therapist. The nutritional recommendations and remedies are the author's own.

Contents

Introduction	4
Dairy	27
Eggs	39
Fruits and Fruit Juices	43
Grains	103
Herbs, Spices, and Seasonings	110
Legumes (Pulses)	130
Meats	138
Mushrooms	156
Nuts and Seeds	161
Poultry	178
Seafood and Fish	188
Treats	246
Vegetables, Non-starchy	248
Vegetables, Starchy	285
Index	302
Select Bibliography	304

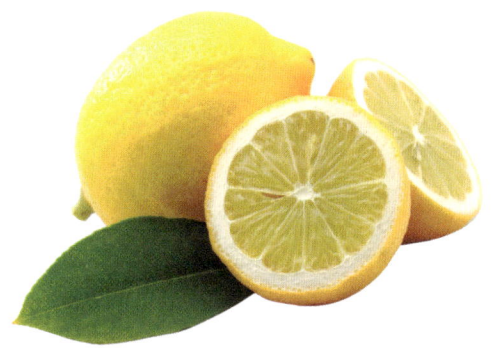

Introduction

"Let food be thy medicine and medicine be thy food."

Hippocrates, the father of medicine

Food is required for life. From the simplest one-celled organism to the most complex of animals—all require a variety of essential nutrients to stay alive and function healthily.

Over the years, a number of diets, both fad and scientifically led, have existed to promote a healthy lifestyle, reduce obesity, and improve well-being. Countless diets and nutrition regimes have come and gone, including, among others, the Paleolithic (Paleo) diet, with its focus on wild foods, the low-carbohydrate Atkins diet, and the nutrition-based, low-carb diet promoted by Dr. Broda Barnes. However, the most crucial element to take from any one of these is the focus on nutrients for health and listening to the needs of your own body. *Foods That Heal* provides a reference to promote health and well-being, as well as to cure ailments and illnesses, nourishing from the inside out. Feel free to read the book from cover to cover, or dip in and out, using the index at the back to guide you. Simple tweaks to your everyday diet could add up to huge changes in your future health!

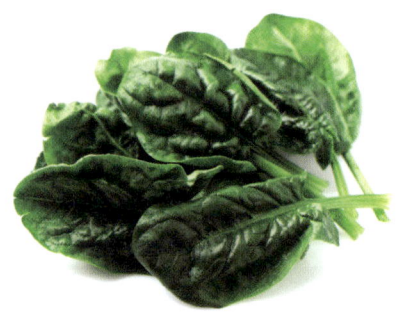
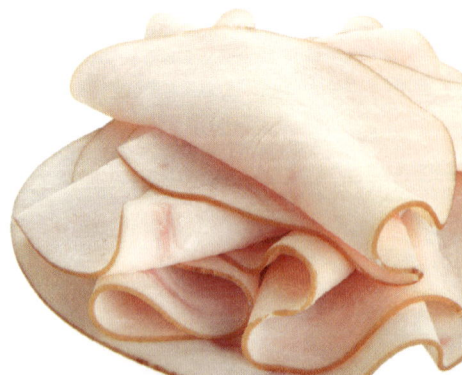

CURRENT U.S. DEPARTMENT OF AGRICULTURE AND U.S. FDA VITAMIN AND MINERAL RECOMMENDATIONS

Micronutrient	Current DV[1]	UL[2]
Vitamin A	900 mcg	3,000 mcg (10,000 IU)
Vitamin C	90 mg	2,000 mg
Calcium	1,300 mg	2,500 mg
Iron	18 mg	45 mg
Vitamin D	20 mcg	100 mcg (4,000 IU)
Vitamin E	15 mg alpha-tocopherol	1,000 mg
Vitamin K	120 mcg	ND
Thiamin	1.2 mg	ND
Riboflavin	1.3 mg	ND
Niacin	16 mg NE	35 mg
Vitamin B6	1.7 mg	100 mg
Folate	400 mcg	1,000 mcg
Vitamin B12	2.4 mcg	ND
Biotin	30 mcg	ND
Pantothenic acid	5 mg	ND
Phosphorus	1,250 mg	4 g
Iodine	150 mcg	1,100 mcg
Magnesium	420 mg	350 mg
Zinc	11 mg	40 mg
Selenium	55 mcg	400 mcg
Copper	0.9 mg	10,000 mcg
Manganese	2.3 mg	11 mg
Chromium	35 mcg	ND
Molybdenum	45 mcg	2,000 mcg
Sodium chloride	2,300 mg	2.3 g
Choline	550 mg	3,500 mg

1 The table lists the daily values (DVs) based on an intake of 2,000 calories for adults and children four or more years of age. The nutrients in the table above are listed in the order in which they are required to appear on a dietary supplement label. This list includes only those nutrients for which a DV has been established.
These levels may prevent serious deficiency diseases such as pellagra, beriberi, and scurvy; however, Dr. Emanuel Cheraskin (1916–2001) demonstrated in the late 1970s that the optimal healthy intake of many of these is far higher. For example, we know now that at least 1,000 mg, and even up to 2,000 mg of vitamin C is far healthier. And in adults at least 5,000 units of vitamin D3 is healthier.

2 The UL is the tolerable upper limit according to the U.S. government.

ANTIOXIDANTS

Antioxidants are essential for optimal health. If you eat a wide variety of real food, especially if 80 percent of your food intake is from the plant kingdom, you may get adequate antioxidants. These compounds help decrease free radical molecules, which damage cells and lead to every known disease. The best way to measure antioxidant capacity is Oxygen Radical Absorbance Capacity (ORAC). The following are the most critical antioxidants:

Anthocyanins—these great health enhancers are abundant in many fresh fruits and vegetables, especially the red, orange, and blue ones.

Ascorbic acid—this is vitamin C, and although ascorbic acid in foods is usually associated with bioflavonoids, Szent-Györgyi (1893–1986), who discovered vitamin C, took 10 grams of ascorbic acid daily. In addition, Linus Pauling (1901–94), an eminent 20th-century scientist, was said to take 25 grams. Bioflavonoids are additional antioxidants, but according to Szent-Györgyi and Linus Pauling, they are not essential, and most research on vitamin C has been done with ascorbic acid. I recommend for adults an average of 2,000 mg or 2 grams daily. In viral infections, I have given IVs with 25 to 50 grams daily for a few days. And when treating cancer patients, I have used up to 100 grams IV daily for two or more weeks.

Carotenoids—this family of yellow, orange, and red compounds includes beta carotene, astaxanthin, and lycopene. They are precursors to vitamin A and are safe at very high doses. I prefer 25,000 units of beta carotene and 4 to 10 mg of astaxanthin daily. If you eat cooked tomatoes three times a week, you will get plenty of carotenoids, including lycopene and lutein. Vitamin C, beta carotene, and vitamin E work synergistically, and all three are essential for a healthy immune system.

CoQ10 (Ubiquinone)—another master immune enhancer, as well as helping to prevent atherosclerosis. It is also available in a slightly different form as ubiquinol, which is much more expensive. Although ubiquinol may be more potent, milligram for milligram, I do not think the cost difference is worthwhile. A minimum of 60 mg daily is essential. If you are unfortunate enough to have been placed on a statin drug, you should take 300 mg of CoQ10 daily, to minimize many of the toxic effects of statins.

Flavinoids—additional antioxidants plentiful in fruits and vegetables.

Polyphenols—the final big category of antioxidants, best obtained from a diet plentiful in fruits and vegetables.

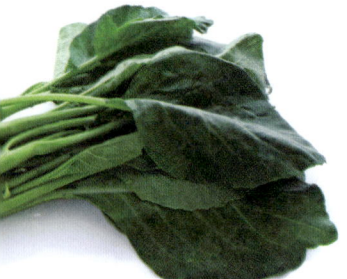
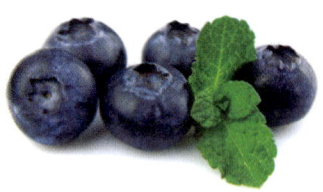

ESSENTIAL VITAMINS

Vitamin A—mostly from fish oils, such as cod liver oil. It is not essential if you get adequate carotenoids in your diet. No more than 5,000 units of vitamin A daily are advised, and I take none, because I get adequate carotenoids. Long-term intakes of 10,000 units of vitamin A can be toxic, and 25,000 units daily will make most people toxic within six months or less—with severe headaches and, essentially, swelling of the brain. Beta carotene, astaxanthin, lycopene and lutein are the antioxidants needed to provide vitamin A.

THE B VITAMINS

All the B vitamins are essential and required for day-to-day metabolism, energy, and function, especially brain function. Although there are recommended daily allowances and minimum daily requirements, there is considerable evidence that, under many stresses, much larger dosages are needed and indeed vital. Personally I think an average intake of 25 mg each of B1, B2, B3, B5, and B6 is wise.

B1, Thiamin—deficiency of B1 leads to beriberi, optic nerve damage, Korsakoff's syndrome, peripheral neuropathy, and heart failure. All animals require B1, which is made in bacteria, fungi, and plants. Interestingly, B1 is one of the few vitamins which can safely be taken in huge dosages, even up to 1,000 mg. Benfotiamine is a derivative of thiamin, that has been particularly useful in painful nerve disorders and is one of the safest energy boosters; 300 mg daily may give a big boost in energy.

B2, Riboflavin—B2 deficiency causes bloodshot eyes, extreme sensitivity to light, irritability of the eye, infections in the mouth and throat, a weak immune system, and sore tongue and lips. It is critical to energy production and to metabolism in general. Interestingly, 400 mg of riboflavin daily has been very helpful for some migraine patients.

B3, Niacin—B3 deficiency leads to pellagra with delusions, diarrhea, inflamed mucous membranes, mental confusion, and scaly, sore skin, as well as increased risk of type 1 diabetes, Alzheimer's disease, atherosclerosis, cataracts, and osteoarthritis. Niacin dilates blood vessels, and even 100 mg may cause significant burning sensations in the skin. On the other hand, 500 mg of timed-release niacin is one of the safest and most effective natural ways to lower cholesterol levels. Another form of niacin, niacinamide or nicotinamide, at dosages of 1,500 mg daily, is helpful in osteoarthritis and can be used in orthomolecular psychiatry at even larger dosages to help some psychoses.

B4—no longer considered a vitamin. Also known as adenine, it is a critical component of DNA and RNA.

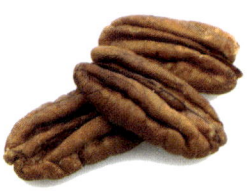

B5, Pantothenic acid—B5 is one of the most popular "folk remedies" used to treat everything from dandruff to gray hair. B5 deficiency mainly leads to general loss of energy, as B5 is critical to proper metabolism of fats, as well as proteins and carbohydrates. In general, true deficiency occurs primarily in alcoholics and individuals on radically deficient diets. Meats, dairy products, and whole grains are all good sources of B5. High dosages of B5 may cause diarrhea, so I would not recommend more than 25 mg daily, except in rare medically supervised situations.

B6, Pyridoxine (also pyridoxyl and pridoxamine)—B6 occurs in nature in much smaller concentrations than B1, B2, and B3. Deficiency is found especially in patients with heart disease, atherosclerosis, premenstrual syndrome, and carpal tunnel syndrome. It works synergistically to assist in magnesium metabolism, and is safe long term at 100 mg per day.

In short-term use, carpal tunnel syndrome responds well to 1,000 mg daily for one month only, 500 mg daily for the second month, and then 100 mg daily. Longer-term use of over 100 mg daily may lead to significant neuropathy.

B7, Biotin—B7 deficiency leads to fatigue, depression, hair loss, nausea, muscle pains, and anemia. Since it is widely available in a variety of foods, deficiency implies a very inadequate diet, or may be found in those who are on some anti-epilepsy drugs.

B8, Inositol—B8 deficiency leads to weakness of the immune system, skin problems, neurological problems, anxiety, depression, polycystic ovaries, psoriasis, hair loss, and fatigue. It is important in cholesterol metabolism and particularly in preventing metabolic syndrome and diabetes. Inositol plus choline makes up lecithin, one of the most critical compounds for nerve function and for memory. Dosages of up to 100 mg of inositol are well tolerated by most people.

B9, Folate (folic acid)—B9 is one of the most critical vitamins, especially during pregnancy, where deficiencies increase the risk of spinal defects and mental retardation in the fetus. In the general population, folate is particularly important in all aspects of brain function and in cholesterol metabolism. Deficiencies also lead to homocysteine increases, and blood levels above 7.5 micromoles per liter are associated with increasing risks of hypertension, heart disease, stroke, and Alzheimer's disease. In the 1970s, Kurt Oster (1909–88) demonstrated that homogenization of milk led to increased cholesterol and markedly increased the need for folate, with some individuals requiring up to 80 mg daily. It is available in 100 mg capsules, which is what I take daily.

B10, PABA (para amino benzoic acid)—B10 deficiency leads to vitiligo, pemphigus, a variety of autoimmune diseases such as scleroderma, infertility, lupus, rheumatic fever, Peyronie's disease, anemia, and headache. Unfortunately, dermatologists have pushed PABA as a sunscreen, thus even the small amount of exposure to sun that most people get does not allow them the benefit of sunlight—making vitamin D3. On the other hand, it is a superb way to assist in tanning and avoiding sunburn; 2,000 mg taken orally, especially when combined with 10 mg of astaxanthin, helps markedly in avoiding sunburn. Obviously, it is still important to increase sun exposure slowly—say an hour or two daily and build up. If you are out for more than four hours in the sun, take a second dose of 2,000 mg.

B11, Salicylic acid—B11 is formed in the body from the amino acid phenylalanine, an essential amino acid. It is critical in both DNA and RNA metabolism. Deficiency of B11 leads to anemia, fatigue, poor appetite, and damage to the skin and small intestine.

B12, Cobalamine (also methylcobalamine)—B12 deficiency leads to pernicious anemia, and severe damage to the spinal cord and brain. B12 is found only in animal protein, and all vegans eventually become anemic if they do not take B12 supplements. B12 absorption requires intrinsic factors found in the stomach; however, increasingly after age 60, many individuals develop a deficiency of intrinsic factors. The mucosa of the mouth (sublingual) may absorb B12 better than the stomach, but many with B12 deficiency require shots of this critical vitamin.

I think a minimum of 1,000 mcg daily is essential, and in some situations where there is general fatigue, up to 5,000 mcg daily is beneficial.

Vitamin C (ascorbic acid)—Vitamin C is one of the most critical vitamins supporting immune health. The paltry 60 mg recommended daily amount is only 6 percent of that which Dr. Emanuel Cheraskin, a pioneer in vitamin requirement research, found optimal over 30 years ago. I personally recommend 2,000 mg daily for adults. Furthermore, vitamin C does not help restore the most important hormone dehydroepiandrosterone (DHEA), which becomes significantly depleted after age 30, so that by age 80 most individuals have less than 10 percent of what they had at age 25. I have found that 2,000 mg of vitamin C plus 1,000 mg of methyl sufonyl sulfate, raises DHEA by an average of 60 percent (the exact range is a 30 to 100 percent increase). On the other hand, a very small percentage of people who take larger doses of vitamin C will develop kidney stones unless they also take 25 mg of B6 daily. Of course, as I have said, I recommend 25 mg of B1, B2, B3, B5, and B6 for all adults. And in viral infections I have given hundreds of IVs of 25 grams of vitamin C with 100 mg of B6, while in cancer treatment I have given many of the patients 100 grams of vitamin C with 200 mg of B6.

Vitamin D3—of all vitamins, D3 is by far the most commonly deficient. This deficiency leads to a weak immune system, osteoporosis, and increases the risk of arteriosclerosis. Vitamin D3 is the vitamin we make when our skin is exposed to sunlight, and to a great extent deficiency occurs because we live in modern-day caves, and even in the short time most people are outside, they are advised to use sunscreen. The minimum healthy level of D3 intake is 2,000 units daily and the safe level is up to 10,000 units daily. I recommend 50,000 units of D3 once a week. This is safe for adults and is far less expensive than taking daily supplements. For children I recommend taking 50,000 units of D3 once a month by age two. Taking this optimal level of D3 cuts the rate of colds and influenza by at least 80 percent. D3 is critical for immune health, bone health and strength, and arterial health. If you take no other supplement, take D3. Incidentally, for some reason, the D vitamin that most physicians recommend by prescription is D2, which is far inferior to D3.

Vitamin E, Tocopherols (also tocotrienols)—in infants, vitamin E deficiency leads to blindness, delayed growth, and physical and mental problems. In children, E deficiency leads to liver disease and severe brain damage. In adults, E deficiency leads to cataracts, anemia, age spots, decreased libido, infertility, atherosclerosis, and muscle, liver, bone marrow, and brain dysfunctions. For many decades we were told only about tocopherols—alpha, delta, and gamma—and the mixture was considered most beneficial. More recently it has become unequivocally proven that tocotrienols, the other limb of the E family, are far more potent. The single best source is annatto seeds, not a food we eat commonly. A mixture of just 100 mg daily of the tocotrienols appears to be optimal. It is important to emphasize that there is significant interaction between vitamins A, C, and E, so that a deficiency in any one of these interferes with optimal function of the others.

CARBOHYDRATES

Carbohydrates consist of sugars and starches, each of which is used by the body to produce energy. On the other hand, if more calories are consumed than are burned, carbohydrates are the major contributor to the obesity epidemic. The major reason for the carbohydrate excess is refined wheat products, table sugar (sucrose), and corn-based fructose. Not one of these three products is natural. Indeed, in general sucrose is primarily made from sugarcane or sugar beets, which are refined to remove all the vitamins and fiber. Thus, intake of these artificial products leads to their robbing the body of its vitamins and minerals in order to metabolize the sugars. I personally have not brought sugar or white flour into my home in many years. And, of course, there is no excuse to bring in fructose, the current favorite of the food industry.

White "enriched" flour and bread are also oxymorons. They have no real nutritional value and do a lot of harm. The bottom line is that we need no added high-carbohydrate foods. Indeed, we could live without any carbohydrates, as we can make all the energy we need from fats and proteins. On the other hand, the healthy vegetables, even those with high starch, and the plethora of wonderful fruits carry with them some of our most essential nutrients, vitamins, minerals, and antioxidants.

My number one recommendation for nutrition is to avoid all fast-food restaurants and all packaged, "refined" foods. If the package lists more than basic real food and a bit of salt, it likely contains many of the toxins listed earlier. In the average grocery store, 60 percent of the "food" is junk, and in fast-food restaurants virtually 100 percent is junk.

Throughout the book, "glycemic load" measurements are provided. The glycemic load is the measurement of the amount of carbohydrate in a serving of food. This is not to be confused with the "glycemic index" measurement, which defines how fast a carbohydrate is released as sugar into the blood after eating.

Glucose (Dextrose)

Most simple sugars are found in two chemical variations, L- and D-, meaning rotated left or right. Glucose is the D-form of the simple monosaccharide responsible for our "blood sugar", the foundation for the Krebs cycle, our energy mechanism, which can use carbohydrates, fats, or amino acids to produce glucose and convert it to citric acid. It is critical that our blood sugar is in the range of 70 to 100 mg/dL when fasting. Ideally, even after a meal, the level should not go above 160 mg/dL. Blood sugar levels below 50 are considered hypoglycemic and can lead to seizures or loss of consciousness. High levels eventually lead to diabetes mellitus, one of the more serious chronic diseases, which leads to increased risks of cancer, hypertension, and stroke. Type 1 diabetes is a disease beginning in childhood or young adulthood, resulting from severe failure of the pancreas. Adult onset or type 2 diabetes is largely the result of excess caloric intake and obesity.

Fructose

Fructose is a much sweeter form of simple sugar, normally found in fruits and honey, but most often as a mixture of dextrose and fructose. High fructose, largely extracted from corn, has become a modern plague, one highly responsible for the obesity epidemic. There are no health benefits to fructose or dextrose when extracted from their natural source.

Sucrose, a disaccharide chemical bonding of glucose and fructose, is almost nonexistent except in sugarcane and sugar beets. Once removed from the cane or beets, sucrose is actually toxic, as it lacks all the vitamins and minerals needed to metabolize it. Although healthy individuals can handle 5 to 7 teaspoons of sucrose fairly well, if they have an otherwise healthy, balanced diet, the average American eats 42 teaspoons daily! It is a major contributor to obesity, heart disease, cancer, and diabetes, and was the first "artificial" food.

Honey consists of a mixture of fructose and dextrose, with various percentages depending on the flower source. Interestingly, it is sweeter than dextrose, fructose, or sucrose, so that total sweetness is achieved with one-third less volume than those sources. Natural raw honey has many advantages over sucrose or fructose or any of the artificial sweeteners. If obtained from local sources, it has local pollen and may help prevent seasonal allergies. It contains a small amount of protein, some B vitamins, and a wide variety of essential minerals, especially potassium—similar to a fruit. Obviously, it should be eaten in moderation. Except for those who are obese or who have diabetes, using, at the most, up to 5 teaspoons of honey daily is reasonable. Incidentally, honey with cinnamon is much healthier than honey alone. Cinnamon is a great source of chromium, essential for the metabolism of carbohydrates.

Of course, the natural source of fructose or dextrose—fruits—also come with vitamins and minerals, unless they have been artificially removed.

Starches

Complex carbohydrates are found in many starchy vegetables, which are fine eaten in moderation because they also provide vitamins, minerals, and fiber. However, starches provide no health benefits.

FATS

Amino acids and carbohydrates have 4 calories per gram of consumption. Fats carry a whopping 9 calories per gram—although as with all foods, there are some that are healthier than others. Fats have long chains of hydrocarbons—carbon molecules with hydrogen molecules. Saturated fats have no open hydrogen bonds. Monounsaturated fats have one open hydrogen bond and are by far the healthiest, but interestingly, if you take in adequate omega-3s and 6s, you can make all the omega-9 fats you need. Polyunsaturated fats have multiple open hydrogen bonds, favorites of the food industry, which delights in hydrogenating or "saturating" them, producing the totally unnatural and toxic trans-fats. Avoid these artificial foods.

Omega-3

Omega-3s are alpha linolenic acid (ALA), eicosapentaenoic acid (EPA), and docosahexaenoic acid (DHA) and are by far the most "essential" fats, as they are anti-inflammatory. They are also among the most critical essential nutrients. Deficiencies lead to low HDL cholesterol and high LDL and triglycerides, and such diverse problems as depression, high blood pressure, atherosclerosis, eclampsia, macular degeneration, schizophrenia, Alzheimer's, and diabetes. The single best source is wild salmon. Grass-fed beef, beefalo, chicken, and turkey are also excellent. Personally, because I eat a lot of wild salmon and grass-fed meats, I take only 1,000 mg of good omega-3s daily. Because of the potential of mercury contamination in salmon, any supplement of omega-3 should be guaranteed to be mercury-free.

Health benefits (helps with or helps to prevent):
- Arthritis
- Asthma
- Attention Deficit Disorder
- Depression
- Diabetes
- Digestion
- Elevated cholesterol
- Hypertension
- Immune strength
- Macular degeneration
- Osteoporosis
- Cancer

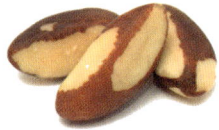

Best sources of omega-3s:
- Wild salmon
- Grass-fed meats and fowl
- Brazil nuts
- Chia seeds
- Flaxseed oil
- Hemp seed oil
- Pumpkin seeds
- Walnut
- Green leafy veggies
- Wheat germ oil

Omega-6

Although omega-6 fats are also essential polyunsaturated fats, the average diet is overloaded with omega-6s, which are found in canola oil, corn oil, peanut oil, safflower oil, soy oil, and sunflower oil, all of which are heavily used by the food industry. I do not recommend any of those oils, as they have a high content of linoleic acid (LA), which is inflammatory. Although LA can be converted to the healthier gamma linoleic acid (GLA), that process is not guaranteed, as many other nutrients are needed for proper conversion. The only good sources of omega-6 are evening primrose oil and blackcurrant seed oil, which naturally contain higher amounts of GLA; however, these can also be inflammatory in high concentrations.

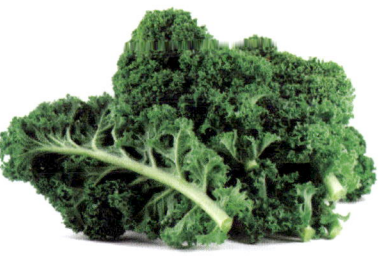

The bottom line is you need a ratio of one to one omega-3s to omega-6s. In this optimal ratio, the health benefits are the same as those listed above for omega-3s.

Best sources of omega-6s:
- Raw nuts and seeds
- Evening primose and blackcurrant seed oil

Omega-9

These are the monounsaturated fats, and are not "essential" fatty acids. If you get adequate omega-3s and omega-6s, you do not need an intake of omega-9s.

Best sources of omega-9s:
- Almonds
- Avocados
- Cashews
- Chia seeds
- Hazelnuts
- Macadamia nuts
- Pecans
- Pistachios
- Olives and olive oil

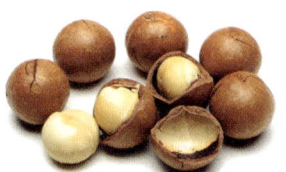
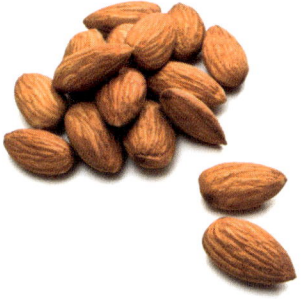

ESSENTIAL AMINO ACIDS

Although most scientific sources state that there are nine essential amino acids, some also consider taurine to be "conditionally" essential. Considering the fact that 84 percent of depressed people are deficient in taurine, I consider it essential. In general, all the essential amino acids are the L-form, that is, rotated on their axis to the left. A few specific examples of D-amino acids will be mentioned. Most amino acids are simple straight "chains" of carbon and nitrogen with attached hydrogen molecules. A few have perpendicular "branches" off to one side.

Histidine

This amino acid is primarily used to make histamine, which reduces sensitivity to allergens. It also enhances uptake of zinc but inhibits absorption of copper. Histidine is critical in stabilizing hemoglobin and protecting against the buildup of carbon monoxide. Levels are usually low in those with fibromyalgia, and deficiency also increases the risk of allergies. Good sources of histidine are pork, cheese, and wheat germ.

Branched Chain Amino Acids: Isoleucine, Leucine, and Valine

These three unique amino acids have branches instead of straight chains of carbon and hydrogen. They are essential for building muscle as well as preventing breakdown of muscle, so they are popular with bodybuilders and heavy exercise enthusiasts. More importantly, they are crucial in protein synthesis, lipid metabolism, and fatty acid metabolism. Interestingly, biotin is essential for the metabolism of both leucine and isoleucine. The branched chain amino acids have been used medically to help prevent breakdown of muscle in bedridden patients, such as in amyotrophic lateral sclerosis, tardive dyskinesia, spinocerebellar degeneration, in patients with kidney failure, and in cancer patients, mostly to help prevent muscle wasting. They may also help fatigue and mental concentration, and have even been given intravenously to help reduce brain swelling as a result of severe liver disease. Good food sources are eggs, seaweed, turkey, chicken, lamb, cheese, and fish.

Lysine

One of the best known amino acids, helpful in treating and preventing herpes simplex or fever blisters, where it is taken with zinc. Interestingly, it also increases the absorption of calcium, so one should not take calcium supplements while taking lysine. Grains are notoriously low in lysine, and thus the usual high-grain diet may well lead to deficiencies. Lysine is essential in the formation of collagen and cartilage, so a deficiency may be involved in osteoarthritic and other joint and spinal disc disorders. Deficiency may also be a significant factor in anxiety, as lysine is an anti-anxiety agent, mainly because it is a serotonin antagonist. Serotonin excess is prominent in severe anxiety, especially when diarrhea is a component of the stress reaction. Deficiency of lysine leads to a significant increase in production of serotonin in the amygdala, a major emotional control center. Dosages of 1,000 mg daily help reduce the frequency of fever blisters in those who are prone to this problem, and during flare-ups up to 3,000 mg may be taken.

Methionine

Methionine is one of the sulfur-containing amino acids and is essential, but without adequate folate, B12, and vitamin C, it creates one of the great health hazards—increased homocysteine, which increases the risk of Alzheimer's, cancer, hypertension, and stroke. In general, methionine is abundant in all the high-protein foods—meats, eggs, and legumes.

Health benefits (helps with or helps to prevent):
- Detoxifying acetaminophen
- Liver detoxification in general
- Wound healing

Phenylalanine

One of the major building blocks of muscle, L-phenylalanine is also essential for adrenal function. Major sources are the proteins—cheese, eggs, fish, milk, meat. Phenylalanine is significantly transformed to tyrosine, one of the most important foundations for making the thyroid hormone, L-Dopa, norepinephrine, and epinephrine.

Phenylketonuria is a genetic defect in which individuals lack the ability to convert phenylalanine to tyrosine and, in this situation, they need tyrosine to assist them, but they are restricted to lifelong avoidance of high-phenylalanine foods. In healthy individuals, tyrosine is not an essential amino acid as it is easily made from phenylalanine.

Health benefits (helps with or helps to prevent):
- ADHD
- Alcohol withdrawal
- Alertness
- Appetite suppressant
- Chronic fatigue
- Cocaine and drug withdrawal
- Heart disease
- Loss of libido
- Narcolepsy
- Pain
- Parkinson's disease
- Premenstrual syndrome
- Schizophrenia
- Vitiligo

In the early 1980s, there was significant interest in D-phenylalanine, which was said to raise beta endorphins because it inhibited enkephalinase, the enzyme that breaks down naturally produced beta endorphins. Thus, there was great interest in using it for depression and for pain. In the long run it seems no better than L-phenylalanine. However, large doses of L-phenylalanine can interfere with dopamine-enhancing drugs that help treat Parkinson's disease and can increase blood pressure, as well as interfere with some antidepressant drugs.

Taurine

As indicated earlier, taurine is not considered "essential" by everyone, but its deficiency is extremely widespread. Taurine cannot be found in vegetables; it occurs only in animal protein. Taurine works to stabilize membrane potential in cells, as does magnesium, and it is often clearly deficient in those suffering from epilepsy, migraines, hypertension, and depression. It is another of the sulfur-containing amino acids. Dosages of up to 6,000 mg daily are safe and well tolerated, although may make some individuals slightly sleepy.

Health benefits (helps with or helps to prevent):
- Anxiety
- Chronic fatigue syndrome
- Depression
- Epilepsy
- Fibromyalgia
- Hypertension
- Migraines

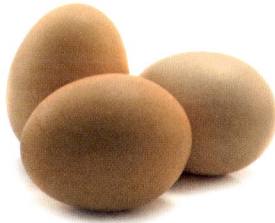

Threonine

Threonine is essential in the production of collagen, elastin, and muscle tissue. It helps build strong bones and tooth enamel, and assists in wound healing. Overall it is important in supporting the cardiovascular system, brain, and immune system. In general, deficiency is found in those with inadequate nutrition and in those with a leaky gut. It aids in the synthesis of glycine and serine that are essential for collagen production. Best sources are complete proteins such as meats and eggs.

Health benefits (helps with or helps to prevent):
- Familial spastic paraparesis
- Post-stroke spasticity
- Possibly multiple sclerosis
- Possibly leaky gut

Tryptophan

Tryptophan is the building block for one of the most critical mood stabilizers: serotonin. However, it is essential to have vitamins B3, B6, and lithium in order to convert tryptophan. In healthy people who wake up easily, tryptophan surges to its highest level within an hour and stays high until late afternoon, when it slowly decreases, reaching its lowest level between 9 and 11 p.m. Melatonin rises abruptly as you get sleepy in the evening and stays high until about 4 a.m. when it begins to fall. It reaches its lowest level when you wake bright eyed and bushy tailed ready for the day. In individuals who do not wake and sleep in the usual rhythm, significant dysfunctions of serotonin/melatonin can lead to a multitude of problems. Although the intermediate stage of conversion to serotonins, 5-hydroxy tryptamine, has been widely promoted, personally I find tryptophan highly superior to 5-HT for optimizing serotonin production.

Health benefits (helps with or helps to prevent):
- Anxiety
- Carbohydrate craving and overeating
- Depression
- Impatience
- Impulsiveness
- Inability to concentrate
- Insomnia
- Poor dream recall
- Weight gain

CONDITIONALLY ESSENTIAL AMINO ACIDS

Arginine

Arginine is truly deficient only in general nutritional deficiency. It is widely available and its major function is conversion to nitric oxide, the essential nutrient every cell needs to function optimally. It is thus important in blood flow, erectile function, and in immune health. It works synergistically with citrulline in large dosages, 5 to 7 grams, to help lower blood pressure. After age 40, that pathway is rapidly diminished, and arginine is primarily used to maintain muscle mass.

Health benefits (helps with or helps to prevent):
- Hypertension, up to age 40
- Maintaining muscle mass
- Male sexual function

Cysteine

Cysteine is usually synthesized in the human body from methionine. However, deficiencies in B12, B6, or folate prevent this normal function and lead to increases in homocysteine, with increasing risks of hypertension, heart disease, stroke, and Alzheimer's disease. In infants, the elderly, and in those with intestinal absorption problems, cysteine may become deficient. Cysteine is sometimes used by athletes to support muscle building, but its major benefit is increased energy; 300 mg in the morning and at noon can be a great boost to those needing extra energy.

N-acetyl cysteine (NAC) is perhaps the most important cysteine function, as it is critical to treat a number of disorders, including acetaminophen toxicity and to enhance overall feelings of energy. Note that acetaminophen is often toxic to the liver and kidneys.

Health benefits (helps with or helps to prevent):
- Acetaminophen toxicity
- Alcoholic liver disease
- Allergic reactions to the anti-epilepsy drug Dilantin®
- Alzheimer's
- Amyotrophic lateral sclerosis
- Angina pectoris
- Bile duct blockage
- High cholesterol
- Homocysteine excess
- Kidney failure

Glutamine

Glutamine is normally produced in the intestines by healthy bacteria. However, it is also needed by the most important intestinal bacteria: probiotics. Dosages of one teaspoon or more three times daily may be helpful.

Health benefits (helps with or helps to prevent):
- ADHD
- Anxiety
- Crohn's disease
- Depression
- Diarrhea
- Immune enhancement, especially in those on chemotherapy
- Nerve pain
- Stomach ulcers
- Ulcerative colitis

Tyrosine

As mentioned under phenylalanine, tyrosine is usually manufactured from that essential amino acid, so the health benefits are primarily in patients with phenylketonuria.

Health benefits (helps with or helps to prevent):
- ADHD
- Alcohol withdrawal
- Alertness
- Appetite suppressant
- Chronic fatigue
- Cocaine and drug withdrawal
- Heart disease
- Loss of libido
- Narcolepsy
- Pain
- Parkinson's disease
- Premenstrual syndrome
- Schizophrenia
- Vitiligo

Glycine

Glycine deficiency is another of those general malnutrition problems, as it is available in all high-protein foods.

Health benefits (helps with or helps to prevent):
- Alcoholism
- Benign prostatic hypertrophy
- Cancer prevention
- Kidney protection after kidney transplant
- Schizophrenia
- Skin ulcers (direct skin application)
- Stroke

Ornithine

Ornithine deficiency is another general malnutrition problem. Ornithine and arginine assist in releasing the growth hormone, especially in those over 50 years of age.

Health benefits (helps with or helps to prevent):
- Athletic performance
- Muscle building
- Glutamine poisoning
- Hepatic encephalopathy
- Wound healing

Proline

Proline is made in the body from glutamine, and is primarily used in making cartilage.

Serine

Normally serine is produced in the body, mainly from glycine. As with all these conditionally essential amino acids, it is deficient primarily where there is a general protein deficiency. The conversion to serine takes place in the kidney, but with protein deficiency, the liver also assists in attempting to produce adequate serine.

Interestingly, apparently the brain converts L-serine to D-serine, which is present in the brain in large quantities. D-serine contributes to the formation of S-adenosylmethionine, the methyl donor, essential for everything from cell proliferation to gene expression, and thus part of the ever-widening study of epigenetics.

NON-ESSENTIAL AMINO ACIDS

Non-essential amino acids are alanine, asparagine, aspartic acid, and glutamic acid. Deficiencies of these amino acids occur only in cases of severe malnutrition.

MINERALS

Calcium
Calcium is essential for maintaining the pH of the blood and for bone strength. Deficiencies lead to bone deformities in children and to osteoporosis in adults. Severe deficiencies in the blood lead to seizures and coma. Significant excesses in calcium lead to kidney stones, calcification of soft tissues, and heart arrhythmias.

Carbon
Carbon is one of the essentials of organic matter, and a building block of carbohydrates, fats, and amino acids.

Chlorine
Chlorine is present in the body as chloride, where blood chloride levels are part of basic electrolytes. It helps keep the amount of fluid inside and outside cells balanced, maintains blood volume, blood pressure, and pH of the blood—ideally 7.4. The amount of chloride in your body comes largely from sodium chloride (salt), and excess is excreted in the urine. Unfortunately, many processed and packaged foods have a significant excess of salt, which can lead to hypertension.

Hydrogen
Hydrogen makes up organic compounds, and is required only in its natural occurrence in fats, amino acids, and carbohydrates.

Magnesium
Second only to calcium in quantity needed, magnesium deficiency is rampant. Indeed, about 80 percent of people are deficient in magnesium, largely because of magnesium-deficient soil. Magnesium is critical in 350 enzymes and largely inside cells, and blood levels need to be finely balanced within a narrow range. It is mainly responsible for the cellular charge on cells; a lower charge makes the cells oversensitive and an excess makes them undersensitive. Much of the body's magnesium is in the bones, which are a chemical bonding of calcium and magnesium, with some protein and boron. You need roughly half as much magnesium daily as you do calcium.

Magnesium is far better absorbed through the skin than orally, if needed as a supplement. Green vegetables and almonds are the best food sources.

Health benefits (helps with or helps to prevent):
- Anxiety
- Atherosclerosis
- Cancer
- Carpal tunnel syndrome
- Depression
- Diabetes
- Epilepsy
- Irregular heartbeat
- Heart attack
- Hypertension
- Muscle cramps
- Osteoporosis
- Pain

Phosphorus
Phosphorus deficiency is only a problem in cases of severe malnutrition, or metabolic disorder. Most foods are loaded with phosphorus. Unfortunately, phosphorus excess is far more common because it is commonly found in soft drinks.

Potassium
Potassium deficiency is largely due to an inadequate intake of vegetables and fruits, which may be deficient themselves because of soil deficiency. Potassium is one of the critical electrolytes for healthy cell function.

Health benefits (helps with or helps to prevent):
- Nerve conduction
- Blood pressure
- Heart rhythm

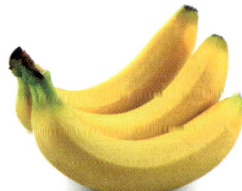

Sodium (Salt)
Sodium is one of the big four electrolytes, critical for overall cellular function. Unfortunately, thanks to the food industry, excess sodium is far too common. In excess it is a major contributor to hypertension. The best way to avoid excess is to avoid processed and packaged foods. Start with fresh foods and make your own meals.

Health benefits (helps with or helps to prevent):
- Balance of fluids
- Contraction/relaxation of muscles
- Transmitting nerve impulses

Sulfur
Sulfur is the third most abundant mineral as a percentage of weight, with major sources coming from the sulfur-containing amino acids: cystine, cysteine, methionine, and taurine. Methylsulfonylmethane (MSM) is another natural and healthy source. Sulfur is essential for glucosamine production, critical

in joint support and S-adenosylmethionine (SAM-e), as well as adrenal function. Interestingly, 90 percent of the most abundant hormone dehydroepiandrosterone (DHEA) is bound to a sulfur molecule. Deficiencies are most likely in vegans, athletes, and some children.

Health benefits (helps with or helps to prevent):
- Allergy
- Arthritis
- Athletic injuries
- Cancer
- Congestive heart failure
- Depression
- Diabetes
- Fibromyalgia
- Interstitial cystitis

TRACE MINERALS

Although required in much smaller amounts, these are just as critical for health.

Boron

Daily requirement: 3 to 12 mg daily. In adults, 9 to 12 mg is ideal.

Health benefits (helps with or helps to prevent):
- Arthritis
- Attention span
- Bone strength
- Estradiol production
- Immune function
- Lipid metabolism
- Memory
- Testosterone production

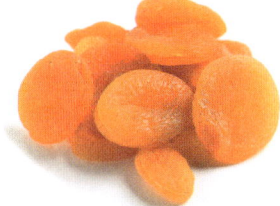

Chromium

Daily requirement: 1,000 mg.

Health benefits (helps with or helps to prevent):
- Bone loss (osteoporosis)
- Diabetes
- Glaucoma
- Lowers total cholesterol
- Increases HDL cholesterol
- Sugar metabolism
- Weight loss

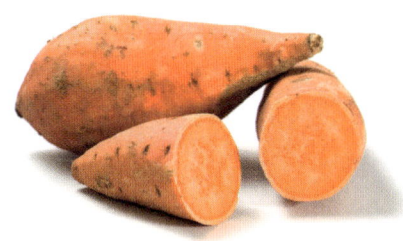

Cobalt

Deficiency can cause pernicious anemia with fatigue, brain damage, memory problems, and spinal cord degeneration. A deficiency is most likely in the vegan diet. Daily requirement: 5 to 8 mg.

Health benefits (helps with or helps to prevent):
- Pernicious anemia

Copper

Daily requirement: 2 mg. An adequate copper to zinc ratio is required within the body for optimal function.

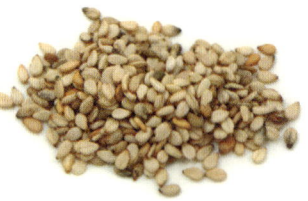

Health benefits (helps with or helps to prevent):
- Arthritis
- Elasticity of arteries
- Inflammation

Iodine

Essential for thyroid function, immune competence, and muscle strength, but deficient in about 80 percent of Americans. Daily requirement: 1.5 to 12.5 mg.

Health benefits (helps with or helps to prevent):
- Brain function
- Energy
- Immune deficiencies
- Overall metabolism

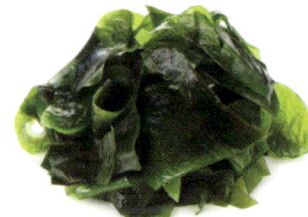

Iron

Essential for blood manufacture. There is a condition called hemochromatosis—iron storage disease—which occurs in about 1 percent of men, in which excessive storage in the liver can cause serious liver failure. Daily requirement: 15 mg.

Health benefits (helps with or helps to prevent):
- Iron-deficient anemia

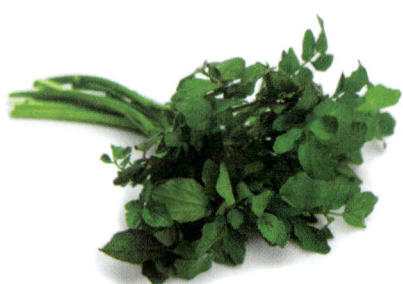

Lithium

Essential for the production of serotonin—deficiencies can cause anxiety and depression. Lithium orotate is the best form. Daily requirement in adults: 15 to 20 mg.

Health benefits (helps with or helps to prevent):
- ADHD
- Anxiety
- Depression
- Protects brain from physical and emotional trauma

Manganese

Deficiency can lead to brain problems and multiple enzyme deficiencies. Excess can lead to a Parkinson's-like problem. Daily requirement: 5 mg.

Health benefits (helps with or helps to prevent):
- Enzyme deficiencies
- Free radical reduction

Molybdenum

Deficiency primarily in those on parenteral feeding (those given IVs rather than food). Daily requirement: 75 mg.

Health benefits (helps with or helps to prevent):
- DHEA production
- Some enzyme functions

Selenium

Deficiencies occur primarily because of soil deficiency. Daily requirement: 100 to 200 mg.

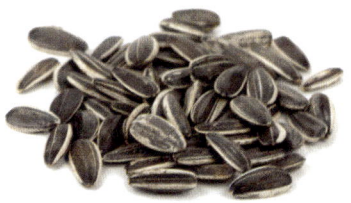

Health benefits (helps with or helps to prevent):
- Immune competence
- Cancer prevention, especially prostate cancer

Silicon

Deficiency leads to bone, hair, skin, nail, arterial wall, and collagen problems. Daily requirement: 20 mg.

Health benefits (helps with or helps to prevent):
- Arterial wall strength
- Bone, skin, and nail health
- Collagen production

Strontium

Deficiency is associated with weak bones. Daily requirement: about 100 mg.

Health benefits (helps with or helps to prevent):
- Osteoporosis

Vanadium

Vanadium deficiency is found in diabetics and hypertensive individuals. Its most common form is vanadyl sulfate. Daily requirement: about 1 mg.

Health benefits (helps with or helps to prevent):
- Cancer prevention
- Diabetes
- Hypertension
- Low blood sugar

Zinc

Zinc deficiency leads to a weak immune system (frequent colds and flu, etc.), diarrhea, hair loss, skin lesions, loss of appetite and anorexia, ADHD, hypertension, diabetes, decreased sense of taste, ulcerative colitis, and enlarged prostate. Daily requirement: 10 to 20 mg.

Health benefits (helps with or helps to prevent):
- Immune strength at all levels
- Overall metabolic balance

TOXIC MINERALS

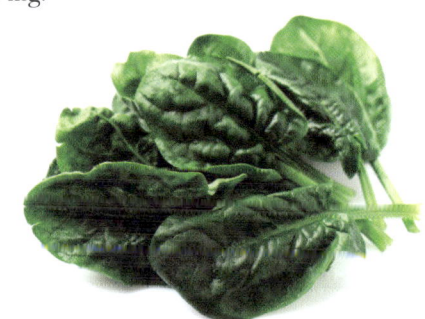

All of the following minerals are toxic and are to be avoided:
- Aluminum
- Arsenic
- Cadmium
- Fluoride
- Lead
- Mercury
- Uranium

ARTIFICIAL AND PROCESSED ADDITIVES

All of the following are not real foods and should be avoided at all times:
- Artificial flavorings
- Aspartame
- High-fructose corn syrup
- Margarine
- Monosodium glutamate
- Monosodium laureate
- Olestra®
- Processed cheese
- Saccharine
- Splenda®
- Textured vegetable protein
- Trans-fats

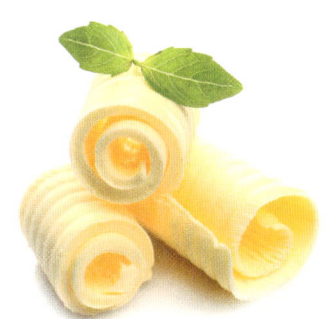

ACID/BASIC BALANCE

The body in general, and the blood especially, needs to maintain a basic pH of 7.4. In general, 80 percent of food should be alkaline-producing and only 20 percent acid-producing.

BEVERAGES

Water

Aside from air, water is the most critical requirement for life itself. Approximately 75 percent of our body is water and, of course, much of the food eaten is also water. The water content of blood is a critical factor in maintaining health. If you are dehydrated, serious illness can occur. Equally, if you have an excess of water, that is also dangerous. The specific gravity of urine is a simple indication of water balance; if the specific gravity is above 1.025 you are beginning to be dehydrated, and if it is below 1.010 you are nearing water oversaturation. The usual recommendation for daily water intake is to drink in ounces half of your body's weight in pounds. So a 150-pound person should drink 75 ounces, though more may be needed.

Equally important is the quality of water. In the U.S. and in many Western countries, municipal water is chlorinated and usually fluoridated. While it is essential that chlorine be used to avoid many infections, I recommend finding a filter that removes chlorine. Fluoride is a toxin and should be avoided.

Bottled water is expensive, and some plastic containers may add polyvinyl chlorides (PVCs) to the water. Finally, to demonstrate the negative effect of microwaving, boil some water in the microwave and boil some in a kettle on the stove. Let them cool and taste the difference. If microwaving can seriously damage the taste of water, imagine what it does to food.

Alcohol

Although not harmful in small amounts—one drink per day for adults—there is no nutritional need for alcohol.

Other healthy beverages include many herbal teas, green tea, and one or two cups of coffee daily. Soft drinks and energy drinks are non-essential for our fluid intake and in the case of energy drinks, may be dangerous.

CULINARY OILS

Healthier oils:
- Almond
- Coconut—also excellent for cooking
- Flaxseed
- Grapeseed
- Hazelnut
- Olive—best overall
- Palm
- Sesame
- Walnut
- Wheat germ

Culinary oils to avoid:
- Canola
- Chicken fat
- Cod liver
- Corn
- Cottonseed
- Lard—most has been artificially hydrogenated
- Peanut
- Safflower
- Sunflower

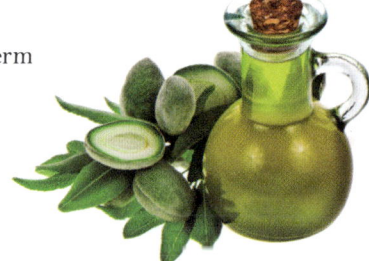

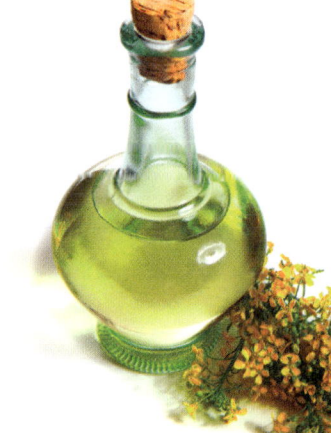

Key to abbreviations used in this book:

g	grams
IU	international units
mcg	micrograms
mg	milligrams
ORAC	oxygen radical absorbance capacity
oz.	ounces
RDV	recommended daily value
tbsp.	tablespoon
tsp.	teaspoon

Dairy

In general, all dairy products are primarily good for quality protein. Eaten in moderation, they provide essential amino acids, many of which are available only from animal protein. They are also a good source of calcium. The fat content is considered a potential problem; however, balanced with foods high in antioxidants, they are an excellent component of good nutrition.

Cheese

Cheeses are an important source of energy, immune-boosting protein, bone-building and tooth-strengthening calcium, and fat, vitamins, and minerals. Eating cheese after a meal has been shown to help prevent tooth decay by forming a protective film on the tooth surface and stimulating the production of saliva, helping to guard against acid damage from other foods. The presence of conjugated linoleic acid (CLA), a muscle-building essential amino acid, has been linked with improved immune function and the prevention of cancer. Vitamin B promotes strong bones, helping to prevent osteoporosis, while vitamin K2 has been connected with maintaining a healthy heart, brain, and bones—good news for cheese lovers!

Cheese contains less lactose than milk and is therefore better tolerated by people suffering from lactose intolerance—as a rule of thumb, the older the cheese, the lower the lactose content. Many people digest goat's milk more easily than cow's milk, so chevre (goat's milk cheese) may provide an option that's lighter on the digestive system. However, in general, cheese is high in saturated fat—if you are trying to control your weight, consider low-fat options, such as low-fat cottage cheese or feta, which have a lower fat content than most cheeses. Most cheese is mildly inflammatory, and high levels of cholesterol and sodium mean it may not be suitable for people with hypertension (high blood pressure). As with all dairy products, cheese provides an excellent component of good nutrition as part of a balanced diet that includes foods high in antioxidants.

NUTRIENTS IN 1 CUBIC INCH OF FULL-FAT CHEDDAR CHEESE:

Calories, 69
Calcium, 121 mg
Carbohydrate, 0.6 g
Cholesterol, 16.8 mg
Fat, 5.7 g
Iron, 0 mg
Magnesium, 4.6 mg
Phosphorus, 77.4 mg
Protein, 4 g
Riboflavin, 0.1 mg
Selenium, 4.8 mcg
Sodium, 111 mg
Vitamin A (RAE), 57.3 mcg
Vitamin B12, 0.2 mcg
Vitamin D, 4.1 IU
Vitamin K, 0.4 mcg
Zinc, 0.6 mg

Glycemic load: 0

NUTRIENTS IN 1 CUBIC INCH OF LOW-FAT CHEDDAR CHEESE:

Calories, 29
Calcium, 70.6 mg
Carbohydrate, 0.3 g
Cholesterol, 3.6 mg
Fat, 1.2 g
Iron, 0.1 mg
Magnesium, 2.7 mg
Phosphorus, 82.3 mg
Protein, 4.2 g
Riboflavin, 0 mg
Selenium, 2.5 mcg
Sodium, 148 mg
Vitamin A (RAE), 10.2 mcg
Vitamin B12, 0.1 mcg
Vitamin K, 0.1 mcg
Zinc, 0.3 mg

Glycemic load: 0

HEALTH AND HEALING BENEFITS:

TEETH AND BONES:

Rich in calcium and vitamin B2, cheese is one of the best foods for keeping teeth healthy and maintaining strong bones.

IMMUNITY:

Essential amino acids in cheese have been linked with improved immune function, therefore lowering the risk of cancer and other diseases.

LACTOSE INTOLERANCE:

Most of the lactose is removed in the cheesemaking process, meaning many cheeses can be enjoyed by those who are lactose intolerant.

RECOMMENDED FOR HELP WITH:

- Healthy teeth and bones
- Immune health
- Cancer prevention

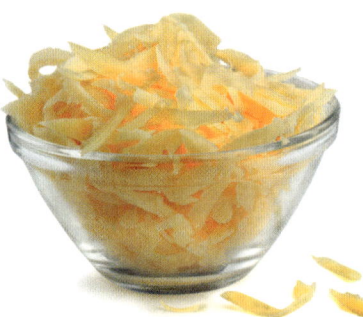

Kefir

An ancient drink originating in the Caucasus mountains, kefir is a fermented milk drink similar to liquid yogurt, made by adding kefir "grains" to a live culture of cow, goat, sheep, or soy milk. It contains probiotic micro-organisms, healthy bacteria that may be beneficial to the gut. Gut-friendly bacteria and yeast consume lactose during the fermentation process, so kefir can provide a suitable option for those who are lactose intolerant. Kefir is packed with immune-boosting proteins, essential minerals, and B vitamins. Kefir products are available in larger grocery stores and health food stores. The nutrients in homemade kefir will vary depending on the type of culture used in fermentation, while nutrients in commercially available products vary by brand.

NUTRIENTS IN 1 CUP OF REGULAR KEFIR
(commercially available pre-bottled product):

Calories, 127
Calcium, 303 mg
Carbohydrate, 18.3 g
Fat, 2.3 g
Protein, 8.8 g
Sugars, 16.9 g
Vitamin A (RAE), 425 mcg
Vitamin D, 2.4 mcg

HEALTH AND HEALING BENEFITS:

DIGESTION:

Probiotic micro-organisms may improve gastrointestinal conditions, helping to reduce the symptoms of irritable bowel syndrome.

HEALTHY BONES AND TEETH:

The high calcium content helps prevent tooth decay and increases bone strength, therefore helping to protect against the onset of osteoporosis.

IMMUNITY:

Certain probiotics have been shown to help regulate immune function.

Glycemic load: 7
Inflammatory index: Mildly inflammatory
RECOMMENDED FOR HELP WITH:

- Irritable bowel syndrome
- Healthy bones
- Immunity

MILK

Milk provides a good source of protein, carbohydrate, and fat, except skim milk, which contains virtually no fat. Milk contains essential amino acids and calcium as well as lactose. Lactose needs to be broken down by the enzyme lactase in the small intestine. Some people do not have sufficient lactase in their system and therefore find milk difficult to digest. This is known as lactose intolerance. For those who suffer from lactose intolerance, alternative lactose-free options are available, including almond milk, coconut milk, and soy milk.

Milk, whole

Contains essential amino acids, the fundamental building blocks of our tissues, important in the development of the brain and nervous system, and the singular component of protein. It's also a good source of bone- and teeth-strengthening calcium. However, it is high in saturated fat, and sugars contribute a large portion of the calories.

NUTRIENTS IN 1 CUP OF WHOLE MILK (with added vitamin D):

Calories, 149
Calcium, 276 mg
Carbohydrate, 12 g
Cholesterol, 24 mg
Fat, 8 g
Protein, 7.7 g
Riboflavin, 0.4 mg
Sodium, 105 mg
Vitamin A (RAE), 112 mcg
Vitamin B12, 1.1 mcg
Vitamin D, 124 IU

Glycemic load: 4
Inflammatory index: Mildly inflammatory

Milk, 2% (low-fat)

A cup of 2% milk contains 3 g less fat than whole, or full-fat milk, yet even low-fat milk is still fairly high in saturated fat.

NUTRIENTS IN 1 CUP OF 2% MILK (with added nonfat milk solids, without added vitamin A):

Calories, 137
Calcium, 350 mg
Carbohydrate, 14 g
Cholesterol, 20 mg
Fat, 5 g
Protein, 9.7 g

Riboflavin, 0.5 mg
Sodium, 145 mg
Vitamin, A (RAE), 41.6 mcg
Vitamin B12, 1 mg
Vitamin C, 2.7 mg

Glycemic load: 4
Inflammatory index: Mildly inflammatory

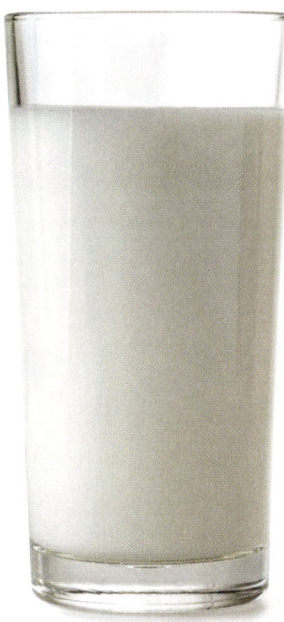

Milk, skim

Low in saturated fat and cholesterol, but sugars contribute a large portion of the calories in skim milk.

NUTRIENTS IN 1 CUP OF SKIM MILK:

Calories, 86
Calcium, 299 mg
Carbohydrate, 12 g
Cholesterol, 5 mg
Protein, 8 g
Riboflavin, 0.5 mg
Sodium, 103 mg
Vitamin A (RAE), 4.9 mcg
Vitamin B12, 1.2 mcg
Vitamin C, 0 mg

Glycemic load: 3
Inflammatory index: Mildly inflammatory

Health and healing benefits of milk:

HEART HEALTH:

Full-fat milk should generally be avoided to reduce the risk of cardiovascular diseases.

TEETH AND BONES:

Studies show that the consumption of milk can prevent tooth decay. Calcium is also essential for maintaining the pH of the blood and for bone strength. Calcium deficiency can lead to bone deformities in children and to osteoporosis in adults.

PREVENTING CANCER:

Calcium and vitamin D may help reduce the risk of colon cancer.

METABOLISM:

Whole milk contains over a quarter of the recommended daily intake of riboflavin (vitamin B2). Vitamin B2 is critical to energy production and to metabolism in general.

RECOMMENDED FOR HELP WITH:

- Prevention of tooth decay
- Osteoporosis
- Metabolism

Almond milk

Made from ground almonds, high in immune-boosting antioxidants and low in cholesterol, almond milk is often used as a lactose-free substitute for cow's milk. It's also dairy-free and therefore suitable for vegans. However, it is lower in protein than cow's milk or soy milk, so you should seek alternative sources of protein if using almond milk as a substitute for these. It's easy to make at home by blending ground almonds with water, or it can be purchased at the supermarket. Its popularity has grown steadily and it is now more widely purchased than soy milk. However, it's not suitable for anyone with a nut allergy.

NUTRIENTS IN 1 CUP OF UNSWEETENED SHELF-STABLE ALMOND MILK:

Calories, 39
Calcium, 482 mg
Carbohydrate, 3 g
Fat, 3 g
Iron, 0.7 mg
Protein, 1 g
Sodium, 189 mg
Vitamin A (RAE), 0 mcg
Vitamin E, 16.6 mg

HEALTH AND HEALING BENEFITS:

WEIGHT LOSS:

A good substitute for cow's milk as it has a very favorable low calorie count.

HEART HEALTH:

An extremely low cholesterol count means almond milk may help prevent cardiovascular diseases.

ANTIOXIDANT:

A good source of antioxidants, which have been linked with the prevention of cancer and lessening the signs of aging.

Glycemic load: 1
RECOMMENDED FOR HELP WITH:

- Heart disease
- Aging skin
- Weight loss
- Cancer prevention

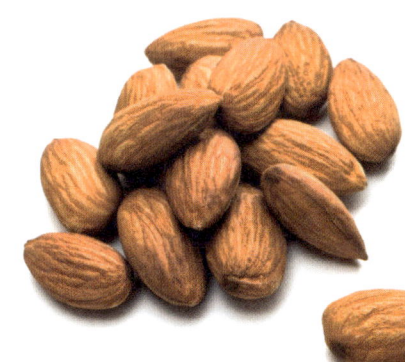

Coconut milk

Not to be confused with coconut water, which is simply the juice extracted from the nut, coconut milk and cream are made in a remarkably similar way to dairy products. The flesh of the coconut is mixed with water, the cream rises to the top and is skimmed off, and the resulting mixture is sieved to produce coconut milk. Rich in fiber and packed with vitamins and minerals, but lactose free, coconut products are suitable for those who are lactose intolerant. Coconut milk is a popular alternative to cow's milk for vegans in everything from baking to milkshakes, although it should be consumed in moderation because of its high fat content as well as its high calorific value.

NUTRIENTS IN 1 CUP OF COCONUT MILK:

Calories, 552
Calcium, 38.4 mg
Carbohydrate, 13 g
Copper, 0.6 mg
Fat, 57 g
Folate, 38.4 mcg
Iron, 3.8 mg
Magnesium, 88.8 mg
Manganese, 2.2 mg
Niacin, 1.8 mg
Phosphorous, 240 mg
Potassium, 631 mg
Protein, 5 g
Selenium, 14.9 mcg
Sodium, 36 mg
Vitamin B6, 0.1 mg
Vitamin C, 6.7 mg
Vitamin E, 0.4 mg
Vitamin K, 0.2 mcg
Zinc, 1.6 mg

HEALTH AND HEALING BENEFITS:

IMMUNE SYSTEM:

A major part of the fat content is lauric acid (also found in mothers' milk), which has been shown to have antibacterial, antiviral, and antifungal properties.

ANEMIA:

One cup of coconut milk contains just under half of your daily recommended value of iron. With such a high iron content, coconut milk helps combat iron deficiency.

HAIR/SKIN:

Vitamin E and the high fat content moisturize hair and skin and can promote hair growth.

Glycemic load: 5
RECOMMENDED FOR HELP WITH:

- Iron-deficient anemia
- Improved digestion
- Immune system
- Good complexion

Goat's milk

Worldwide, a larger amount of goat's milk is consumed than cow's milk. Many children in the United States have an allergy to cow's milk. This allergic reaction is caused by a protein known as alpha-s1-casein—goat's milk contains significantly less of this protein. Goat's milk also tends to be more easily digestible as it contains very little lactose. However, those who are lactose intolerant should check with a nutritionist to determine whether goat's milk is right for them. It's also a good source of essential amino acids, the fundamental building blocks of our tissues, important to the development of the brain and nervous system, and the singular component of protein.

NUTRIENTS IN 1 CUP OF GOAT'S MILK:

Calories, 168
Fat, 10 g
Calcium, 327 mg
Carbohydrate, 11 g
Cholesterol, 27 mg
Copper, 0.1 mg
Folate, 2.4 mcg
Iron, 0.1 mg
Magnesium, 34.2 mg
Niacin, 0.7 mg
Pantothenic acid, 0.8 mg
Phosphorus, 271 mg
Potassium, 498 mg
Protein, 9 g
Riboflavin, 0.3 mg
Selenium, 3.4 mcg
Sodium, 122 mg
Vitamin A (RAE), 139 mcg
Vitamin B6, 0.1 mg
Vitamin B12, 0.2 mcg
Vitamin C 3.2 mg
Vitamin D, 29.3 IU
Zinc, 0.7 mg

HEALTH AND HEALING BENEFITS:

BONES AND TEETH:

The high calcium content helps prevent tooth decay and increases bone strength, therefore helping to protect against the onset of osteoporosis.

DIGESTIVE SYSTEM:

Many people are able to digest goat's milk more easily than cow's milk.

BLOOD PRESSURE:

Potassium helps maintain healthy blood pressure.

Glycemic load: 3
Inflammatory index: Mildly inflammatory
RECOMMENDED FOR HELP WITH:

- Blood pressure
- Strong bones
- Healthy teeth

Soy milk

Soy milk is made by grinding soybeans and mixing with boiling water. It's high in health-boosting essential fatty acids, fiber, protein, minerals, and vitamins. A good lactose-free alternative to cow's milk, it contains no cholesterol and is higher in antioxidants. It's also a good source of bone-strengthening calcium. Soy milk has been associated with weight loss and reducing the risk of cancer. It also contains phytoestrogens, which have been linked to alleviating post-menopausal symptoms.

NUTRIENTS IN 1 CUP OF SOY MILK:

Calories, 131
Calcium, 60.7 mg
Carbohydrate, 6 g
Copper, 0.3 mg
Fat, 1 g
Folate, 43.7 mcg
Magnesium, 60.7 mg
Manganese, 0.5 mg
Pantothenic acid, 0.9 mg
Protein, 2 g
Riboflavin, 0.2 mg
Selenium, 11.7 mcg
Sodium, 37 mg
Thiamin, 0.1 mg
Vitamin K, 7.3 mcg

HEALTH AND HEALING BENEFITS:

LACTOSE INTOLERANCE:

Lactose free, making it suitable for those suffering from lactose intolerance.

MENOPAUSE:

Phytoestrogens are thought to help alleviate post-menopausal symptoms.

CANCER PREVENTION:

A good source of free-radical-zapping antioxidants, which have been linked with reducing the risk of cancer.

OSTEOPOROSIS:

Phytoestrogen can help with the absorption of calcium, preventing the loss of bone mass and contributing to healthy bones.

Glycemic load: 2
Inflammatory index: Mildly inflammatory
RECOMMENDED FOR HELP WITH:

- Post-menopausal syndrome
- Weight loss
- Cancer prevention

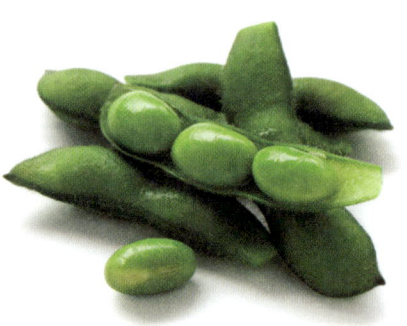

Yogurt, plain

Yogurt contains essential amino acids, the fundamental building blocks of our tissues, important to the development of the brain and nervous system, and the singular component of protein. It's also a good source of probiotic micro-organisms, healthy bacteria that may be beneficial to the gut. Certain probiotics have been shown to help regulate immune function and improve gastrointestinal (GI) problems such as constipation, diarrhea, and irritable bowel syndrome. Yogurt is also rich in bone-building calcium and phosphorus. However, it is high in saturated fat, so enjoy in moderation.

NUTRIENTS IN 1 CONTAINER (6 OZ.) OF PLAIN, WHOLE MILK YOGURT:

Calories, 104
Calcium, 206 mg
Carbohydrate, 8 g
Fat, 6 g
Phosphorus, 162 mg
Protein, 6 g
Riboflavin, 0.2 mg
Sugars, 8 g
Vitamin A (RAE), 45.9 mcg
Vitamin B12, 0.6 mcg
Vitamin C, 0.9 mg
Vitamin E, 0.1 mg
Vitamin K, 0.3 mcg

HEALTH AND HEALING BENEFITS:

GI HEALTH:

Probiotic micro-organisms may improve gastrointestinal conditions, helping to reduce the symptoms of irritable bowel syndrome.

BONES AND TEETH:

The high calcium content helps prevent tooth decay and increases bone strength, therefore helping to protect against the onset of osteoporosis.

The phosphorus content regulates the production of calcium and is an essential part of the production of skeletal tissue.

EYES, MOUTH, AND IMMUNITY:

Riboflavin (vitamin B2) boosts the health of eyes, mouth, throat, and overall immunity. Riboflavin deficiency causes bloodshot eyes, sensitivity to light, infections in the mouth and throat, a weak immune system, and sore tongue and lips. It is critical to energy production and to metabolism in general.

Glycemic load: 3
Inflammatory index: Mildly inflammatory
RECOMMENDED FOR HELP WITH:

- Irritable bowel syndrome
- Strong bones and teeth
- Immunity

Yogurt, Greek

Greek yogurt is traditionally made by straining the yogurt to remove the whey, resulting in a thick, creamy yogurt with less sugar, more protein, and fewer carbohydrates than regular yogurt. It's a powerhouse of quality protein, and a good source of bone-building calcium, tissue-building essential amino acids, and probiotic micro-organisms, healthy bacteria that may be beneficial to the gut. However, it is high in saturated fat, and it's worth noting that levels of protein, sugar, and added ingredients will vary according to the brand. Check the label—the main ingredients should be active live culture and milk. Some products miss out the straining process and use added thickeners and proteins such as modified corn starch and whey concentrates instead.

NUTRIENTS IN 1 CONTAINER (6 OZ.) OF GREEK YOGURT:

Calories, 165
Calcium, 170 mg
Carbohydrate, 7 g
Fat, 9 g
Protein, 15 g
Sugars, 7 g
Vitamin A (RAE), 3.4 mcg

HEALTH AND HEALING BENEFITS:

GI HEALTH:

Probiotic micro-organisms may improve gastrointestinal conditions, helping to reduce the symptoms of irritable bowel syndrome.

HEALTHY BONES AND TEETH:

The high calcium content helps prevent tooth decay and increases bone strength, therefore helping to protect against the onset of osteoporosis.

IMMUNITY:

Certain probiotics have been shown to help regulate immune function.

Glycemic load: 1
Inflammatory index: Mildly inflammatory
RECOMMENDED FOR HELP WITH:

- Irritable bowel syndrome
- Strong bones and teeth
- Immunity

Eggs

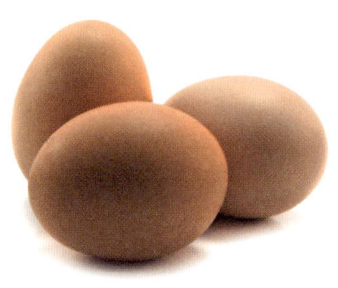

As with dairy products, eggs contain an ideal mixture of essential amino acids. The high cholesterol in eggs is at least partially counteracted by the lecithin in the yolk; be careful not to overcook the yolk, though, as this will destroy the lecithin. Eggs are an excellent source of nutrition for most individuals; however, they are not suitable for those with an egg allergy or familial hypercholesterolemia. If you suffer from high cholesterol, consult your doctor about egg consumption.

EGGS, CHICKEN

This is the most commonly eaten type of egg, and one of the best complete proteins, supplying all essential amino acids. Just two eggs supply the daily recommended amount of vitamin B12.

NUTRIENTS IN 1 MEDIUM WHOLE FRESH RAW CHICKEN EGG:

Calories, 71
Calcium, 26.5 mg
Fat, 5 g
Iron, 0.9 mg
Phosphorus, 95.5 mg
Potassium, 67 mg
Protein, 6.3 g
Riboflavin, 0.2 mg
Selenium, 15.8 mcg
Vitamin A (RAE), 73 mcg
Vitamin B12, 0.6 mcg
Vitamin D, 17.5 IU

Glycemic load: 0
Inflammatory index: Moderately inflammatory

Eggs, boiled

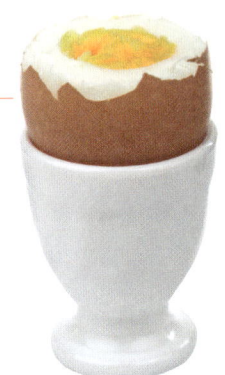

Eggs are one of the best complete proteins, with all essential amino acids. Because no fat is used in preparing boiled eggs, they are generally lower in calories and fat than scrambled, baked, or fried eggs, which use fats in the cooking process.

NUTRIENTS IN 1 LARGE HARD-BOILED EGG:

Calories, 77
Calcium, 25 mg
Fat, 5 g
Iron, 0.6 mg
Phosphorus, 86 mg
Potassium, 63 mg
Protein, 6.3 g
Riboflavin, 0.3 mg
Selenium, 15.4 mcg
Vitamin A (RAE), 74.5 mcg
Vitamin B12, 0.6 mg

Glycemic load: 0
Inflammatory index: Moderately inflammatory

Eggs, poached

Like soft- and hard-boiled eggs, poached eggs are generally lower in calories and fat than scrambled, baked, or fried eggs.

NUTRIENTS IN 1 MEDIUM POACHED EGG:

Calories, 71
Calcium, 26.5 mg
Fat, 5 g
Iron, 0.6 mg
Phosphorus, 86 mg
Potassium, 63 mg
Protein, 6.3 g
Riboflavin, 0.3 mg
Selenium, 15.4 mcg
Vitamin A (RAE), 87.9
Vitamin B12, 0.6 mcg

Glycemic load: 0
Inflammatory index: Mildly inflammatory

Eggs, scrambled

While scrambled eggs, like other types of cooked egg, are a good source of protein, riboflavin, and selenium, they are also high in saturated fat, very high in cholesterol, and contain trans fat.

NUTRIENTS IN 1 LARGE SCRAMBLED EGG:

Calories, 102
Calcium, 43.3 mg
Fat, 7 g
Iron, 0.7 g
Phosphorus, 104 mg
Potassium, 84.2 g

Protein, 6.8 g
Riboflavin, 0.3 mg
Selenium, 13.7 mcg
Vitamin A (RAE), 96.3
Vitamin B12, 0.5 mcg
Vitamin D, 20.7 IU

Glycemic load: 0
Inflammatory index: Moderately inflammatory

Eggs, whole fried

Be sure to use olive oil or coconut oil for frying. While fried eggs, like other types of cooked eggs, are a good source of protein, riboflavin, and selenium, they're also high in saturated fat, and very high in cholesterol.

NUTRIENTS IN 1 MEDIUM FRIED EGG:

Calories, 90
Calcium, 27.1 mg
Fat, 7 g
Iron, 0.9 mg
Phosphorus, 95.7 mg
Potassium, 67.6 mg

Protein, 6.3 g
Riboflavin, 0.2 mg
Selenium, 15.7 mcg
Vitamin A (RAE), 100.5 mcg
Vitamin B12, 0.6 mcg
Vitamin D, 17.0 IU

Glycemic load: 0
Inflammatory index: Mildly inflammatory

Duck eggs

Duck eggs are alkalizing, with anti-cancer properties. They are a good source of folate and vitamin B12, which contribute to healthy brain function. One duck egg contains over half (63%) of your recommended daily value of vitamin B12, which helps maintain healthy red blood cells and contributes to neurological health. Duck eggs are richer in protein than chicken eggs, but are also higher in cholesterol.

NUTRIENTS IN 1 LARGE DUCK EGG:

Calories, 130
Calcium, 44.8 mg
Fat, 10 g
Folate, 56.0 mcg
Iron, 2.7 mg
Phosphorus, 154 mg
Potassium, 155 mg
Protein, 9 g
Riboflavin, 0.3 mg
Selenium, 25.5 mcg
Vitamin A (RAE), 136 mcg
Vitamin B12, 3.8 mcg

Glycemic load: 0
Inflammatory index: Moderately inflammatory

HEALTH AND HEALING BENEFITS OF EGGS:

EYES, MOUTH, AND IMMUNITY:

Riboflavin (vitamin B2) boosts the health of eyes, mouth, throat, and overall immunity. Riboflavin deficiency causes bloodshot eyes, sensitivity to light, infections in the mouth and throat, a weak immune system, and sore tongue and lips. It is critical to energy production and to metabolism in general.

ANTIOXIDANT:

Eggs are a very good source of the antioxidant mineral selenium. Antioxidants are essential for optimal health. These compounds help decrease free radical molecules, which damage cells and lead to every known disease. For people who avoid fish, shellfish, and mushrooms—other good sources of selenium—eggs provide an important source.

RECOMMENDED FOR HELP WITH:

- Cataract prevention
- Acne
- Immunity

Fruits and fruit juices

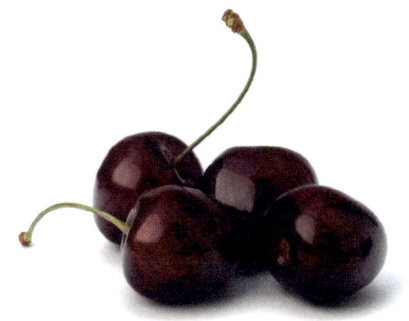

Fruits have numerous health benefits, and all except plums, rhubarb, and cranberries are alkalizing foods. They also contain high levels of antioxidants, including vitamins A, C, and E, and a wide variety of anthocyanins, flavonoids, and polyphenols. However, many fruits provide most of their calories from sugars, so do eat in moderation. Different types of the same fruit (such as sweet cherries and black cherries) and different preparations of the same fruit (such as fresh mango and dried mango) can have varying nutrients and health benefits. Fruits and fruit juices are a delicious—and easily portable—means of adding vitamins and minerals to your diet.

Acai

Often called a superfood, acai berries are a purple palm fruit native to South America. Mainly available in concentrate or capsule form, acai can also be made into drinks and foods. Acai provides exceptionally high levels of antioxidants and was traditionally used to combat aging and assist in weight loss. Acai berries have a multitude of health benefits, including strengthening immunity, reducing inflammation, improving heart health, and potentially protecting against cancer. The fiber in acai maintains digestive health and bowel regularity, and has been found to help reduce the risk of diabetes, high cholesterol, and gastrointestinal disease. Some people can have allergic reactions to acai; test a small amount first.

NUTRIENTS IN 1 CUP OF ACAI JUICE:

Calories, 125
Carbohydrate, 28.8 g
Dietary fiber, 4 g
Folate, 25 mcg
Niacin, 1 mg
Pantothenic acid, 0.4 mg
Protein, 0.8 g
Riboflavin, 0.2 mg
Sugar, 20.8 g
Thiamin, 0.1 mg
Vitamin B6, 0.2 mg
Vitamin B12, 0.3 mcg
Vitamin C, 20 mg

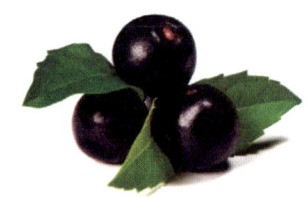

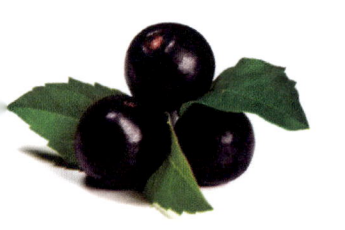

HEALTH AND HEALING BENEFITS:

IMMUNITY:

Vitamin C provides a huge boost to the immune system, and riboflavin aids in the production of antibodies.

STRONG MUSCLES AND BONES:

Protein helps build and repair bones, tissues, hormones, and body chemicals.

BLOOD HEALTH:

Vitamins B6 and B12 maintain healthy red blood cells and improve their ability to carry oxygen to cells around the body. Low levels of B12 lead to anemia and potential damage to the spinal cord and brain. Vitamin B6 deficiency is found in people with heart disease, premenstrual syndrome, atherosclerosis, and carpal tunnel syndrome. Fiber helps to lower cholesterol.

HEART HEALTH:

Thiamin helps ensure the healthy functioning of the heart. Vitamin B12 promotes a strong heart and red blood cells.

ENHANCED BRAIN FUNCTION:

Vitamin B6 is crucial to brain function and is believed to help stabilize mood. Folate is important for all aspects of brain function, and is especially important during pregnancy for reducing the risk of spinal and mental defects in the fetus. It may also help protect against Alzheimer's.

DIGESTIVE HEALTH:

The dietary fiber and carbohydrates aid digestive health and help you feel fuller faster. They also maintain bowel regularity and reduce the risk of diabetes, high cholesterol, and gastrointestinal disease. Folate improves the metabolism of fat.

Glycemic load: 1
Inflammatory Index: Anti-inflammatory

RECOMMENDED FOR HELP WITH:

- Immunity
- Heart health
- Reduces cholesterol
- Digestive health
- Blood health
- Enhanced brain function

Acerola

Acerola are dark red, cherrylike fruits that grow in hot climates. According to the USDA, acerola provide more vitamin C than other food sources—reputedly up to 13 times more in acerola juice than orange juice. Acerola can be found as supplements or juices, and less commonly as fresh fruit, syrups, or preserves. Acerola are low in calories, fat-free, and provide dietary fiber and vitamin A.

NUTRIENTS IN 1 CUP OF ACEROLA:

Calories, 31
Dietary fiber, 1.1 g
Magnesium, 17.6 mg
Niacin, 0.4 mg
Omega-3 fatty acids, 43 mg
Omega-6 fatty acids, 45 mg
Pantothenic acid, 0.3 mg
Phosphorus, 10.8 mg
Potassium, 143 mg
Vitamin A (RAE), 37.2 mcg
Vitamin C, 1,650 mg

HEALTH AND HEALING BENEFITS:

IMMUNITY:

Vitamin C provides a boost to the immune system.

HEART HEALTH:

Omega-3 and -6 and vitamin A protect against stroke, heart disease, and diabetes, and lower blood pressure.

STRONG MUSCLES AND BONES:

Protein helps build and repair bones, tissues, hormones, and body chemicals. Phosphorus assists healthy bone formation.

BRAIN FUNCTION:

Omega-3 and -6 enhance brain function and are believed to aid memory.

GOOD INTERNAL HEALTH:

Potassium keeps the organs in good working order.

JOINT HEALTH:

Fatty acids and magnesium reduce joint inflammation.

HEALTHY SKIN:

Vitamin A helps prevent acne.

TISSUE REGENERATION:

Vitamin A is central to tissue regeneration, and fatty acids and protein assist in cellular regeneration.

DIGESTIVE HEALTH:

The dietary fiber aids digestive health and reduces cholesterol.

Glycemic load: 0
Inflammatory index: Strongly anti-inflammatory

RECOMMENDED FOR HELP WITH:

- Immunity
- Heart health
- Reduces cholesterol
- Tissue regeneration
- Joint health
- Healthy skin

Apple

Apples are one of the most popular fruit snacks. They are delicious, and rich in antioxidants, vitamins, and minerals. The antioxidants in apples prevent disease and strengthen the immune system, fighting bone disease and inflammation. Apples are low in calories but rich in fiber, promoting digestion. The carbohydrates and sugar in apples are good for quick energy. Apples have been recommended for acid reflux, and some people swear eating an apple dispels migraines.

NUTRIENTS IN 1 MEDIUM APPLE, RAW:

Calories, 95
Calcium, 10.9 mg
Carbohydrate, 25.1 g
Dietary fiber, 4.4 g
Omega-3 fatty acids, 16 mg
Omega-6 fatty acids, 78 mg
Phosphorus, 20 mg
Potassium, 195 mg
Sugars, 18.9 g
Vitamin C, 8.4 mg
Vitamin K, 4 mcg

HEALTH AND HEALING BENEFITS:

INTERNAL HEALTH:

Potassium keeps the organs in good working order.

HEART AND BLOOD HEALTH:

Omega-3 and -6 protect against heart disease and stroke, and lower blood pressure. Vitamin K is important to the blood, such as regulating clotting, and menstrual flow and pain.

IMMUNITY:

Vitamin C provides a huge boost to the immune system.

JOINT HEALTH:

Fatty acids reduce joint inflammation.

ENERGY:

Carbohydrates are important for energy production.

BRAIN FUNCTION:

Omega-3 and -6 enhance brain function and are believed to aid memory.

STRONG BONES:

Calcium, phosphorus, and vitamin K assist healthy bone formation.

DIGESTIVE HEALTH:

The dietary fiber aids digestive health and reduces cholesterol, helping you feel fuller faster.

Glycemic load: 9
Inflammatory index: Anti-inflammatory

RECOMMENDED FOR HELP WITH:

- Immunity
- Heart health
- Strong bones
- Reduces inflammation
- Energy
- Digestive health

Apple juice

Although it does not contain the fiber and pectin of whole apples, apple juice is an alkalizing drink. Like fresh apples, the carbohydrates in apple juice provide a boost of energy. Vitamin C is essential for immune health, and potassium maintains the good condition of organs. However, apple juice often has a high sugar content, so should be drunk in moderation.

Apricot

Apricots are small orange fruits that are native to China, but are now found all over the world as fresh fruit, dried fruit, and preserves. Apricots are very low in saturated fat, sodium, and cholesterol, and area good source of dietary fiber. However, most of the calories come from sugars. Apricots are packed with beta-carotene for heart health and are a good source of vitamins A, C, E, and K, as well as potassium. Apricots provide health benefits for the immune system, vision, skin, and bone strength. The fiber content is good for digestion. Dried apricots are also nutrition-packed and easier to transport, but if you suffer from asthma, avoid those with sulfites.

NUTRIENTS IN 1 APRICOT:

Calories, 17
Dietary fiber, 1 g
Magnesium, 3.5 mg
Niacin, 0.2 mg
Omega-6 fatty acids, 27 mg
Pantothenic acid, 0.1 mg
Phosphorus, 8.1 mg
Potassium, 90.6 mg
Protein, 0.5 g
Sugars, 3.2 g
Vitamin A (RAE), 33.6 mcg
Vitamin C, 3.5 mg
Vitamin E, 0.3 mg
Vitamin K, 1.2 mcg

HEALTH AND HEALING BENEFITS:

MUSCLES AND BONES:

Protein helps build and repair bones, tissues, hormones, and body chemicals. Phosphorus and magnesium assist healthy bone formation. Vitamin K maintains healthy bones.

HEART AND BLOOD HEALTH:

Omega-6 regulates blood pressure and, with vitamin A, helps prevent cardiovascular disease. Beta-carotene promotes heart health, supported by vitamins C and E, and potassium. Vitamin K is important to matters related to the blood, such as regulating clotting, and menstrual flow and pain.

IMMUNITY:

Vitamins C and E, and omega-6 provide a huge boost to the immune system.

GOOD INTERNAL HEALTH:

Potassium keeps the organs in good working order.

TISSUE REGENERATION:

Vitamins A and E are central to tissue regeneration, and fatty acids and protein assist in cellular regeneration.

JOINT HEALTH:

Fatty acids and magnesium reduce joint inflammation.

ENHANCED BRAIN FUNCTION:

Omega-6 is integral to brain function.

VISION:

Vitamin E reduces the risk of cataracts and macular degeneration and maintains eye health.

DIGESTIVE HEALTH:

The dietary fiber aids digestive health and maintains bowel regularity. Vitamin E improves metabolism.

HEALTHY SKIN:

Vitamin A helps prevent acne and maintains healthy skin.

Glycemic load: 1
Inflammatory index:
Anti-inflammatory

RECOMMENDED FOR HELP WITH:

- Supports immunity
- Heart and blood health
- Digestive health and bowel regularity
- Healthy skin
- Improved vision, reducing risk of macular degeneration
- Strong bones
- Tissue regeneration

Avocado

Considered a superfood, avocados are grown in warm climates around the world. They minimize the negative effects of more inflammatory meals and contain healthy fats. They are also extremely low in sodium and cholesterol and a good source of dietary fiber, but high in calories, so should be eaten in moderation. Avocados support the body's absorption of vitamins and minerals, and strengthen immunity. Avocados are rich in fatty acids that are crucial to both brain development and heart health. Vitamin K and folate maintain healthy blood cells, and avocados are also believed to promote healthy skin.

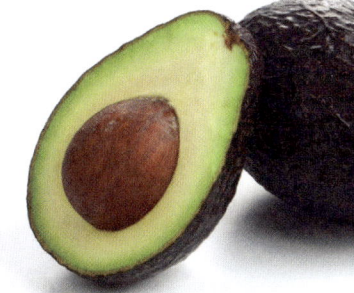

NUTRIENTS IN 1 AVOCADO:

Calories, 322
Carbohydrate, 17.1 g
Dietary fiber, 13.5 g
Folate, 163 mcg
Omega-3 fatty acids, 223 mg
Omega-6 fatty acids, 3,395 mg
Pantothenic acid, 2.8 mg
Potassium, 975 mg
Protein, 4 g
Sugars, 1.3 g
Vitamin B6, 0.5 mg
Vitamin K, 42.2 mcg

HEALTH AND HEALING BENEFITS:

HEART HEALTH:

Fatty acids and protein help protect the body against stroke, heart disease, and diabetes, and lower blood pressure. Vitamin C and potassium promote heart health. Folate reduces the risk of heart disease and hypertension.

MUSCLES AND BONES:

Protein helps build and repair bones, tissues, hormones, and body chemicals.

BLOOD HEALTH:

Vitamin B6 maintains healthy red blood cells. Vitamin B6 deficiency is found in people with heart disease, premenstrual syndrome, atherosclerosis, and carpal tunnel syndrome. Vitamin K is important to matters related to the blood, such as regulating clotting, and menstrual flow and pain.

ENHANCED BRAIN FUNCTION:

Omega-3 and -6 are integral to brain function. Folate is important for all aspects of brain function, and is especially important during pregnancy for reducing the risk of spinal and mental defects in the fetus. It may also help protect against Alzheimer's.

GOOD INTERNAL HEALTH:

Potassium keeps the organs in good working order.

IMMUNITY:

Vitamin C and omega-6 provide a huge boost to the immune system.

DIGESTIVE HEALTH:

The dietary fiber aids digestive health and maintains bowel regularity.

HEALTHY SKIN:

The nutrients and fatty acids maintain healthy skin.

Glycemic load: 2
Inflammatory index: Anti-inflammatory

RECOMMENDED FOR HELP WITH:

- Heart and blood health
- Strong bones
- Enhanced brain function
- Immunity
- Healthy skin
- Digestive health
- Developing fetus during pregnancy

Banana

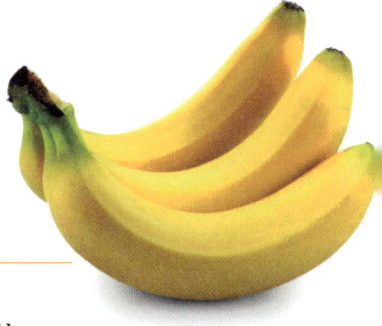

The USDA reports that Americans eat more than ten pounds of bananas per person per year. Bananas are often babies' first solid food. Carbohydrates provide energy, and potassium eases muscle cramps and digestion, including an upset stomach.

NUTRIENTS IN 1 MEDIUM BANANA:

Calories, 105
Carbohydrate, 26.9 g
Dietary fiber, 3.1 g
Magnesium, 31.9 mg
Manganese, 0.3 mg
Omega-6 fatty acids, 54 mg
Phosphorus, 26 mg
Potassium, 422 mg
Sugars, 14.4 g
Vitamin A (RAE) 3.5 mcg
Vitamin B6, 0.4 mg
Vitamin C, 10.3 mg

HEALTH AND HEALING BENEFITS:

BLOOD HEALTH:

Vitamin B6 maintains healthy red blood cells. Vitamin C and potassium promote heart health.

HEART HEALTH:

Omega-6 regulates blood pressure and heart health.

BRAIN FUNCTION AND MOOD:

Omega-6 and vitamin B6 aid brain function, mood, and sleep.

JOINT HEALTH:

Omega-6 and magnesium reduce joint inflammation.

INTERNAL HEALTH:

Potassium maintains organs.

IMMUNITY:

Vitamin C and omega-6 boost immunity.

MUSCLES:

Potassium is good for easing muscle cramps.

HEALTHY SKIN:

Vitamin A and manganese promote healthy skin.

DIGESTIVE HEALTH:

Carbohydrates, fiber, and potassium aid digestive health, calming the stomach and reducing the symptoms of gastro-esophageal reflux disease. They also maintain bowel regularity and reduce the risk of diabetes, high cholesterol, and gastrointestinal disease.

ENERGY:

Carbohydrates and magnesium are a great source of energy.

Glycemic load: 13
Inflammatory index: Anti inflammatory

RECOMMENDED FOR HELP WITH:

- Heart and blood health
- Brain function
- Immunity
- Healthy skin
- Easing muscle cramps
- Joint health
- Energy

Blackberries

Blackberries are rich in antioxidants and very low in sodium, cholesterol, and saturated fat, and are seen as useful for weight loss. Blackberries are great for optimal health and can be eaten as a snack on their own or added to salads and cereal. Fiber maintains healthy digestion and cholesterol, and the high vitamin C is great for boosting the immune system.

NUTRIENTS IN 1 CUP OF BLACKBERRIES:

Calories, 62
Carbohydrate, 13.8 g
Dietary fiber, 7.6 g
Folate, 36 mcg
Manganese, 0.9 mg
Omega-3 fatty acids, 135 mg
Omega-6 fatty acids, 268 mg
Sugars, 7 g
Vitamin C, 30.2 mg
Vitamin E, 1.7 mg
Vitamin K, 28.5 mcg

HEALTH AND HEALING BENEFITS:

HEART AND BLOOD HEALTH:

Omega-3 helps protect the body against stroke, heart disease, and diabetes. Omega-6 regulates blood pressure. Vitamin K is important to matters related to the blood, such as regulating clotting, and menstrual flow and pain. Vitamin E reduces cardiovascular disease, and folate reduces the risk of heart disease and hypertension.

ENHANCED BRAIN FUNCTION:

Omega-3 and -6 are integral to brain function and may aid memory. Folate is important for all aspects of brain function, and is especially important during pregnancy for reducing the risk of spinal and mental defects in the fetus. It may also help protect against Alzheimer's.

IMMUNITY:

Vitamins C and E provide a huge boost to the immune system.

DIGESTIVE HEALTH:

Fiber and carbohydrates aid digestive health and, alongside vitamin E, reduce cholesterol, helping you feel fuller faster, thereby aiding weight loss. They also calm diarrhea.

Glycemic load: 3
Inflammatory index: Anti-inflammatory

RECOMMENDED FOR HELP WITH:

- Heart health
- Reducing cholesterol
- Enhanced brain function
- Immunity
- Digestive health
- Calms diarrhea
- Developing fetus during pregnancy

Blueberries

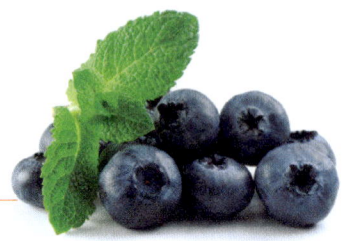

Considered the powerhouse of the fruits, commercial blueberries contain more antioxidants than any other commonly grown fruit—and wild blueberries are even higher in antioxidants than commercial blueberries. Blueberries contain optimal amounts of anthocyanins, hydroxycinnamic acids, hydrobenzoic acids, flavanoids, and other phenol-related polynutrients. Blueberries provide a multitude of healing benefits—from brain function, mood, and memory, to heart and skin health, strengthened immunity, bone strength, and purported cancer protection. Plus, they are great as a snack or as a healthful addition to cereals and desserts.

NUTRIENTS: IN 1 CUP OF BLUEBERRIES:

Calories, 84
Calcium, 8.9 mg
Carbohydrate, 21.5 g
Dietary fiber, 3.6 g
Folate, 8.9 mcg
Magnesium, 8.9 mg
Manganese, 0.5 mg
Niacin, 0.6 mg
Omega-3 fatty acids, 86 mg
Omega-6 fatty acids, 130 mg
Phosphorus, 17.8 mg
Potassium, 114 mg
Protein, 1.1 g
Sugars, 14.7 g
Vitamin C, 14.4 mg
Vitamin E, 0.8 mg
Vitamin K, 28.6 mcg

HEALTH AND HEALING BENEFITS:

HEART AND BLOOD HEALTH:

Omega-3 helps protect the body against stroke, heart disease, and diabetes. Omega-6 regulates blood pressure. Vitamin K is important in matters related to the blood, such as regulating clotting, and menstrual flow and pain. Vitamin E reduces cardiovascular disease, and folate reduces the risk of heart disease and hypertension.

BONES AND MUSCLES:

Protein helps build and repair bones, tissues, hormones, and body chemicals. Vitamin K, phosphorus, and magnesium support calcium in maintaining strong bones.

EYE HEALTH:

Vitamin A and lutein promote eye health, protecting against cataracts and macular degeneration.

HEALTHY SKIN:

Manganese and fatty acids promote healthy skin.

IMMUNITY:

Vitamins C and E provide a huge boost to the immune system.

ENHANCED BRAIN FUNCTION:

Omega-3 and omega-6 enhance brain function and are believed to aid memory and prevent neurodegenerative diseases. Folate is important for all aspects of brain function, and is especially important during pregnancy for reducing the risk of spinal and mental defects in the fetus. It may also help protect against Alzheimer's.

DIGESTIVE HEALTH:

The dietary fiber and carbohydrates aid digestive health and, alongside vitamin E, reduce cholesterol, helping you feel fuller faster.

CANCER PROTECTION:

Antioxidants and vitamin E protect against cancer, and pancreatic cancer in particular.

Glycemic load: 11
Inflammatory index: Anti-inflammatory

RECOMMENDED FOR HELP WITH:

- Heart health
- Healthy blood flow
- Enhanced brain function
- Strong bones
- Eye health
- Healthy skin
- Immunity
- Digestive health
- Possible cancer protection

Cantaloupe

Cantaloupe is a large melon with pale green skin and sweet, orange flesh. It is one of the most popular melons in the United States. Cantaloupe is low in cholesterol, sodium, and saturated fat. However, many of the calories come from sugar. Cantaloupe is a source of vitamins A and C and carotenoids for eye health.

NUTRIENTS IN 1 WEDGE OF MEDIUM CANTALOUPE (AROUND 1/8 OF FRUIT):

Calories 24
Carbohydrate, 5.6 g
Folate, 14.5 mcg
Magnesium, 8.3 mg
Omega-3 fatty acids, 32 mg
Omega-6 fatty acids, 24 mg
Potassium, 184 mg
Sugars, 5.4 g
Vitamin A (RAE), 117 mcg
Vitamin C, 25.3 mg
Vitamin K, 1.7 mcg

HEALTH AND HEALING BENEFITS:

HEART AND BLOOD HEALTH:

Omega-3 and -6 protect against heart disease and stroke, and lower blood pressure. Vitamin K is important to the blood, such as regulating clotting, and menstrual flow and pain, and folate reduces the risk of heart disease and hypertension.

STRONG BONES:

Protein and magnesium help build and maintain bones.

EYE HEALTH:

Carotenoids promote eye health, protecting against cataracts and macular degeneration.

IMMUNITY:

Vitamin C provides a huge boost to the immune system.

ENHANCED BRAIN FUNCTION:

Omega-3 and 6 are integral to brain function and may aid memory. Folate is important for all aspects of brain function, and is especially important during pregnancy for reducing the risk of spinal and mental defects in the fetus. It may also help protect against Alzheimer's.

TISSUE REGENERATION:

Vitamin A is central to tissue regeneration, and fatty acids assist in cellular regeneration.

Glycemic load: 4
Inflammatory index: Anti-inflammatory

RECOMMENDED FOR HELP WITH:

- Heart health
- Healthy blood flow
- Enhanced brain function
- Tissue regeneration
- Strong bones
- Eye health
- Immunity

CHERRIES

Cherries vary in color from light red to deep purple and range in flavor from sweet to tart. But all cherries are rich in antioxidants and loaded with nutrients; sour cherries trump even blueberries in this field. Cherries are ideal as a snack or flavorful addition to salads and desserts—because of their sweet flavor, they can be substituted for sugar-laden treats. Cherries are high in water and low in calories, which keeps you fuller for longer, and the fiber helps with digestion and weight loss. Cherries contain melatonin, which helps regulate sleep cycles, and the vitamin and mineral content promotes healthy bones and strong immunity. Dried cherries provide slightly less nutrients than listed below.

Sour cherries

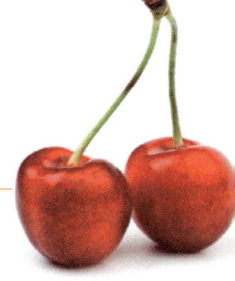

NUTRIENTS IN 1 CUP OF SOUR CHERRIES:

Calories, 52
Calcium, 16.5 mg
Carbohydrate, 12.6 g
Dietary fiber, 1.7 g
Folate, 8.2 mcg
Magnesium, 9.3 mg
Omega-3 fatty acids, 45 mg
Omega-6 fatty acids, 47 mg
Potassium, 178 mg
Sugars, 8.7 g
Vitamin A (RAE), 65.9 mcg
Vitamin C, 10.3 mg
Vitamin K, 2.2 mcg

Glycemic load: 3
Inflammatory index: Anti-inflammatory

Sweet cherries

NUTRIENTS IN 1 CUP OF SWEET CHERRIES:

Calories, 87
Calcium, 17.9 mg
Dietary fiber, 2.9 g
Folate, 5.5 mcg
Omega-3 fatty acids, 36 mg
Omega-6 fatty acids, 37 mg
Phosphorus, 29 mg
Potassium, 306 mg
Sugars, 17.7 g
Vitamin C, 9.7 mg
Vitamin K, 2.9 mcg

Glycemic load: 3
Inflammatory index: Anti-inflammatory

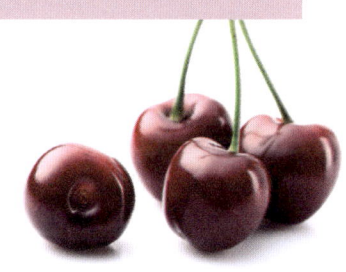

Tart cherry juice

Tart cherry juice is one of the best sources of antioxidants, with more ORACS (Oxygen Radical Absorbance Capacity) than any other food except cocoa nibs. Cherry juice provides both vitamin A and vitamin C, but black cherry juice has been found to contain higher traces of these vitamins than tart cherry juice, although it also contains more sugar. Tart cherry juice provides a wide range of healing benefits, including reducing hypertension, lowering cholesterol, and preventing gout. Both types of cherry juice have been found to reduce inflammation and help in managing arthritis pain, but tart cherry juice provides greater benefit in this area.

HEALTH AND HEALING BENEFITS:

HEART AND BLOOD HEALTH:

Omega-3 helps protect the body against stroke, heart disease, and diabetes. Omega-6 regulates blood pressure. Vitamin K is important to matters related to the blood, such as regulating clotting, and menstrual flow and pain, and folate reduces the risk of heart disease and hypertension.

BONES AND MUSCLES:

Calcium builds strong bones, supported by phosphorus, magnesium, and vitamin K.

EYE HEALTH:

Vitamin A promotes eye health, protecting against cataracts and macular degeneration.

HEALTHY SKIN:

Vitamin A and manganese promote healthy skin.

IMMUNITY:

Vitamin C provides a huge boost to the immune system.

ENHANCED BRAIN FUNCTION:

Omega-3 and 6 enhance brain function and are believed to aid memory and prevent neurodegenerative diseases. Folate is important for all aspects of brain function, and is especially important during pregnancy for reducing the risk of spinal and mental defects in the fetus. It may also help protect against Alzheimer's.

DIGESTIVE HEALTH:

The dietary fiber and carbohydrates aid digestive health and reduce cholesterol, helping you feel fuller faster and aiding in weight loss.

GOUT:

The anthocyanins in cherries reduce the pain and swelling of gout.

SLEEP:

Melatonin helps regulate sleep cycles.

RECOMMENDED FOR HELP WITH:

- Heart health
- Strong bones
- Eye health
- Healthy skin
- Immunity
- Enhanced brain function
- Digestive health
- Weight loss
- Reduced risk of gout
- Regulated sleep patterns

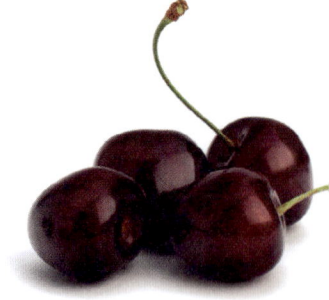

Coconut, raw

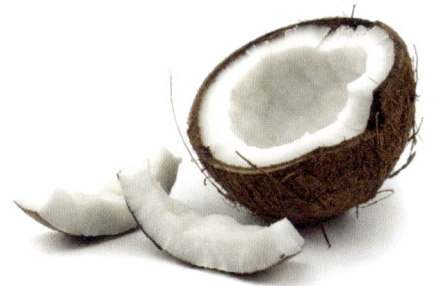

Coconut contains quality fat that is superior to most animal fat. Coconut is rich in antioxidants and high in fiber, copper, vitamin C, and manganese, strengthening bones, the immune system, and blood cells.

Coconut is used in foods, drinks, and cosmetics, and can be purchased as fresh coconut, shredded, dried, coconut milk, coconut oil, and coconut water.

NUTRIENTS IN 1 CUP OF SHREDDED COCONUT:

Calories, 283
Carbohydrate, 12.2 g
Copper, 0.3 mg
Dietary fiber, 7.2 g
Iron, 1.9 mg
Manganese, 25.6 mg
Omega-6 fatty acids, 293 mg
Phosphorus, 90.4 mg
Potassium, 285 mg
Protein, 2.7 g
Saturated fat, 23.8 g
Selenium, 8.1 mcg
Sugars, 5 g
Vitamin C, 2.6 mg

HEALTH AND HEALING BENEFITS:

IMMUNITY:

Coconut has anti-viral properties. Vitamin C, iron, and omega-6 boost immunity. Selenium aids immunity.

ENERGY:

Copper and protein are key to energy production.

JOINT HEALTH:

Omega-6 and selenium reduce joint inflammation.

HEART AND BLOOD HEALTH:

Omega-6 regulates blood pressure and reduces cholesterol. Iron maintains healthy red blood cells and improves their ability to carry oxygen to cells around the body. Growing children and adolescents, as well as menstruating, pregnant, or lactating women, have an increased need for iron. Copper aids iron absorption.

ENHANCED BRAIN FUNCTION:

Omega-6 is integral to brain function and may aid memory.

BONES AND MUSCLES:

Protein and phosphorus help build and maintain strong bones.

DIGESTIVE HEALTH:

Fiber aids digestive health.

Glycemic load: 6
Inflammatory index: Anti-inflammatory

RECOMMENDED FOR HELP WITH:

- Immunity
- Energy
- Joint health
- Heart health
- Reduced cholesterol
- Anemia deficiency
- Enhanced brain function
- Strong bones
- Digestive health

Coconut oil

Coconut oil is an excellent source of medium-chain fatty acids, among the healthiest of all dietary fats.

CRANBERRIES

Cranberries have a long history, including their use by Native Americans as traditional remedies and food. When choosing cranberries, the U.S. Centers for Disease Control and Prevention recommend cranberries that are darker in color, shiny, plump, and able to bounce, in order to garner the most benefit. Cranberries are well known as a remedy for urinary tract infections, but they are also great at maintaining gastrointestinal health, maintaining heart health, and preventing kidney stones. Cranberries are high in antioxidants and vitamin C to boost the immune system and fight colds. Because of fresh cranberries' limited season, dried cranberries are a good option, but have more sugar and less vitamin C than fresh.

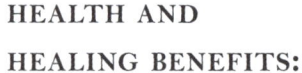

Cranberries, raw

NUTRIENTS IN 1 CUP OF CRANBERRIES:

Calories, 46
Carbohydrate, 12 g
Dietary fiber, 3.6 g
Manganese, 0.3 mg
Omega-3 fatty acids, 22 mg
Omega-6 fatty acids, 33 mg
Potassium, 80 mg
Sugars, 4.3 g
Vitamin C, 14 mg
Vitamin E, 1.3 mg
Vitamin K, 5 mcg

HEALTH AND HEALING BENEFITS:

URINARY TRACT HEALTH:

Cranberries are a well-known remedy for urinary tract infections (UTIs).

IMMUNITY:

Vitamins C and E provide a huge boost to mmunity.

HEART AND BLOOD HEALTH:

Omega-3 helps protect the body against stroke, heart disease, and diabetes. Omega-6 regulates blood pressure. Vitamin K is important in matters related to the blood, such as regulating clotting, and menstrual flow and pain, and vitamin E reduces cardiovascular disease.

HEALTHY SKIN:

Manganese and fatty acids promote healthy skin.

ENHANCED BRAIN FUNCTION:

Omega-3 and -6 enhance brain function and are believed to aid memory.

DIGESTIVE HEALTH:

Cranberries maintain gastrointestinal health. The dietary fiber and carbohydrates aid digestive health and, alongside vitamin E, reduce cholesterol, helping you feel fuller faster.

KIDNEYS:

Cranberries help prevent kidney stones.

Glycemic load: 5
Inflammatory index: Anti-inflammatory

RECOMMENDED FOR HELP WITH:

- Immunity
- Heart health
- Healthy blood flow
- Healthy skin
- Enhanced brain function
- Digestive health
- Urinary tract infections
- Kidney stones

Cranberry juice, unsweetened

Cranberry juice often contains sweeteners—choose one with little added sugar. This juice strengthens immunity and urinary health.

Currants

Currants are a type of berry found in North America, Europe, and Asia. They can be red, black, or white, and each has a different flavor. Currants are low in calories and fat free. Rich in antioxidants and iron, currants have up to four times more vitamin C than oranges. White currants are slightly sweeter than red or black and often made into preserves and desserts. Red currants are the tartest in flavor and in jelly form serve as a traditional condiment in the UK.

Currants, black

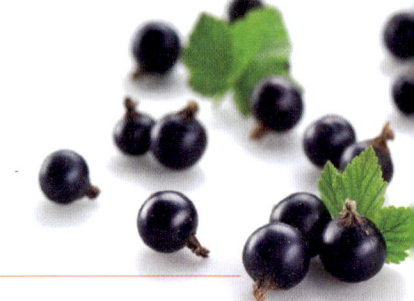

NUTRIENTS IN 1 CUP OF BLACK CURRANTS:

Calories, 71
Calcium, 61.6 mg
Carbohydrate, 17.2 g
Iron, 1.7 mg
Magnesium, 26.9 mg
Manganese, 0.3 mg
Omega-3 fatty acids, 81 mg
Omega-6 fatty acids, 120 mg
Phosphorus, 66.1 mg
Potassium, 361 mg
Vitamin C, 203 mg

HEALTH AND HEALING BENEFITS:

IMMUNITY:

Vitamin C and iron provide a boost to the immune system.

STRONG BONES:

Calcium builds strong bones, while phosphorus and magnesium maintain health.

HEART AND BLOOD HEALTH:

Omega-3 helps protect the body against stroke, heart disease, and diabetes. Omega-6 regulates blood pressure. Iron maintains healthy red blood cells and improves their ability to carry oxygen to cells around the body. Growing children and adolescents, as well as menstruating, pregnant, or lactating women, have an increased need for iron.

JOINT HEALTH:

Omega-6 and magnesium reduce joint inflammation.

HEALTHY SKIN:

Manganese and fatty acids promote healthy skin.

ENHANCED BRAIN FUNCTION:

Omega-3 and -6 may aid memory.

Glycemic load: 3
Inflammatory index: Anti-inflammatory

RECOMMENDED FOR HELP WITH:

- Immunity
- Heart health
- Strong bones
- Joint health
- Healthy skin
- Enhanced brain function

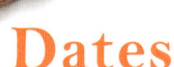

Dates

Dates are the fruit of the date palm tree, which grows in warm climates around the world. The dates most commonly found in the United States are Medjool or Deglet Noor, both of which are packed with nutrients. Dates are an excellent source of dietary fiber, keeping digestion regular and leaving you feeling fuller for longer. The potassium level of dates is high—great for building muscle and maintaining

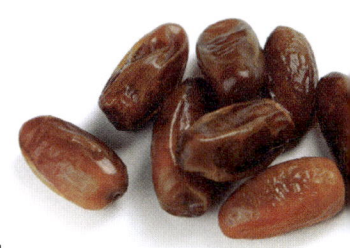

organ function. Magnesium boosts energy and helps regulate blood pressure. However, dates are high in calories and energy density, so eat these—and all dried fruit—in moderation.

NUTRIENTS IN 1 CUP OF CHOPPED DEGLET NOOR DATES:

Calories, 415
Carbohydrate, 110 g
Copper, 0.3 mg
Dietary fiber, 11.8 g
Magnesium, 63.2 mg
Manganese, 0.4 mg
Phosphorus, 91.1 mg
Potassium, 964 mg
Protein, 3.6 g
Sugars, 93.2 g
Vitamin B6, 0.2 mg

HEALTH AND HEALING BENEFITS:

DIGESTIVE HEALTH:

The dietary fiber, carbohydrates, and potassium aid digestive health and reduce cholesterol, leaving you feeling fuller for longer. They also maintain bowel regularity, ease constipation, as well as reducing the risk of diabetes, high cholesterol, and gastrointestinal disease.

GOOD INTERNAL HEALTH:

Potassium keeps the organs in good working order.

HEART AND BLOOD HEALTH:

Omega-3 helps protect the body against stroke, heart disease, and diabetes. Omega-6 regulates blood pressure. Magnesium also regulates blood pressure. Vitamin B6 strengthens blood. Vitamin B6 deficiency is found in people with heart disease, premenstrual syndrome, atherosclerosis, and carpal tunnel syndrome.

ENERGY:

Copper and magnesium play a key role in energy production.

HEALTHY SKIN:

Manganese and fatty acids promote healthy skin.

ENHANCED BRAIN FUNCTION AND MOOD:

Omega-3 and -6 enhance brain function and are believed to aid memory. Vitamin B6 plays an integral part in brain function and helps stabilize mood.

STRONG BONES AND MUSCLES:

Phosphorus and magnesium maintain healthy bones. Potassium helps build strong muscles.

JOINT HEALTH:

Omega-6 and magnesium reduce joint inflammation.

Glycemic load: 77
Inflammatory index: Mildly anti-inflammatory

RECOMMENDED FOR HELP WITH:

- Digestive health
- Easing constipation
- Reduced cholesterol
- Heart health
- Strong bones and muscles
- Energy
- Joint health
- Healthy skin
- Mood stabilizer

Elderberries, black

Elderberries grow in both hemispheres, though they are more common in the Northern. The berries are dark purple or red and are made into drinks, preserves, syrups, and teas. Elderberries have a long history as a traditional remedy. Today, they are used to boost immunity, and research is being carried out on their potential as a flu treatment. They may also help weight loss and cholesterol. Always cook elderberries before eating.

NUTRIENTS IN 1 CUP OF BLACK ELDERBERRIES:

Calories, 106
Calcium, 55.1 mg
Carbohydrate, 26.7 g
Dietary fiber, 10.2 g
Iron, 2.3 mg
Omega-3 fatty acids, 123 mg
Omega-6 fatty acids, 235 mg
Potassium, 406 mg
Vitamin A (RAE), 43.5 mcg
Vitamin B6, 0.3 mg
Vitamin C, 52.2 mg

HEALTH AND HEALING BENEFITS:

HEART AND BLOOD HEALTH:

Omega-3 and -6 protect against stroke, heart disease, and diabetes and lower blood pressure and cholesterol. Iron maintains and oxygenates healthy red blood cells.

STRONG BONES:

Calcium builds strong bones.

EYE HEALTH:

Vitamin A promotes eye health, protecting against cataracts and macular degeneration.

IMMUNITY:

Vitamin C and iron boost immunity and may protect against flu.

GOOD INTERNAL HEALTH:

Potassium maintains organs.

ENHANCED BRAIN FUNCTION AND MOOD:

Omega-3 and -6 and vitamin B6 enhance brain function, aid memory, and help stabilize mood.

Glycemic load: 11
Inflammatory index: Anti-inflammatory

RECOMMENDED FOR HELP WITH:

- Heart health
- Reduced cholesterol
- Strong bones
- Eye health
- Healthy skin
- Immunity, which may include flu
- Mood stabilizer
- Weight loss
- Gout

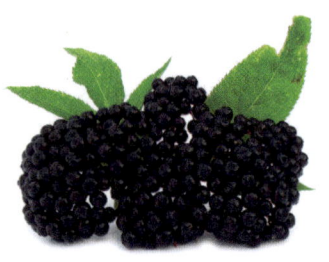

DIGESTIVE HEALTH:

The dietary fiber, carbohydrates, and potassium aid digestive health and reduce cholesterol, helping you feel fuller faster and aiding in weight loss.

GOUT:

The antioxidants reduce the pain of gout.

HEALTHY SKIN:

Vitamin A and fatty acids promote healthy skin.

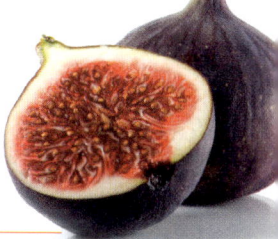

Figs

Figs are a delicious, sweet-tart fruit that are grown in warm climates. Figs are rich in antioxidants and are eaten both fresh and dried. Figs provide a healthy amount of dietary fiber and carbohydrates, making them great for digestive health and bowel regularity, and good in moderation for weight management. Fresh figs can be eaten whole as a snack or added to salads and other dishes. Because of fresh figs' seasonability, dried figs are a good year-round alternative and provide nearly the same amount of vitamins and minerals as fresh.

NUTRIENTS IN 1 MEDIUM FIG:

Calories, 37
Calcium, 17.5 mg
Carbohydrate, 9.6 g
Dietary fiber, 1.5 g
Magnesium, 8.5 mg
Omega-6 fatty acids, 72 mg
Potassium, 116 mg
Sugars, 8.2 g
Vitamin A (RAE), 3.5 mcg
Vitamin K, 2.4 mcg

HEALTH AND HEALING BENEFITS:

DIGESTIVE HEALTH:

Fiber, carbohydrates, and potassium aid digestion and reduce cholesterol, also easing constipation. Magnesium assists healthy metabolism.

GOOD INTERNAL HEALTH:

Potassium maintains organs.

STRONG BONES:

Vitamin K and magnesium support calcium in maintaining strong bones.

Glycemic load: 3
Inflammatory index: Mildly anti-inflammatory

RECOMMENDED FOR HELP WITH:

- Digestive health
- Easing constipation
- Reducing cardiovascular disease
- Strong bones
- Healthy skin
- Enhanced brain function

HEART AND BLOOD HEALTH:

Omega-6 regulates blood pressure, and vitamin A helps prevent cardiovascular disease. Vitamin K is important in matters related to the blood, such as regulating clotting, and menstrual flow and pain.

HEALTHY SKIN:

Vitamin A and fatty acids promote healthy skin.

ENHANCED BRAIN FUNCTION:

Omega-6 enhances brain function and may aid memory.

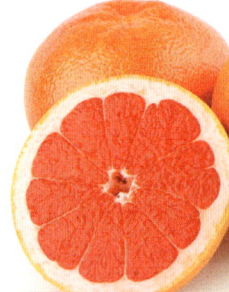

GRAPEFRUIT

The botanical name of grapefruit translates to "paradise citrus," and it's no wonder when you consider the vitamin-filled beauty of this fruit. Grapefruits come in pink, red, or white, each with varying degrees of sweet or tart flavor. All types are low in calories and high in fiber, as well as providing a wealth of fatty acids, vitamins C and A, and calcium. Grapefruit is known as an immunity booster, cholesterol-reducer, metabolism-increaser, and potentially a cancer-preventer as well. Some medications, including statins, may not react well with grapefruit; for any concerns, discuss with your doctor.

Grapefruit (pink and red)

Red and pink grapefruit have higher levels of vitamin A than their white counterpart. They are also sweeter.

NUTRIENTS IN ½ PINK/RED GRAPEFRUIT:

Calories, 52
Calcium, 27.1 mg
Carbohydrate, 13.2 g
Folate, 16 mcg
Magnesium, 11.1 mg
Omega-3 fatty acids, 10 mg
Omega-6 fatty acids, 36 mg
Phosphorus, 22.1 mg
Potassium, 166 mg
Sugars, 8.5 g
Vitamin A (RAE), 71.3 mcg
Vitamin C, 38.4 mg

Glycemic load: 3
Inflammatory index: Anti-inflammatory

64 　FOODS THAT HEAL

Grapefruit (white)

Referred to as both "white" and "yellow," this grapefruit has a tarter taste and marginally more vitamin C than pink/red.

NUTRIENTS IN ½ WHITE GRAPEFRUIT:

Calories, 39
Calcium, 14.2 mg
Carbohydrate, 9.9 g
Folate, 11.8 mcg
Magnesium, 10.6 mg
Omega-3 fatty acids, 6 mg
Omega-6 fatty acids, 22 mg
Phosphorus, 9.4 mg
Potassium, 175 mg
Sugars, 8.6 g
Vitamin A (RAE), 2.4 mcg
Vitamin C, 39.3 mg

Glycemic load: 2
Inflammatory index: Anti-inflammatory

Grapefruit juice (pink)

Pink grapefruit juice is high in antioxidants and, in particular, lycopene, which has anti-tumor properties.

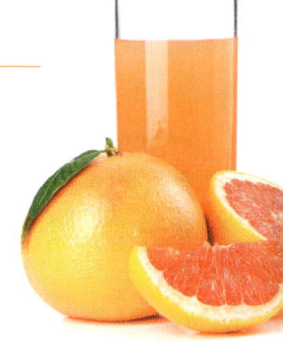

GRAPES

Grapes are grown around the world, from the United States to China, and Chile to South Africa. They come in a wide variety of colors and flavors and can be eaten raw, turned into juice and wine, and added to salads. Grapes are low in calories and a great replacement for a sugary treat; they help you maintain a healthy weight by filling up on fewer calories. All grapes contain antioxidants—in particular, resveratrol, which is higher in dark-skinned grapes than in white, and fights inflammation and heart disease. Grapes also provide good dietary fiber and help with bowel regularity, plus vitamins A, C, and K.

Grapes (green)

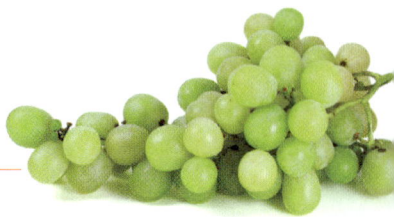

While lower in resveratrol than darker-skinned grapes, these grapes (called both white and green) are still loaded with antioxidants and vitamins and are often a more popular choice for children.

Grapes (red)

Red grapes, also known as black, are a richer source of the antioxidant resveratrol than green grapes.

NUTRIENTS IN 1 CUP OF RED OR GREEN GRAPES:
(Only shared nutritional data is available for red and green grapes.)

Calories, 104
Carbohydrate, 27.3 g
Omega-3 fatty acids, 17 mg
Omega-6 fatty acids, 56 mg
Sugars, 23.4 g
Vitamin C, 4.8 mg
Vitamin K, 22 mcg

HEALTH AND HEALING BENEFITS OF GRAPES:

JOINT HEALTH:

The antioxidant resveratrol and fatty acids fight inflammation.

IMMUNITY:

With antiviral properties, the antioxidants, vitamin C, and iron boost the immune system and fight illness.

HEART AND BLOOD HEALTH:

Omega-3, omega-6, and protein help protect the body against stroke, heart disease, and diabetes, and lower blood pressure. Vitamin C promotes heart health. Vitamin K is important to matters related to the blood, such as regulating clotting, and menstrual flow and pain. Resveratrol prevents heart disease.

Glycemic load: 12
Inflammatory index: Anti-inflammatory

RECOMMENDED FOR HELP WITH:

- Reducing cardiovascular disease
- Joint health
- Immunity
- Enhanced brain function, including memory
- Weight loss
- Easing constipation

ENHANCED BRAIN FUNCTION AND MOOD:

Vitamin C and iron provide a huge boost to the immune system and fight illness.

DIGESTIVE HEALTH:

Carbohydrates aid digestive health and reduce cholesterol, helping you feel fuller faster and aiding in weight loss, while also easing constipation.

STRONG BONES:

Vitamin K helps maintain strong bones.

Grape juice

Grape juice is rich in antioxidants and good for the heart. The most common grape found in grape juice is the Concord.

NUTRIENTS IN 1 CUP OF GRAPE JUICE (UNSWEETENED):

Calories, 152
Carbohydrate, 37 g
Dietary fiber, 1 g
Iron, 0.6 mg
Magnesium, 25.3 mg
Manganese, 0.6 mg
Omega-3 fatty acids, 13 mg
Omega-6 fatty acids, 43 mg
Phosphorus, 35.4 mg
Potassium, 263 mg
Protein, 1 g
Sugars, 36 g
Vitamin B6, 0.1 mg
Vitamin C, 0.25 mg

HEALTH AND HEALING BENEFITS:

DIGESTIVE HEALTH:

The dietary fiber and carbohydrates aid digestive health and reduce cholesterol, helping you feel fuller faster and aiding in weight loss. They also ease constipation and maintain bowel regularity.

BLOOD HEALTH:

Iron maintains healthy red blood cells and improves their ability to carry oxygen to cells around the body. Growing children and adolescents, as well as menstruating, pregnant, or lactating women, have an increased need for iron. Vitamin B6 strengthens blood. Vitamin B6 deficiency is found in people with heart disease, premenstrual syndrome, atherosclerosis, and carpal tunnel syndrome.

ENERGY:

Magnesium and protein are key to energy production.

STRONG BONES AND MUSCLES:

Protein helps build and repair bones, tissues, hormones, and body chemicals. Phosphorus and magnesium maintain strong bones. Potassium helps build strong muscles and is good for easing muscle cramps.

HEART AND BLOOD HEALTH:

Omega-3, omega-6, and protein help protect the body against stroke, heart disease, and diabetes, and lower blood pressure. Vitamin C and potassium promote heart health. Fiber helps lower cholesterol.

Glycemic load: 17
Inflammatory index: Anti-inflammatory

ENHANCED BRAIN FUNCTION AND MOOD:

Fatty acids and vitamin B6 are integral to brain function and may aid memory and stabilize mood.

HEALTHY SKIN:

Manganese and fatty acids promote healthy skin and help prevent acne.

IMMUNITY:

Vitamin C and iron provide a huge boost to the immune system. Riboflavin aids in the production of antibodies.

JOINT HEALTH:

Omega-6 and magnesium reduce joint inflammation.

GOOD INTERNAL HEALTH:

Potassium keeps the organs in good working order.

RECOMMENDED FOR HELP WITH:

- Digestive health
- Weight loss
- Easing constipation and maintaining bowel regularity
- Immunity
- Heart and blood health
- Joint health
- Enhanced brain function
- Strong bones
- Healthy skin

GUAVA

Guava is a tropical fruit that remains rare in mainstream grocery stores, but its growing popularity means it can now be found in many health food stores. Guava originated in Central and South America and is now grown in a range of warmer regions. Guava comes in different types, including pineapple and strawberry, with the common guava also called the green apple guava. It can be eaten raw, cooked, or as nectars and preserves. This seed-abundant fruit is an excellent source of vitamins A and C, as well as carbohydrates and fiber. This makes guava good for the digestive system and assists in appetite control, as well as boosting bone strength and immunity. Some pediatric specialists believe guava is a rich nutrient source for nursing mothers.

Pineapple guava, also known as feijoa or guavasteen, is rich in antioxidants and folate. It is oval with green skin and cream flesh. Strawberry guava provides an excellent source of vitamin C and potassium. The skin and flesh are a reddish-purple.

Guava (common)

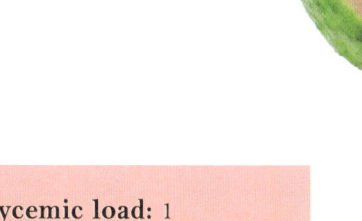

NUTRIENTS IN 1 COMMON GUAVA:

Calories, 37
Carbohydrate, 7.9 g
Copper, 0.1 mg
Dietary fiber, 3 g
Folate, 27 mcg
Omega-3 fatty acids, 62 mg
Omega-6 fatty acids, 158 mg
Potassium, 229 mg
Protein, 1.4 g
Sugars, 4.9 g
Vitamin A (RAE), 17 mcg
Vitamin C, 125 mg

HEALTH AND HEALING BENEFITS:

DIGESTIVE HEALTH:

Fiber and carbohydrates aid digestive health and reduce cholesterol, helping you feel fuller faster and aiding appetite control, as well as easing constipation and calming diarrhea. They also maintain bowel regularity. Folate improves fat metabolism.

HEART HEALTH:

Omega-3, omega-6, and protein help protect the body against stroke, heart disease, and diabetes, and lower blood pressure. Folate reduces the risk of heart disease and hypertension. Vitamin C and potassium promote heart health.

IMMUNITY:

With anti-viral properties, the antioxidants and vitamin C boost the immune system and fight illness.

ENHANCED BRAIN FUNCTION:

Omega-3 and -6 and folate enhance brain function and may aid memory. Folate is especially important during pregnancy for the fetus and may also help protect against Alzheimer's.

INTERNAL HEALTH:

Potassium maintains organs.

TISSUE REGENERATION:

Vitamin A is central to tissue regeneration, and fatty acids assist in cellular regeneration.

MUSCLES:

Potassium helps build strong muscles and eases muscle cramps.

Glycemic load: 1
Inflammatory index: Anti-inflammatory

RECOMMENDED FOR HELP WITH:

- Digestive health
- Reducing cholesterol
- Weight loss
- Easing constipation and calming diarrhea
- Immunity
- Developing fetus during pregnancy and nutrient source for nursing
- Enhanced brain function
- Strong muscles
- Healthy skin and eyes

Guava nectar

As guavas are seasonal, guava nectar is a good alternative, as it's an excellent source of vitamins A and C, but should be consumed in moderation. Like the fresh fruit, guava nectar is rich in fiber and vitamin C, as well as vitamin A.

Honeydew

Honeydew is a type of muskmelon. It is sweet and juicy and often eaten raw as a snack or dessert. The nutrients promote immunity and skin health. Some people can have a melon allergy. If your lips feel numb, consult a doctor.

NUTRIENTS IN 1 WEDGE OF MEDIUM HONEYDEW (ABOUT 1/8 OF FRUIT):

Calories, 58
Calcium, 9.6 mg
Carbohydrate, 14.5 g
Folate, 30.4 mcg
Magnesium, 0.04 mg
Omega-3 fatty acids, 53 mg
Omega-6 fatty acids, 42 mg
Phosphorus, 17.6 mg
Potassium, 365 mg
Sugars, 13 g
Vitamin A (RAE), 4.8 mcg
Vitamin C, 28.8 mg
Vitamin K, 4.6 mcg

HEALTH AND HEALING BENEFITS:

IMMUNITY:

With anti-viral properties, the antioxidants and vitamin C boost the immune system and fight illness.

HEALTHY SKIN:

Vitamin A and fatty acids promote healthy skin.

BONES AND MUSCLES:

Vitamin K, phosphorus, and magnesium support calcium in maintaining strong bones. Potassium helps build strong muscles and eases cramps.

ENHANCED BRAIN FUNCTION:

Omega-3 and -6 and folate enhance brain function and may aid memory. Folate is especially important during pregnancy for the fetus.

Glycemic load: 9
Inflammatory index: Anti-inflammatory

RECOMMENDED FOR HELP WITH:

- Immunity
- Healthy skin
- Reducing risk of cardiovascular disease
- Strong bones and muscles
- Enhanced brain function
- Digestive health

HEART AND BLOOD HEALTH:

Omega-3, omega-6, and protein help protect the body against stroke, heart disease, and diabetes, and lower blood pressure. Folate reduces the risk of heart disease and hypertension, while vitamin C and potassium promote heart health. Vitamin K is important in matters related to the blood, such as regulating clotting, and menstrual flow and pain.

DIGESTIVE HEALTH:

Carbohydrates aid digestive health and reduce cholesterol. Folate improves the metabolism of fat.

Kiwifruit

The kiwifruit (often simply "kiwi") is a delicate, small fruit with brownish-green, fuzzy skin and bright green flesh. Kiwifruit are often peeled and eaten raw or added to fruit salads or desserts. On their own, kiwifruit are an alkalizing food that provide a huge dose of vitamin C, as well as being a good source of carbohydrates, vitamins A and E, potassium, and lutein. As a result, this fruit strengthens immunity, improves eye health, prevents cardiovascular disease, and keeps the organs in good condition.

NUTRIENTS IN 1 KIWIFRUIT:

Calories, 42
Calcium, 23.5 mg
Carbohydrate, 10.1 g
Dietary fiber, 2.1 g
Folate, 17.2 mcg
Omega-3 fatty acids, 29 mg
Omega-6 fatty acids, 170 mg
Potassium, 215 mg
Sugars, 6.2 g

Vitamin A (RAE), 2.8 mcg
Vitamin C, 64 mg
Vitamin E, 1 mg
Vitamin K, 27.8 mcg

Glycemic load: 5
Inflammatory index: Anti-inflammatory

HEALTH AND HEALING BENEFITS:

IMMUNITY:

Vitamins C and E provide a huge boost to the immune system.

HEART AND BLOOD HEALTH:

Omega-3 and -6 help protect the body against stroke, heart disease, and diabetes, and lower blood pressure. Vitamins C and E, and potassium reduce cardiovascular disease, while folate reduces the risk of heart disease and hypertension. Vitamin K is important in matters related to the blood, such as regulating clotting, and menstrual flow and pain.

STRONG BONES:

Vitamin K supports calcium in maintaining strong bones.

STRONG MUSCLES AND TISSUE:

Potassium helps build strong muscles and eases muscle cramps. Vitamin A is central to tissue regeneration, and fatty acids assist in cellular regeneration.

CANCER PROTECTION:

Antioxidants and vitamin E protect against cancer.

INTERNAL HEALTH:

Potassium maintains organs.

HEALTHY SKIN:

Vitamin A and fatty acids promote healthy skin.

EYE HEALTH:

Vitamin A and lutein promote eye health, protecting against cataracts and macular degeneration.

ENHANCED BRAIN FUNCTION:

Omega-3 and omega-6 are integral to brain function and may aid memory. Folate is important for all aspects of brain function, and is especially important during pregnancy for reducing the risk of spinal and mental defects in the fetus. It may also help protect against Alzheimer's.

DIGESTIVE HEALTH:

The dietary fiber and carbohydrates aid digestive health, easing indigestion and calming diarrhea, and, alongside vitamin E, reduce cholesterol. Folate and vitamin E improve metabolism.

RECOMMENDED FOR HELP WITH:

- Immunity
- Heart health
- Strong bones and muscles
- Eye health
- Healthy skin
- Enhanced brain function
- Reducing cholesterol
- Improving metabolism
- Developing fetus during pregnancy
- Possible cancer protection

Lemon

Lemons are not commonly eaten raw, but with the nutritional punch they provide whole, you may think again! However, even by adding its juice or pulp to drinks and dishes, your body is still absorbing this fruit's mighty offerings. Lemons and their juice are an excellent source of vitamin C. The skin provides a huge dose of vitamin C, so for added immune strength, try adding zest the next time you're cooking with lemons. Lemon and honey is a great simple recipe for sore throats.

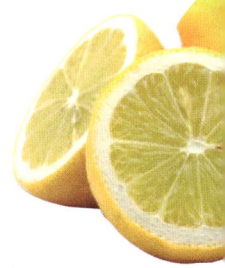

NUTRIENTS IN 1 SMALL LEMON:

Calories, 17
Calcium, 15.1 mg
Carbohydrate, 5.4 g
Dietary fiber, 1.6 g
Magnesium, 4.6 mg
Omega-3 fatty acids, 15 mg
Omega-6 fatty acids, 37 mg
Potassium, 80 mg
Vitamin C, 30.7 mg

HEALTH AND HEALING BENEFITS:

IMMUNITY:

With antiviral properties, the antioxidants, vitamin C, and iron boost the immune system and fight illness.

BONES AND MUSCLES:

Magnesium supports calcium in maintaining strong bones. Potassium builds muscles.

BLOOD HEALTH:

Iron maintains healthy red blood cells and improves their ability to carry oxygen to cells. Growing children and adolescents, as well as menstruating, pregnant, or lactating women, have an increased need for iron. Copper assists iron absorption.

DIGESTIVE HEALTH:

Fiber and carbohydrates aid digestive health as well as easing constipation.

INTERNAL HEALTH:

Potassium keeps the organs in good working order.

HEART HEALTH:

Fatty acids, vitamin C, and potassium protect against stroke, heart disease, and diabetes, and lower blood pressure.

ENHANCED BRAIN FUNCTION:

Omega-3 and -6 are integral to brain function and may aid memory.

Glycemic load: 1
Inflammatory index: Anti-inflammatory

RECOMMENDED FOR HELP WITH:

- Immunity
- Colds and illnesses
- Strong bones
- Digestive health
- Easing constipation
- Reducing risk of cardiovascular disease
- Blood health
- Enhanced brain function

Lemongrass

Nicknamed "fevergrass," lemongrass is a type of grass native to Asia. Lemongrass was traditionally used to quell fevers and fight infection. The anti-inflammatory properties help to reduce nausea, relieve dyspepsia, and aid digestion.

NUTRIENTS IN 1 TBSP. OF LEMONGRASS:

Calories, 5
Calcium, 3.1 mg
Carbohydrate, 1.2 g
Copper, 0 mg
Folate, 3.6 mcg
Iron, 0.4 mg
Magnesium, 2.9 mg
Manganese, 0.3 mg
Omega-3 fatty acids, 1 mg
Omega-6 fatty acids, 7 mg
Phosphorus, 4.9 mg
Potassium, 34.7 mg
Vitamin C, 0.1 mg
Zinc, 0.1 mg

FRUITS AND FRUIT JUICES

HEALTH AND HEALING BENEFITS:

DIGESTIVE HEALTH:

Carbohydrates aid digestive health and reduce cholesterol, helping you feel fuller faster, aiding weight loss, reducing nausea, and relieving dyspepsia. Folate metabolizes fat.

HEART AND BLOOD HEALTH:

Omega-3 and -6 protect against stroke, heart disease, and diabetes, and lower blood pressure. Potassium and vitamin C promote heart health, while folate reduces the risk of heart disease and hypertension.

BLOOD HEALTH:

Iron and copper maintain healthy red blood cells and improve their ability to carry oxygen to cells. Growing children and adolescents, as well as menstruating, pregnant, or lactating women, have an increased need for iron.

IMMUNITY:

Vitamin C, iron, and zinc boost the immune system.

ENERGY:

Copper and magnesium are key to energy production.

BONES AND MUSCLES:

Phosphorus and magnesium support calcium in maintaining strong bones. Potassium helps build strong muscles and eases muscle cramps.

ENHANCED BRAIN FUNCTION:

Omega-3 and -6 are integral to brain function and may aid memory. Folate is important for all aspects of brain function, and is especially important during pregnancy. It may also help protect against Alzheimer's.

JOINT HEALTH:

Omega-6 and magnesium reduce joint inflammation.

Glycemic load: 3
Inflammatory index: Anti-inflammatory

RECOMMENDED FOR HELP WITH:

- Digestive health
- Reducing nausea
- Heart health
- Bones and muscles
- Immunity
- Energy
- Enhanced brain function
- Developing fetus during pregnancy

Lime

This small citrus fruit is rich in antioxidants and an excellent source of vitamin C, and one lime contains 22% of the average RDV for adults—great for boosting immunity and fighting illness. Citrus fruits are recommended as a remedy for chemotherapy patients and others experiencing dramatic changes in taste.

NUTRIENTS IN 1 LIME:

Calories, 20
Calcium, 22.1 mg
Carbohydrate, 7 g
Dietary fiber, 1.9 g
Folate, 5.4 mcg
Iron, 0.4 mg
Omega-3 fatty acids, 13 mg
Omega-6 fatty acids, 24 mg
Pantothenic acid, 0.1 mg
Phosphorus, 12.1 mg
Potassium, 68.3 mg
Vitamin C, 19.5 mg

HEALTH AND HEALING BENEFITS:

IMMUNITY:

With antiviral properties, the antioxidants, vitamin C, and iron boost the immune system and fight illness.

HEART AND BLOOD HEALTH:

Omega-3 and -6 help protect the body against stroke, heart disease, and diabetes, and lower blood pressure. Folate reduces the risk of heart disease and hypertension, while vitamin C and potassium promote heart health. Iron maintains healthy red blood cells and improves their ability to carry oxygen to cells. Growing children and adolescents, as well as menstruating, pregnant, or lactating women, have an increased need for iron.

BONES AND MUSCLES:

Calcium and phosphorus build and maintain strong bones. Potassium helps build muscle.

INTERNAL HEALTH:

Potassium keeps the organs in good working order.

ENHANCED BRAIN FUNCTION:

Omega-3 and -6 are integral to brain function and may aid memory. Folate is important for all aspects of brain function, and is especially important during pregnancy.

DIGESTIVE HEALTH:

The dietary fiber and carbohydrates aid digestive health and reduce cholesterol. Folate improves the metabolism of fat.

Glycemic load: 2
Inflammatory index: Anti-inflammatory

RECOMMENDED FOR HELP WITH:

- Chemotherapy patients
- Immunity
- Bones and muscles
- Heart health
- Reduces cholesterol
- Brain function
- Developing fetus during pregnancy
- Digestive health

Lychee

Native to Asia, the lychee (or litchi) was once considered an aphrodisiac. Distinctive in appearance, this alkalizing food has bumpy pink skin, juicy white flesh, and a floral aroma. It can be found in Asian grocery stores and health food stores. It is loaded with vitamin C and provides a huge boost to immune function. The polyphenols have been found to combat obesity and prevent liver disease.

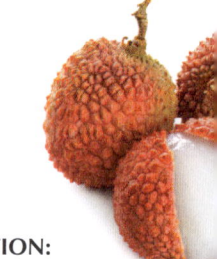

NUTRIENTS IN 1 LYCHEE:

Calories, 6
Carbohydrate, 1.6 g
Folate, 1.3 mcg
Magnesium, 1 mg
Niacin, 0.1 mg
Omega-3 fatty acids, 6 mg
Omega-6 fatty acids, 6 mg
Phosphorus, 3 mg
Potassium, 16.4 mg
Sugars, 1.5 g
Vitamin C, 6.9 mg

HEALTH AND HEALING BENEFITS:

ENERGY:

Magnesium and niacin are key to energy production.

DIGESTIVE HEALTH:

Carbohydrates aid digestive health and reduce cholesterol, helping you feel fuller faster and, with polyphenols, help combat obesity. Folate improves fat metabolism.

IMMUNITY:

Vitamin C boosts immunity.

INTERNAL HEALTH:

Polyphenols help prevent liver disease. Potassium keeps the organs in good working order.

BONES AND MUSCLES:

Phosphorus and magnesium maintain strong bones, while potassium builds strong muscles.

JOINT HEALTH:

Omega-6 and magnesium reduce joint inflammation.

HEART AND BLOOD HEALTH:

Omega-3 and omega-6 help protect the body against stroke, heart disease, and diabetes, and lower blood pressure. Vitamin C and potassium promote heart health, while folate reduces the risk of heart disease and hypertension.

ENHANCED BRAIN FUNCTION:

Omega-3 and -6 and folate enhance brain function and may aid memory.

Glycemic load: 1
Inflammatory index: Anti-inflammatory

RECOMMENDED FOR HELP WITH:

- Immunity
- Protection against liver disease
- Digestive health
- Combating obesity
- Energy
- Heart health
- Strong bones and muscles
- Joint health

Mandarin (satsuma)

The mandarin, or satsuma, looks like a small orange. It is commonly understood to be the same as the tangerine, although some retailers distinguish the two by skin color. Mandarins provide 80% of your vitamin C RDV, boosting immunity, and the fiber is important for weight loss and cholesterol reduction. Studies suggest the juice can help protect against liver cancer.

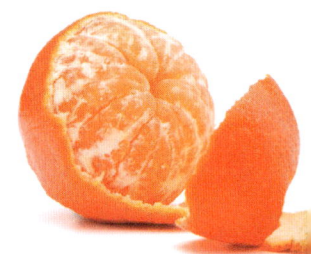

NUTRIENTS IN 1 MEDIUM MANDARIN:

Calories, 47
Calcium, 32.6 mg
Carbohydrate, 11.7 g
Dietary fiber, 1.6 g
Folate, 14.1 mcg
Omega-3 fatty acids, 16 mg
Omega-6 fatty acids, 42 mg
Potassium, 146 mg
Sugars, 9.3 g
Vitamin A (RAE), 29.9 mcg
Vitamin C, 23.5 mg

HEALTH AND HEALING BENEFITS:

IMMUNITY:

With antiviral properties, the antioxidants and vitamin C boost immunity.

DIGESTIVE HEALTH:

Fiber and carbohydrates aid digestive health and reduce cholesterol, helping you feel fuller faster and aiding in weight loss. Folate improves the metabolism of fat.

BONES, MUSCLES, AND TISSUE:

Calcium builds strong bones, while potassium builds muscle. Vitamin A is central to tissue regeneration, and fatty acids assist cellular regeneration.

EYE HEALTH:

Vitamin A promotes eye health, protecting against cataracts and macular degeneration.

HEALTHY SKIN:

Vitamin A and fatty acids promote healthy skin.

INTERNAL HEALTH:

Potassium maintains organs.

ENHANCED BRAIN FUNCTION:

Omega-3 and -6 are integral to brain function and may aid memory. Folate is important for brain function, and is especially important during pregnancy for the fetus.

HEART AND BLOOD HEALTH:

Omega-3 and -6 help protect the body against stroke, heart disease, and diabetes, and lower blood pressure. Vitamin C and potassium promote heart health, while folate reduces the risk of heart disease and hypertension.

CANCER PROTECTION:

The juice may help protect against liver cancer.

Glycemic load: 1
Inflammatory index: Anti-inflammatory

RECOMMENDED FOR HELP WITH:

- Digestive health
- Reducing cholesterol
- Immunity
- Heart health
- Bones and muscles
- Healthy skin and eyes
- Enhanced brain function

Mango, raw

Mangoes are large fruits with a stone, covered in reddish-green skin, with juicy yellow flesh. They are a rich source of antioxidants, providing high levels of vitamins A, C, and E for immune strength, healthy skin and eyes, and cardiovascular health, and they are known to reduce symptoms of gastritis.

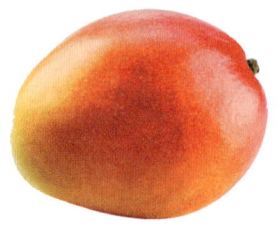

NUTRIENTS IN 1 RAW MANGO:

Calories, 202
Carbohydrate, 50.4 g
Dietary fiber, 5.4 g
Folate, 144 mcg
Magnesium, 33.6 mg
Niacin, 2.3 mg
Omega-3 fatty acids, 171 mg
Omega-6 fatty acids, 64 mg
Phosphorus, 47 mg
Potassium, 564 mg
Sugars, 46 g
Vitamin A (RAE), 181 mcg
Vitamin C, 122 mg
Vitamin E, 3 mg
Vitamin K, 14.1 mcg

HEALTH AND HEALING BENEFITS:

IMMUNITY:

With antiviral properties, the antioxidants and vitamin C boost the immune system and fight illness.

EYE HEALTH:

Vitamin A promotes eye health, protecting against cataracts and macular degeneration.

HEALTHY SKIN:

Vitamin A and fatty acids promote healthy skin.

HEART AND BLOOD HEALTH:

Omega-3 and -6, potassium, and vitamins C and E protect against stroke, heart disease, and diabetes and lower blood pressure. Folate reduces the risk of hypertension, and vitamin K is important to blood health, such as regulating clotting.

BONES, MUSCLES, AND TISSUE:

Vitamin K, phosphorus, and magnesium maintain strong bones. Potassium helps build strong muscles. Vitamin A is central to tissue regeneration, and fatty acids assist in cellular regeneration.

INTERNAL HEALTH:

Potassium maintains organs.

ENERGY:

Magnesium and niacin are key to energy production. Vitamin E boosts stamina.

ENHANCED BRAIN FUNCTION:

Omega-3 and -6 are integral to brain function and may aid memory. Folate is important for all aspects of brain function, and is especially important during pregnancy for the fetus. It may also help protect against Alzheimer's disease.

DIGESTIVE HEALTH:

Fiber and carbohydrates aid digestive health and, with vitamin E, reduce cholesterol, as well as reducing gastritis. Folate and vitamin E improve metabolism.

CANCER PROTECTION:

Antioxidants and vitamin E protect against cancer.

Glycemic load: 28
Inflammatory index: Anti-inflammatory

RECOMMENDED FOR HELP WITH:

- Immunity
- Eye health
- Healthy skin
- Blood health
- Strong bones and muscles
- Energy
- Enhanced brain function
- Digestive health, reducing gastritis
- Possible cancer protection

Mango, dried

Dried mango is an energy-boosting snack packed with vitamin A, but it does contain more sugar than the fresh fruit. Dried mango is recommended for help with immunity, energy, digestion, and healthy eyes and skin.

Mango nectar, canned

While higher in calories and sugars than fresh mango, mango nectar is still a great source of vitamins A and C. Look for nectar without added sugar.

Nectarine

Nectarines belong to the same species as peaches. The dietary fiber and low calories assist with weight loss, and because of their sweet taste, nectarines are an ideal replacement for sugary treats. Nectarines are an alkalizing food with vitamins A and C, and potassium. Like peaches and plums, they can cause an allergic reaction in those suffering from birch-pollen allergies.

NUTRIENTS IN 1 MEDIUM NECTARINE:

Calories, 63
Carbohydrate, 15.1 g
Magnesium, 12.8 mg
Niacin, 1.6 mg
Omega-3 fatty acids, 3 mg
Omega-6 fatty acids, 158 mg
Phosphorus, 36.9 mg
Potassium, 285 mg
Sugars, 11.2 g
Vitamin A (RAE), 24.1 mcg
Vitamin C, 7.7 mg
Vitamin K, 3.1 mcg

HEALTH AND HEALING BENEFITS:

DIGESTIVE HEALTH:

Carbohydrates aid digestion and reduce cholesterol, helping you feel fuller faster and aiding in weight loss.

IMMUNITY:

With antiviral properties, the antioxidants and vitamin C boost immunity.

SKIN AND EYE HEALTH:

Vitamin A and fatty acids promote healthy skin. Vitamin A promotes eye health, protecting against cataracts and macular degeneration.

HEART AND BLOOD HEALTH:

Omega-3 and -6 help protect against stroke, heart disease, and diabetes, and lower blood pressure. Vitamin K is important in matters related to the blood, such as regulating clotting, and menstrual flow and pain. Vitamin C and potassium promote heart health.

BONES, MUSCLES, AND TISSUE:

Vitamin K, phosphorus, and magnesium maintain strong bones, while potassium helps build strong muscles and eases cramps. Vitamin A is central to tissue regeneration, and fatty acids assist cellular regeneration.

INTERNAL HEALTH:

Potassium maintains organs.

ENERGY:

Magnesium and niacin are key to energy production.

ENHANCED BRAIN FUNCTION:

Omega-3 and -6 are integral to brain function.

Glycemic load: 5
Inflammatory index: Anti-inflammatory

RECOMMENDED FOR HELP WITH:

- Immunity
- Digestive health
- Weight loss
- Skin and eye health
- Heart health
- Bones and muscles
- Energy
- Enhanced brain function

Olives

Both green and black olives are a good source of vitamins and nutrients. The difference in color is down to preparation methods and black olives being left longer on the vine. Green olives are picked before they are ripe, and both are soaked in lye and brine. However, they are high in antioxidants and omega fatty acids, and provide fiber and vitamins A and E, protecting against cardiovascular disease, high cholesterol, and arthritis. Green olives contain more sodium, and black olives are slightly higher in calories. Because of the sodium content, olives should be eaten in moderation.

NUTRIENTS IN 1 LARGE CANNED OLIVE:

Calories, 5
Calcium, 3.9 mg
Carbohydrate, 0.3 g
Copper, 0 mg
Dietary fiber, 0.1 g
Iron, 0.3 mg
Omega-6 fatty acids, 28 mg
Sodium, 32.3 mg
Vitamin A (RAE), 0.8 mcg
Vitamin E, 0.1 mg

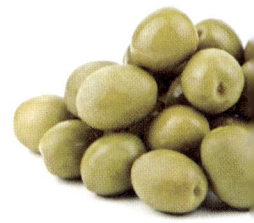

HEALTH AND HEALING BENEFITS:

DIGESTIVE HEALTH:

The fiber and carbohydrates aid digestive health and, alongside vitamin E, reduce cholesterol. Vitamin E improves metabolism.

JOINT HEALTH:

Omega-6 and magnesium reduce joint inflammation, helping with arthritis.

BONES AND TISSUE:

Calcium builds strong bones. Vitamin A is central to tissue regeneration.

ENERGY:

Copper and magnesium are key to energy production, while vitamin E boosts stamina.

SKIN AND EYE HEALTH:

Vitamin A and fatty acids promote healthy skin and help prevent acne. Vitamin A promotes eye health, protecting against cataracts and macular degeneration.

HEART AND BLOOD HEALTH:

Omega-3 and -6 help protect against stroke, heart disease, and diabetes, and lower blood pressure. Vitamin E reduces cardiovascular disease. Iron maintains healthy red blood cells and improves their ability to carry oxygen to cells.

IMMUNITY:

Iron and vitamin E boost immunity.

ENHANCED BRAIN FUNCTION:

Omega-3 and -6 are integral to brain function and may aid memory.

Glycemic load: 0
Inflammatory index: Anti-inflammatory

RECOMMENDED FOR HELP WITH:

- Heart health
- Digestive health
- Reducing cholesterol
- Skin and eye health
- Reducing inflammation and arthritis
- Strong bones and tissue
- Immunity
- Energy
- Enhanced brain function
- Possible cancer protection

Orange

Originating in Asia, oranges are an incredibly popular citrus fruit, believed to be the most cultivated fruit in the world. Oranges are rich in antioxidants, best known as an excellent source of vitamin C. Due to their carbohydrates, they are a good source of energy and maintain metabolism—a great snack for weight control. Fiber protects against cardiovascular disease and aids digestion. Vitamins A and C, and thiamin promote healthy skin and cell regeneration. Like other citrus fruit, oranges are acidic, which can cause damage to your tooth enamel and, in rare cases, trigger an allergic reaction. Consult your dentist or doctor if symptoms develop.

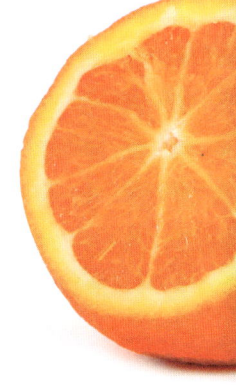

NUTRIENTS IN 1 ORANGE (AVERAGE OF ALL VARIETIES):

Calories, 62
Calcium, 52.4 mg
Carbohydrate, 15.5 g
Dietary fiber, 3.1 g
Folate, 39.3 mcg
Magnesium, 13.1 mg
Omega-3 fatty acids, 9 mg
Omega-6 fatty acids, 24 mg
Potassium, 237 mg
Sugars, 12.2 g
Vitamin C, 69.7 mg
Vitamin A (RAE), 14.4 mcg

HEALTH AND HEALING BENEFITS:

IMMUNITY:

With antiviral properties, the antioxidants and vitamin C boost the immune system and fight illness.

ENERGY:

Carbohydrates and magnesium provide energy.

DIGESTIVE HEALTH:

The dietary fiber and carbohydrates aid digestive health and reduce cholesterol, helping you feel fuller faster and aiding in weight loss. Folate improves the metabolism of fat.

HEART HEALTH:

Omega-3 and -6 help protect against stroke, heart disease, and diabetes, and lower blood pressure. Vitamin C and potassium promote heart health, while folate reduces the risk of heart disease and hypertension.

BONES AND MUSCLES:

Calcium and magnesium build and support strong bones, while potassium helps build muscle and eases cramps.

EYE HEALTH:

Vitamin A promotes eye health, protecting against cataracts and macular degeneration.

HEALTHY SKIN:

Vitamin A and fatty acids promote healthy skin and help prevent acne.

TISSUE REGENERATION:

Vitamin A is central to tissue regeneration, and fatty acids assist in cellular regeneration.

INTERNAL HEALTH:

Potassium keeps the organs in good working order.

ENHANCED BRAIN FUNCTION:

Omega-3 and -6 are integral to brain function and may aid memory. Folate is important for brain function, and is especially important during pregnancy for reducing the risk of spinal and mental defects in the fetus. It may also help protect against Alzheimer's.

Glycemic load: 5
Inflammatory index: Anti-inflammatory

RECOMMENDED FOR HELP WITH:

- Immunity and fighting colds and illnesses
- Energy
- Digestive health
- Weight loss
- Heart health
- Strong bones and muscles
- Skin and eye health
- Tissue regeneration
- Enhanced brain function
- Developing fetus during pregnancy

Orange juice

Orange juice is one of the most popular fruit juice in North America and Europe. It is rich in antioxidants, full of vitamins and minerals, and comes in a wide array of brands and styles. A whole orange packs more nutritional punch than juice, and fresh-squeezed orange juice more than from concentrate—but neither juice type provides much fiber. Vitamins C and A boost immunity and skin health. Large amounts of juice can cause weight gain and damage oral health.

NUTRIENTS IN 1 CUP OF FRESH-SQUEEZED ORANGE JUICE:

Calories, 112
Calcium, 27.3 mg
Carbohydrate, 26 g
Copper, 0.1 mg
Dietary fiber, 0.5 g
Folate, 74.4 mcg
Magnesium, 27.3 mg
Niacin, 1 mg
Omega-3 fatty acids, 27 mg
Omega-6 fatty acids, 72 mg
Pantothenic acid, 0.5 mg
Phosphorus, 42.2 mg
Potassium, 496 mg
Protein, 2 g
Riboflavin, 0.1 mg
Sugars, 21 g
Thiamin, 0.2 mg
Vitamin A (RAE), 24.8 mcg
Vitamin B6, 0.1 mg
Vitamin C, 124 mg

HEALTH AND HEALING BENEFITS:

HEALTHY SKIN:

Vitamin A and fatty acids promote healthy skin.

JOINT HEALTH:

Omega-6 and magnesium reduce joint inflammation.

DIGESTIVE HEALTH:

Carbohydrates aid digestive health and reduce cholesterol. They also maintain bowel regularity and reduce the risk of diabetes and gastrointestinal disease. Folate improves the metabolism of fat.

HEART AND BLOOD HEALTH:

Omega-3, omega-6, and protein help protect against stroke, heart disease, and diabetes, and lower blood pressure. Vitamin C, potassium, and thiamin promote heart health, while folate reduces the risk of heart disease and hypertension. Vitamin B6 strengthens blood.

IMMUNITY:

With antiviral properties, the antioxidants and vitamin C boost immunity and fight illness.

EYE HEALTH:

Vitamin A promotes eye health, protecting against cataracts and macular degeneration.

BONES, MUSCLES, AND TISSUE:

Protein helps build and repair bones and tissues. Magnesium and phosphorus support calcium in maintaining strong bones. Potassium

Glycemic load: 12
Inflammatory index: Anti-inflammatory

helps build strong muscles and eases muscle cramps. Vitamin A is central to tissue regeneration, and fatty acids assist in cellular regeneration.

ENHANCED BRAIN FUNCTION AND MOOD:

Omega-3, omega-6, and vitamin B6 are integral to brain function and may aid memory, as well as stabilizing mood. Folate is important for brain function, and is especially important during pregnancy for reducing the risk of spinal and mental defects in the fetus. It may also help protect against Alzheimer's.

INTERNAL HEALTH:

Potassium keeps the organs in good working order.

ENERGY:

Copper, magnesium, niacin, and protein are key to energy production.

RECOMMENDED FOR HELP WITH:

- Immunity and fighting colds and illnesses
- Eye and skin health
- Reducing inflammation
- Reducing cholesterol
- Reducing risk of cardiovascular disease
- Strong bones and muscles
- Energy
- Enhanced brain function, including memory and mood
- Developing fetus during pregnancy

Papaya

The papaya is a tropical tree-growing fruit originating from Central America. Outside of the Americas, it is occasionally called "pawpaw," "papaw," or "red papaya." Papayas are sweet and juicy and tend to have pinkish-red flesh. It can be cut up and eaten straight, or added to salads and desserts. Papayas are rich in antioxidants and provide a huge amount of vitamin C, as well as vitamin A and potassium, contributing to strong immunity and healthy skin, bones, and body functions. The digestive enzymes contribute to digestive health, including reducing the symptoms of gastritis. The antioxidant lycopene reduces the risk of cardiovascular disease and, with vitamin A, macular degeneration.

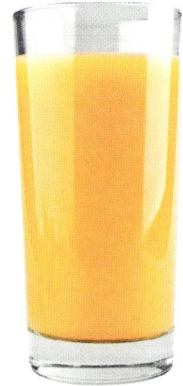

NUTRIENTS IN 1 SMALL PAPAYA:

Calories, 68
Calcium, 31.4 mg
Carbohydrate, 17 g
Dietary fiber, 2.7 g
Folate, 58.1 mcg
Magnesium, 33 mg
Omega-3 fatty acids, 74 mg
Omega-6 fatty acids, 17 mg
Potassium, 286 mg
Sugars, 12.3 g
Vitamin A (RAE), 73.8 mcg
Vitamin C, 95.6 mg
Vitamin E, 0.5 mg
Vitamin K, 4.1 mcg

HEALTH AND HEALING BENEFITS:

DIGESTIVE HEALTH:

Fiber, digestive enzymes, and carbohydrates aid digestive health and, alongside vitamin E, reduce cholesterol, reducing symptoms of gastritis. They also maintain bowel regularity and reduce the risk of diabetes and gastrointestinal disease. Folate and vitamin E improve metabolism.

IMMUNITY:

Antioxidants and vitamins C and E boost immunity.

HEART AND BLOOD HEALTH:

Omega-3 and -6 help protect against stroke, heart disease, and diabetes, and lower blood pressure. Vitamin K is important to matters related to the blood, such as regulating clotting, and menstrual flow and pain. Vitamins C and E and potassium promote heart health, boosted by lycopene, while folate reduces the risk of heart disease and hypertension.

Glycemic load: 10
Inflammatory index: Anti-inflammatory

RECOMMENDED FOR HELP WITH:

- Immunity
- Reducing symptoms of gastritis
- Reducing cardiovascular disease
- Eye health
- Healthy skin
- Strong bones and tissue
- Improved stamina
- Enhanced brain function
- Developing fetus during pregnancy
- Possible cancer protection

Passion fruit

Passion fruit, or purple granadilla, is a tropical fruit that is native to South America. The fruit is small and round, with purple skin and sweet-tasting, yellow, seed-filled flesh. It can be eaten on its own or turned into juices, smoothies, sauces, and desserts. Passion fruit is an alkalizing food that provides fiber and vitamins C and A. Both passion fruit and its flower contain a sedative compound called harman, used as a traditional remedy for insomnia and anxiety.

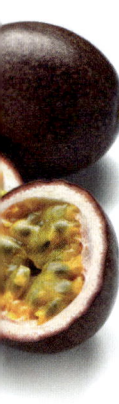

NUTRIENTS IN 1 PASSION FRUIT:

Calories, 18
Carbohydrate, 4.2 g
Dietary fiber, 1.9 g
Iron, 0.3 mg
Magnesium, 5.2 mg
Niacin, 0.3 mg
Omega-6 fatty acids, 74 mg
Phosphorus, 12.2 mg
Potassium, 62.6 mg
Protein, 0.4 g
Sugars, 2 g
Vitamin A (RAE), 11.5 mcg
Vitamin C, 5.4 mg

HEALTH AND HEALING BENEFITS:

IMMUNITY:

With antiviral properties, the antioxidants, vitamin C, and iron boost the immune system and fight illness.

BONES, MUSCLES, AND TISSUE:

Protein helps build and repair bones and tissue. Phosphorus and magnesium maintain strong bones, and potassium helps build strong muscles and eases muscle cramps. Vitamin A is central to tissue regeneration, and fatty acids assist in cellular regeneration.

HEART AND BLOOD HEALTH:

Omega-3, omega-6, and protein help protect against stroke, heart disease, and diabetes, and lower blood pressure. Vitamin C and potassium promote heart health. Iron maintains healthy red blood cells and improves their ability to carry oxygen to cells around the body. Growing children and adolescents, as well as menstruating, pregnant, or lactating women, have an increased need for iron.

EYE HEALTH:

Vitamin A promotes eye health, protecting against cataracts and macular degeneration.

HEALTHY SKIN:

Vitamin A and fatty acids promote healthy skin and prevent acne.

INTERNAL HEALTH:

Potassium maintains organs.

ENERGY:

Magnesium, niacin, and protein are key to energy production.

STRESS AND SLEEP:

The compound harman has traditionally been used as a remedy for insomnia and anxiety.

DIGESTIVE HEALTH:

Fiber and carbohydrates aid digestive health and reduce cholesterol. They also maintain bowel regularity and reduce the risk of diabetes and gastrointestinal disease.

ENHANCED BRAIN FUNCTION AND MOOD:

Omega-3 and -6 are integral to brain function and may aid memory.

JOINT HEALTH:

Omega-6, magnesium, and selenium reduce joint inflammation.

Glycemic load: 1
Inflammatory index: Anti-inflammatory

RECOMMENDED FOR HELP WITH:

- Immunity
- Insomnia and anxiety
- Heart health
- Strong bones and joint health
- Eye and skin health
- Energy
- Digestive health

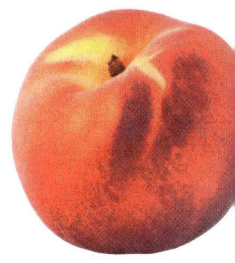

PEACH

Peaches are soft, fuzzy fruit that originated from China. They are related to nectarines and plums. Peaches are delicious when eaten fresh, but with their limited season they can also be enjoyed in canned form throughout the year. Peaches can be eaten raw, or prepared as preserves, juices, sauces, and desserts. Peaches are antioxidant-rich and a good source of vitamins A and C, boosting immunity and skin health, and contain potassium and calcium for strong bones and organs. Fiber and carbohydrates promote digestive health. Peaches can provide a good alternative to sugary treats but should be eaten in moderation due to their sugar content. Dried peaches are higher in sugar than raw.

Peach (fresh)

This is the best nutrient source for peaches, but is only available during summer.

NUTRIENTS IN 1 MEDIUM FRESH PEACH:

Calories, 59
Calcium, 9 mg
Carbohydrate, 14.3 g
Dietary fiber, 2.3 g
Magnesium, 13.5 mg
Niacin, 1.2 mg
Omega-3 fatty acids, 3 mg
Omega-6 fatty acids, 126 mg
Phosphorus, 30 mg
Potassium, 285 mg
Sugars, 12.6 g
Vitamin A (RAE), 24 mcg
Vitamin C, 9.9 mg
Vitamin E, 1.1 mg
Vitamin K, 3.9 mcg

Glycemic load: 5
Inflammatory index: Mildly inflammatory

Peach (canned)

Canned peaches tend to be skinless, which limits their fiber. The preserving process also increases the sugar content. However, canned peaches still provide vitamins A and C. If eating commercially canned peaches, look for "no sugar added" on the label.

HEALTH AND HEALING BENEFITS:

IMMUNITY:

With antiviral properties, the antioxidants and vitamins C and E boost the immune system and fight illness.

BONES, MUSCLES, AND TISSUE:

Vitamin K, phosphorus, and magnesium support calcium in maintaining strong bones. Potassium helps build strong muscles and eases muscle cramps. Vitamin A is central to tissue regeneration, and fatty acids assist in cellular regeneration.

HEART AND BLOOD HEALTH:

Omega-3 and -6 help protect against stroke, heart disease, and diabetes, and lower blood pressure. Vitamins C and E, and potassium promote heart health. Vitamin K is important in matters related to the blood, such as regulating clotting, and menstrual flow and pain.

DIGESTIVE HEALTH:

The dietary fiber and carbohydrates aid digestive health and, alongside vitamin E, reduce cholesterol. They also maintain bowel regularity and reduce the risk of diabetes and gastrointestinal disease. Vitamin E improves metabolism.

EYE AND SKIN HEALTH:

Vitamin A promotes eye health, protecting against cataracts and macular degeneration. Vitamin A and fatty acids promote healthy skin and help prevent acne.

INTERNAL HEALTH:

Potassium keeps the organs in good working order.

ENERGY:

Magnesium and niacin are key to energy production, while vitamin E boosts stamina.

CANCER PROTECTION:

Antioxidants and vitamin E protect against cancer.

ENHANCED BRAIN FUNCTION:

Omega-3 and -6 are integral to brain function and may aid memory.

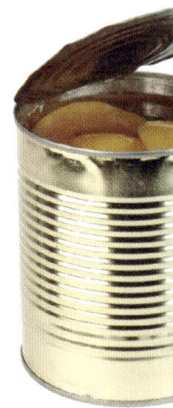

> **RECOMMENDED FOR HELP WITH:**
> - Immunity
> - Digestive health
> - Strong bones and tissue
> - Heart health
> - Eye and skin health
> - Energy
> - Brain function
> - Possible cancer protection

Peach nectar (canned)

Peach nectar is an alkalizing juice that is good for digestive troubles, including easing constipation. It provides vitamins and nutrients, but be aware of the sugar content and drink in moderation.

Pear

There are believed to be more than 3,000 types of pears, including Asian, Anjou, Bartlett (the most popular in the United Stated), Bosc, Comice, Conference (considered the most popular in the UK), and European (or common). Pears are an alkalizing food that can be eaten raw, baked, or poached, and added to salads and desserts. Pears are rich in carbohydrates, fiber, and potassium, making them a great energy snack that is also good for digestive health and good body function, including easing constipation.

NUTRIENTS IN 1 MEDIUM PEAR, RAW:

Calories, 101
Calcium, 16 mg
Carbohydrate, 27.1 g
Dietary fiber, 5.5 g
Folate, 12.5 mcg
Omega-6 fatty acids, 166 mg
Phosphorus, 21.4 mg
Potassium, 206 mg
Sugars, 17.4 g
Vitamin C, 7.7 mg
Vitamin K, 7.8 mcg

HEALTH AND HEALING BENEFITS:

ENERGY:

Carbohydrates and protein make pears a good energy boost.

IMMUNITY:

Vitamin C boosts the immune system.

DIGESTIVE HEALTH:

The dietary fiber and carbohydrates aid digestive health and reduce cholesterol, as well as easing constipation. They also maintain bowel regularity and reduce the risk of diabetes and gastrointestinal disease.

HEART AND BLOOD HEALTH:

Omega-6, vitamin C, and potassium promote heart health, while folate reduces the risk of heart disease and hypertension. Vitamin K is important in matters related to the blood, such as regulating clotting, and menstrual flow.

BONES AND MUSCLES:

Vitamin K and phosphorus support calcium in maintaining strong bones. Potassium helps build strong muscles.

INTERNAL HEALTH:

Potassium keeps the organs in good working order.

Glycemic load: 8
Inflammatory index: Anti-inflammatory

RECOMMENDED FOR HELP WITH:

- Immunity
- Digestive health
- Easing constipation
- Energy boost
- Heart and blood health
- Strong bones and muscles

Pear, dried

Higher in sugar and calories than fresh pears, it should be eaten in moderation. However, it remains an alkalizing food that provides fiber and carbohydrates.

PINEAPPLE

Pineapple is a large tropical fruit with tufted leaves that grows from a tree of the bromeliad family in many warm regions worldwide. It is named for its resemblance to a pine cone. Pineapples are an alkalizing food and are low in fat, cholesterol free, and provide manganese and vitamin C, exceptional for skin, digestive health, and immunity. They may also reduce the risk of heart disease, stroke, and gout. The enzyme bromelain may treat arthritis, sinusitis, and digestive troubles. The acid can cause a tingling sensation in your mouth. If it is more severe, consult a doctor about possible allergies.

Pineapple (fresh)

Fresh pineapple is an alkalizing food that provides a good energy boost, as well as promoting skin, eye, and immune system strength.

NUTRIENTS IN 1 CUP OF FRESH PINEAPPLE CHUNKS:

Calories, 83
Calcium, 21.4 mg
Carbohydrate, 21.6 g
Dietary fiber, 2.3 g
Folate, 29.7 mcg
Magnesium, 19.8 mg
Manganese, 1.5 mg
Niacin, 0.8 mg
Omega-3 fatty acids, 28 mg
Omega-6 fatty acids, 38 mg
Pantothenic acid, 0.4 mg
Potassium, 180 mg
Sugars, 16.3 g
Vitamin C, 78.9 mg

HEALTH AND HEALING BENEFITS:

DIGESTIVE HEALTH:

The dietary fiber and carbohydrates aid digestive health and reduce cholesterol. They also maintain bowel regularity and reduce the risk of diabetes and gastrointestinal disease. The enzyme bromelain eases digestive trouble.

IMMUNITY:

Antioxidants and vitamin C boost the immune system and fight illness.

HEALTHY SKIN:

Manganese and fatty acids promote healthy skin and help prevent acne.

HEART AND BLOOD HEALTH:

Omega-3 and -6 help protect against stroke, heart disease, and diabetes, and lower blood pressure. Vitamin C and potassium promote heart health, while folate reduces the risk of heart disease and hypertension.

JOINT HEALTH:

Omega-6 and magnesium reduce joint inflammation, and the enzyme bromelain reduces arthritis. Anthocyanins reduce the pain and swelling of gout.

SINUS TROUBLE:

The enzyme bromelain eases sinusitis.

BONES AND MUSCLES:

Calcium and magnesium build and support strong bones. Potassium helps build strong muscles and eases muscle cramps.

INTERNAL HEALTH:

Potassium keeps the organs in good working order.

ENERGY:

Magnesium and niacin are key to energy production.

ENHANCED BRAIN FUNCTION AND MOOD:

Omega-3 and -6 are integral to brain function and may aid memory.

Glycemic load: 14
Inflammatory index: Anti-inflammatory

RECOMMENDED FOR HELP WITH:

- Immunity
- Healthy skin
- Heart health
- Reducing inflammation from arthritis and gout
- Easing sinusitis
- Energy
- Enhanced brain function

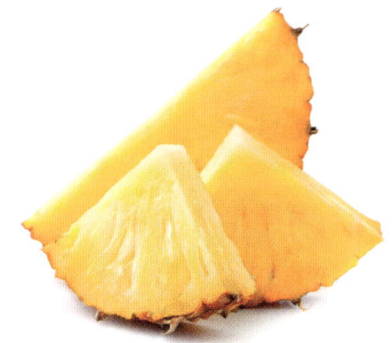

Pineapple juice (unsweetened)

Pineapple juice is also an alkalizing food with digestion-promoting qualities. Ensure you choose the unsweetened, preservative-free variety, or you will be adding high levels of unwanted sugar to your diet.

PLUM

Plums are small, juicy fruit with purple skin and yellow flesh, closely related to peaches and nectarines. Plums are low in calories and a good source of fiber, which makes them great for weight management. Plus, their sweet flavor makes them a suitable alternative to sugary snacks. Plums are rich in antioxidants and a good source of vitamins C and A, important for immunity, cellular repair, and bone and eye health. Like peaches and nectarines, plums can cause an allergic reaction in those suffering from birch-pollen allergies.

Plum (fresh)

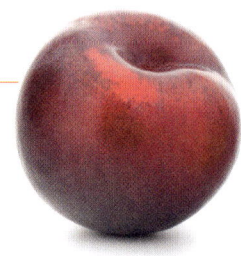

Fresh plums are rich in antioxidants and a good source of fiber. One whole plum has roughly thirty calories.

NUTRIENTS IN 1 PLUM:

Calories, 30
Calcium, 4 mg
Carbohydrate, 7.5 g
Dietary fiber, 0.9 g
Niacin, 0.3 mg
Potassium, 104 mg
Sugars, 6.6 g
Vitamin A (RAE), 11.2 mcg
Vitamin C, 6.3 mg
Vitamin K, 4.2 mcg

HEALTH AND HEALING BENEFITS:

DIGESTIVE HEALTH:

The dietary fiber and carbohydrates aid digestive health and reduce cholesterol, helping you feel fuller faster and aiding in weight loss. They also maintain bowel regularity and reduce the risk of diabetes and gastrointestinal disease.

IMMUNITY:

With antiviral properties, the antioxidants and vitamin C boost the immune system and fight illness.

Glycemic load: 3
Inflammatory index: Anti-inflammatory

RECOMMENDED FOR HELP WITH:

- Dietary health
- Weight loss
- Immunity
- Healthy skin and eyes
- Heart and blood health
- Strong bones and tissue
- Tissue regeneration

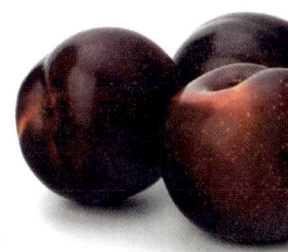

BONES, MUSCLES, AND TISSUE:

Calcium and vitamin K build and maintain strong bones. Potassium helps build strong muscles and eases muscle cramps. Vitamin A is central to tissue regeneration, and fatty acids assist in cellular regeneration.

HEART AND BLOOD HEALTH:

Vitamin C and potassium promote heart health, while vitamin K is important in matters relating to the blood, such as regulating clotting, and menstrual flow and pain.

INTERNAL HEALTH:

Potassium keeps the organs in good working order.

EYE AND SKIN HEALTH:

Vitamin A promotes eye health, protecting against cataracts and macular degeneration, and promotes healthy skin.

Prune (dried plum)

Prunes are rich in antioxidants and a good source of fiber, and their digestive benefit of curing constipation is their best-known trait. However, prunes also provide iron and copper, good for healthy blood.

NUTRIENTS IN 3 PITTED PRUNES:

Calories, 72
Calcium, 12.9 mg
Carbohydrate, 19.2 g
Copper, 0.1 mg
Iron, 0.3 mg
Magnesium, 12.3 mg
Manganese, 0.1 mg
Niacin, 0.6 mg
Omega-6 fatty acids, 13 mg
Phosphorus, 20.7 mg
Potassium, 219.6 mg
Protein, 0.7 g
Vitamin A (RAE), 11.7 mcg
Vitamin B6, 0.1 mg

HEALTH AND HEALING BENEFITS:

DIGESTIVE HEALTH:

Carbohydrates aid digestion and reduce cholesterol, helping you feel fuller faster, aiding weight loss, maintaining regularity, and reducing diabetes risk.

BLOOD HEALTH:

Iron maintains and oxygenates healthy red blood cells. Copper aids iron absorption. Vitamin B6 strengthens blood.

Glycemic load: 8
Inflammatory index: Anti-inflammatory

RECOMMENDED FOR HELP WITH:

- Digestive health
- Easing constipation
- Blood and heart health
- Strong bones and tissue
- Healthy eyes and skin
- Immunity
- Energy
- Enhanced brain function
- Joint health

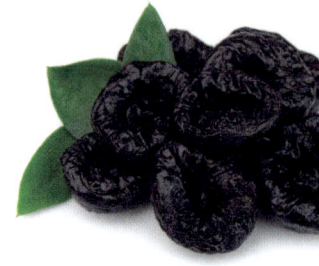

ENERGY:

Copper, magnesium, niacin, and protein are key to energy production.

HEART HEALTH:

Omega-6, protein, and potassium promote heart health and help protect against stroke, heart disease, and diabetes, and lower blood pressure.

BONES, MUSCLES, AND TISSUE:

Protein helps build and repair bones and tissues. Potassium builds strong muscles and eases muscle cramps. Vitamin A is central to tissue regeneration, and fatty acids assist in cellular regeneration.

HEALTHY SKIN:

Vitamin A, manganese, and fatty acids promote healthy skin and help prevent acne.

INTERNAL HEALTH:

Potassium maintains organs.

EYE HEALTH:

Vitamin A promotes eye health, protecting against cataracts and macular degeneration.

IMMUNITY:

Vitamin C and iron boost immunity.

ENHANCED BRAIN FUNCTION AND MOOD:

Fatty acids and vitamin B6 are integral to brain function and may aid memory, also stabilizing mood.

JOINT HEALTH:

Omega-6 and magnesium reduce joint inflammation.

POMEGRANATE

Some religious scholars believe that pomegranates were the original forbidden fruit in the Garden of Eden. These gorgeous purple-red fruit, and their seeds, pack a considerable amount of nutrients. This superfood boasts an impressive level of antioxidants, plus vitamins C and K, and potassium, for immunity, cellular repair, and blood health, as well as for maintaining prostate health. The seeds alone contain fiber, but it is a personal preference whether to eat them alongside the fruit itself.

Pomegranate (fresh)

Fresh pomegranates may be messy to eat and more expensive than many other fruit, but their vitamin and mineral super status certainly makes them worth it.

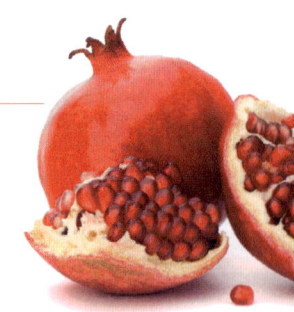

**NUTRIENTS IN
1 POMEGRANATE:**

Calories, 234
Calcium, 28.2 mg
Carbohydrate, 52.7 g
Dietary fiber, 11.3 g
Folate, 107 mcg
Magnesium, 33.8 mg
Omega-6 fatty acids, 223 mg
Phosphorus, 102 mg
Potassium, 666 mg
Protein, 4.7 g
Sugars, 38.6 g
Vitamin C, 28.8 mg
Vitamin K, 46.2 mcg

HEALTH AND HEALING BENEFITS:

IMMUNITY:

With antiviral properties, the antioxidants and vitamin C boost the immune system.

HEART AND BLOOD HEALTH:

Fatty acids and protein help protect against stroke, heart disease, and diabetes, and lower blood pressure. Vitamin C and potassium promote heart health, while folate reduces the risk of heart disease and hypertension. Vitamin K is important in matters related to the blood, such as regulating clotting, and menstrual flow.

PROSTATE HEALTH:

Pomegranates boost the health of the prostate in men.

BONES AND MUSCLES:

Vitamin K, protein, phosphorus, and magnesium support calcium in maintaining strong bones. Potassium helps build strong muscles and eases muscle cramps.

INTERNAL HEALTH:

Potassium keeps the organs in good working order.

DIGESTIVE HEALTH:

Fiber and carbohydrates aid digestive health and reduce cholesterol. They also maintain bowel regularity and reduce the risk of diabetes and gastrointestinal d isease. Folate improves fat metabolism.

ENHANCED BRAIN FUNCTION:

Folate is important for brain function, and is especially important during pregnancy for reducing the risk of spinal and mental defects in the fetus. It may also help protect against Alzheimer's.

JOINT HEALTH:

Omega-6, magnesium, and selenium reduce joint inflammation.

Glycemic load: 18
Inflammatory index: Anti-inflammatory

RECOMMENDED FOR HELP WITH:

- Immunity
- Heart and blood health
- Improves prostate health in men
- Strong bones and muscles
- Digestive health
- Enhanced brain function
- Joint health

Pomegranate juice

Pomegranate juice reduces the risk of cardiovascular disease, is beneficial for prostate health, and promotes sexual health for men in particular. The USDA ranks pomegranate juice as the fifth-strongest antioxidant. However, it may interact badly with some medications, so consult your doctor if necessary.

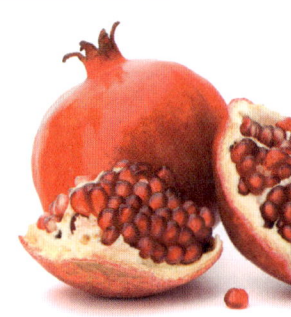

Raspberries

Raspberries come in a beautiful array of colors, including pale gold, red, purple, blue, and black. Red and black are the most common. Raspberries are rich in vitamin C and manganese and packed with antioxidants. These berries are also a good source of fiber, omega fatty acids, and vitamin K. In all, raspberries are good for the heart and blood, as well as important for the immune system and bone strength, and a purifier for the skin.

NUTRIENTS IN 1 CUP OF RASPBERRIES:

Calories, 64
Calcium, 30.8 mg
Carbohydrate, 14.6 g
Copper, 0.1 mg
Dietary fiber, 8 g
Folate, 25.8 mcg
Iron, 0.8 mg
Magnesium, 27.1 g
Manganese, 0.8 mg
Omega-3 fatty acids, 155 mg
Omega-6 fatty acids, 306 mg
Potassium, 186 mg
Protein, 1.5 g
Sugars, 5.4 g
Vitamin C, 32.2 mg
Vitamin E, 1.1 mg
Vitamin K, 9.6 mcg

HEALTH AND HEALING BENEFITS:

HEART HEALTH:

Omega-3, omega-6, and protein help protect against stroke, heart disease, and diabetes, and lower blood pressure. Vitamins C and E, and potassium promote heart health and reduce the risk of cardiovascular disease, while folate reduces the risk of heart disease and hypertension.

DIGESTIVE HEALTH:

The dietary fiber and carbohydrates aid digestive health and, alongside vitamin E, reduce cholesterol, helping you feel fuller faster and aiding in weight loss. They also maintain bowel regularity and reduce the risk of diabetes and gastrointestinal disease. Vitamin E and folate improve metabolism.

ENHANCED BRAIN FUNCTION AND MOOD:

Omega-3 and -6 are integral to brain function and may aid memory. Folate is important for all aspects of brain function, and is especially important during pregnancy for reducing the risk of spinal and mental defects in the fetus. It may also help protect against Alzheimer's.

BLOOD HEALTH:

Vitamin K is important in matters relating to the blood, such as regulating clotting, and menstrual flow and pain. Iron maintains healthy red blood cells and improves their ability to carry oxygen to cells around the body. Growing children and adolescents, as well as menstruating, pregnant, or lactating women, have an increased need for iron. Copper assists with iron absorption.

IMMUNITY:

With antiviral properties, the antioxidants, vitamins C and E, and iron boost the immune system and fight illness.

BONES AND MUSCLES:

Protein helps build and repair bones, tissues, hormones, and body chemicals.
    Vitamin K and magnesium support calcium in maintaining strong bones. Potassium helps build strong muscles and eases muscle cramps.

HEALTHY SKIN:

Manganese and fatty acids promote healthy skin and help prevent acne.

INTERNAL HEALTH:

Potassium keeps the organs in good working order.

ENERGY:

Copper, magnesium, and protein are key to energy production, while vitamin E boosts stamina.

CANCER PROTECTION:

Antioxidants and vitamin E protect against cancer.

JOINT HEALTH:

Omega-6 and magnesium reduce joint inflammation.

Glycemic load: 4
Inflammatory index: Anti-inflammatory

RECOMMENDED FOR HELP WITH:

- Immunity
- Digestive health
- Weight loss and improved metabolism
- Blood and heart health
- Strong bones and muscles
- Healthy skin
- Energy
- Enhanced brain function and memory
- Developing fetus during pregnancy
- Possible cancer protection
- Joint health

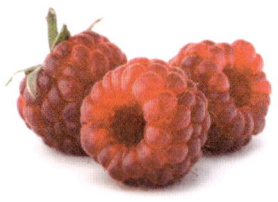

Rhubarb

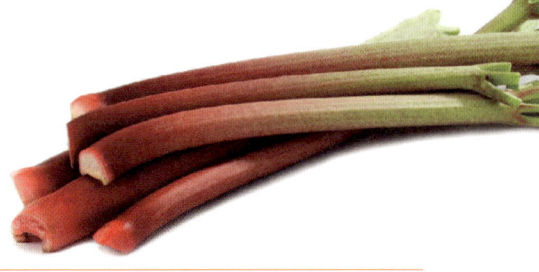

Rhubarb provides fiber, antioxidants, and vitamin K, great for digestive, heart, and blood health. Rhubarb also provides calcium for bone strength, and lutein, which protects against cataracts and macular degeneration. Due to its laxative qualities, use it in moderation. Significant overuse of rhubarb can also potentially cause kidney stones and uterine contractions.

NUTRIENTS IN 1 CUP OF DICED RAW RHUBARB STALKS:

Calories, 26
Calcium, 105 mg
Carbohydrate, 5.5 g
Dietary fiber, 2.2 g
Omega-6 fatty acids, 121 mg
Potassium, 351 mg
Vitamin A (RAE), 6.1 mcg
Vitamin C, 9.8 mg
Vitamin K, 35.7 mcg

HEALTH AND HEALING BENEFITS:

IMMUNITY:

With antiviral properties, the antioxidants and vitamin C boost the immune system.

HEART AND BLOOD HEALTH:

Fatty acids, potassium, and vitamin C promote heart health, reduce the risk of cardiovascular disease and diabetes, and lower blood pressure. Vitamin K is important in matters relating to the blood, such as regulating clotting, and menstrual flow.

BONES AND MUSCLES:

Vitamin K supports calcium in maintaining strong bones. Potassium helps build strong muscles and eases cramps.

EYE HEALTH:

Vitamin A and lutein promote eye health, protecting against cataracts and macular degeneration.

HEALTHY SKIN:

Vitamin A and fatty acids promote healthy skin.

GOOD INTERNAL HEALTH:

Potassium keeps the organs in good working order.

DIGESTIVE HEALTH:

Fiber and carbohydrates aid digestive health and reduce cholesterol. They also maintain regularity and reduce the risk of diabetes and gastrointestinal disease.

TISSUE REGENERATION:

Vitamin A is central to tissue regeneration, and fatty acids assist in cellular regeneration.

Glycemic load: 1
Inflammatory index: Anti-inflammatory

RECOMMENDED FOR HELP WITH:

- Heart and blood health
- Strong bones and muscles
- Easing muscle cramps
- Eye health
- Healthy skin
- Immunity
- Digestive health
- Tissue regeneration

Rose hips

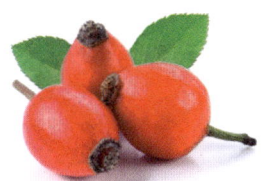

Rose hips have many times more vitamin C than oranges, although the amount is dependent on freshness. Rose hips aid the immune system and protect against arthritis. They may disrupt blood sugar regulation in diabetics.

NUTRIENTS IN 1 CUP OF ROSE HIPS:

Calories, 206
Calcium, 215 mg
Carbohydrate, 48.5 g
Dietary fiber, 30.6 g
Magnesium, 87.6 mg
Manganese, 1.3 mg
Potassium, 545 mg
Sugars, 3.3 g
Vitamin A (RAE), 276 mcg
Vitamin C, 541 mg
Vitamin E, 7.4 mg
Vitamin K, 32.9 mcg

HEALTH AND HEALING BENEFITS:

JOINT HEALTH:

Rose hips help reduce the inflammation of arthritis.

HEALTHY SKIN:

Vitamin A and manganese promote healthy skin and help prevent acne. Vitamin A is central to tissue regeneration, and fatty acids assist in cellular regeneration.

IMMUNITY:

With antiviral properties, the antioxidants and vitamin C boost the immune system.

HEART AND BLOOD HEALTH:

Vitamins C and E, and potassium promote heart health. Vitamin K is important in matters relating to the blood, such as regulating clotting, and menstrual flow and pain.

BONES AND MUSCLES:

Vitamin K and magnesium support calcium in building and maintaining strong bones. Potassium helps build strong muscles and eases cramps.

EYE HEALTH:

Vitamin A promotes eye health, protecting against cataracts and macular degeneration.

INTERNAL HEALTH:

Potassium maintains organs.

DIGESTIVE HEALTH:

Carbohydrates and fiber aid digestive health and, with vitamin E, reduce cholesterol. They also maintain bowel regularity and reduce the risk of diabetes and gastrointestinal disease. Vitamin E improves metabolism.

CANCER PROTECTION:

Antioxidants and vitamin E protect against cancer.

Glycemic load: 30
Inflammatory index: Anti-inflammatory

RECOMMENDED FOR HELP WITH:

- Skin health and tissue regeneration
- Reducing inflammation associated with arthritis
- Immunity
- Heart and blood health
- Bones and muscles
- Eye health
- Digestive health
- Possible cancer protection

Strawberries

Strawberries are an alkalizing food that is loaded with folate, important for brain function, especially for the developing fetus during pregnancy. Additionally, strawberries are a great source of immune-boosting vitamin C, organ-maintaining potassium, and digestion-calming fiber. Due to potential allergic reactions, some doctors recommend not feeding strawberries to babies.

NUTRIENTS IN 1 CUP OF WHOLE STRAWBERRIES:

Calories, 46
Calcium, 23 mg
Carbohydrate, 11.1 g
Dietary fiber, 2.9 g
Folate, 34.6 mcg
Manganese, 0.6 mg
Omega-3 fatty acids, 94 mg
Omega-6 fatty acids, 130 mg
Potassium, 220 mg
Sugars, 7 g
Vitamin C, 84.7 mg

HEALTH AND HEALING BENEFITS:

DIGESTIVE HEALTH:

Fiber and carbohydrates aid digestive health and reduce cholesterol. They also maintain bowel regularity and reduce the risk of diabetes and gastrointestinal disease. Folate improves fat metabolism.

IMMUNITY:

With antiviral properties, the antioxidants and vitamin C boost the immune system.

HEART AND BLOOD HEALTH:

Omega-3 and -6 help protect against stroke, heart disease, and diabetes, and lower blood pressure. Vitamin C and potassium promote heart health, while folate reduces the risk of heart disease and hypertension.

BONES AND MUSCLES:

Calcium builds strong bones. Potassium helps build muscle.

ENHANCED BRAIN FUNCTION:

Omega-3 and -6 are integral to brain function and may aid memory. Folate is important for all aspects of brain function, and is especially important during pregnancy. It may also help protect against Alzheimer's.

HEALTHY SKIN:

Manganese and fatty acids promote healthy skin.

INTERNAL HEALTH:

Potassium maintains organs.

Glycemic load: 3
Inflammatory index: Anti-inflammatory

RECOMMENDED FOR HELP WITH:

- Immunity
- Digestive health
- Heart and blood health
- Healthy skin
- Enhanced brain function
- Developing fetus during pregnancy

TANGERINE

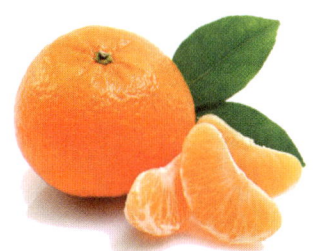

Tangerine is often used as another name for the mandarin orange, although some retailers differentiate between the two based on skin color (with darker-skinned mandarins sold as tangerines in the United States), and is sometimes considered the generic term for the mandarin. Regardless of nomenclature, tangerines are high in vitamin C, boosting the immune system and combating illness, and dietary fiber, assisting with weight loss and reducing cholesterol. This fruit is believed to help protect against liver cancer. In the UK, tangerines are traditional Christmas stocking fillers, and in China, a symbol of happiness and prosperity.

See "Mandarin" entry.

Watermelon

In North America, nothing signifies summer like juicy wedges of watermelon—and this green-skinned, pink-fleshed melon is growing in popularity elsewhere, too. Because of its high water content, watermelon is a healthy, very low-calorie fruit that can be eaten raw (cut into wedges), served in salads, or even grilled. Watermelon provides vitamins A and C, and potassium, as well as moderate fiber and carbohydrates. The color comes from the compound lycopene, which reduces the risk of heart disease and cancers. Most seeds are spat out, but they can be roasted for a healthful treat, providing protein and magnesium.

NUTRIENTS IN 1 WEDGE OF WATERMELON (ABOUT 1/16 OF FRUIT):

Calories, 86
Carbohydrate, 21.6 g
Magnesium, 28.6 mg
Omega-6 fatty acids, 143 mg
Pantothenic acid, 0.6 mg
Potassium, 320 mg
Sugars, 17.7 g
Vitamin A (RAE), 80.1 mcg
Vitamin C, 23.2 mg

HEALTH AND HEALING BENEFITS:

HEART AND BLOOD HEALTH:

Omega-6, vitamin C, and potassium promote heart health and reduce the risk of cardiovascular disease, and lycopene also reduces the risk of heart disease.

BONES AND MUSCLES:

Magnesium maintains strong bones, and potassium helps build strong muscles.

EYE HEALTH:

Vitamin A promotes eye health, protecting against cataracts and macular degeneration.

HEALTHY SKIN:

Vitamin A and fatty acids promote healthy skin and help prevent acne.

GOOD INTERNAL HEALTH:

Potassium keeps the organs in good working order.

IMMUNITY:

With antiviral properties, the antioxidants and vitamin C boost the immune system and fight illness.

DIGESTIVE HEALTH:

Carbohydrates aid digestive health and reduce cholesterol, acting as a natural diuretic. They also maintain bowel regularity and reduce the risk of diabetes and gastrointestinal disease.

JOINT HEALTH:

Omega-6 and magnesium reduce joint inflammation.

TISSUE REGENERATION:

Vitamin A is central to tissue regeneration, and fatty acids assist in cellular regeneration.

CANCER PROTECTION:

Lycopene helps protect against cancers.

Glycemic load: 16
Inflammatory index: Anti-inflammatory

RECOMMENDED FOR HELP WITH:

- Heart and blood health
- Reducing cardiovascular disease
- Strong bones and muscles
- Eye health
- Healthy skin
- Immunity
- Digestive health
- Bladder problems, by acting as a natural diuretic
- Joint health
- Tissue regeneration
- Possible cancer protection

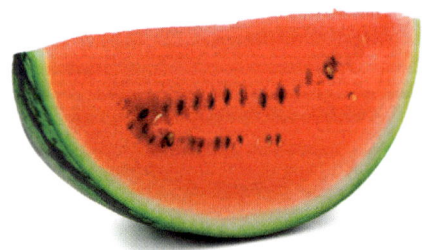

Grains

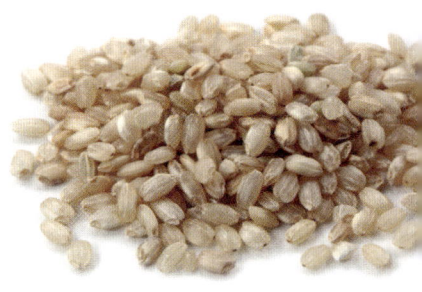

Over the course of the past 10,000 years, grains—bread, cereals, rice, pasta, noodles—have increasingly been consumed, and even recommended, as the staff of life. Unfortunately, since the twentieth century, genetic modifications have increased the gluten content of wheat, and with new technology has come even greater changes. In general, wheat, rye, barley, and spelt contain naturally occurring gluten, and there is good evidence that some oats have been contaminated with gluten. Gluten-free grains include corn, rice, amaranth, millet, buckwheat, quinoa, sorghum, and teff; however, over the past few decades the vast majority of corn has also been significantly genetically modified.

Bran flakes

Packed full of fiber, many breakfast cereals contain bran flakes, which are high in fiber and therefore beneficial for those prone to constipation. However, they also contain gluten and should be avoided by celiacs. Bran flakes are low in fats and sugars and high in immune-boosting vitamin A and metabolism-boosting iron, but these amounts can vary, so it's worth checking individual products.

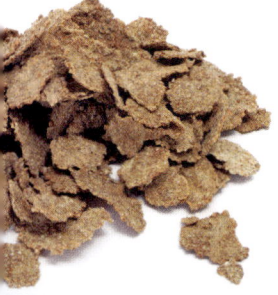

NUTRIENTS IN ¾ CUP OF BRAN FLAKES:

Calories, 96
Calcium, 6.8 mg
Carbohydrate, 24 g
Dietary fiber, 5 g
Iron, 8.1 mg
Protein, 3 g
Sodium, 220 mg
Sugars, 6 g
Total fat, 1 g
Vitamin A (RAE), 225 mcg

HEALTH AND HEALING BENEFITS:

CHOLESTEROL REDUCTION:

The high content of dietary fiber can reduce cholesterol, reduce the risk of diabetes, and minimize weight problems.

BLOOD OXYGENATION:

The iron content prevents anemia, enabling your red blood cells to carry more oxygen around the body in the form of hemoglobin.

IMMUNITY:

Vitamin A is important for the immune system, inhibiting bacteria and viruses from taking hold, and preventing the production of DNA in cancerous cells.

Glycemic load: 10
Inflammatory index:
  Mildly inflammatory

RECOMMENDED FOR HELP WITH:

- Cholesterol
- Diabetes
- Immune health

Granola

A high-protein breakfast cereal with a low glycemic load. Granola is a general term covering cereals which feature oats as their main ingredient. Look for varieties which are high in fiber to aid digestion, and low in added sugar and fat. Better still, make your own. Low in cholesterol and sodium, granola is also a good source of vitamin E (alpha tocopherol), known for its antioxidant properties. Nutrients vary between products, as demonstrated below.

NUTRIENTS IN ½ CUP OF GRANOLA:

	Product A	Product B
Calories	266	225
Carbohydrate	38 g	34 g
Dietary fiber	3 g	7 g
Protein	7 g	6 g
Sodium	19 mg	118 mg
Sugars	12 g	11 g
Total fat	10 g	9 g

Glycemic load: 31
Inflammatory index:
  Moderately inflammatory

RECOMMENDED FOR HELP WITH:

- High blood pressure
- Anemia
- Osteoporosis

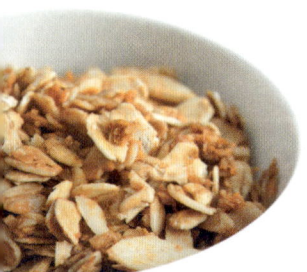

HEALTH AND HEALING BENEFITS:

DIGESTION:

Fiber helps move food through your digestive system. Additionally, getting more fiber in your diet lowers blood cholesterol levels, prevents constipation, and helps you feel full faster.

OSTEOPOROSIS:

The manganese content of cereals is important for the formation of connective tissues and bones, and calcium absorption.

DIABETES AND ANEMIA:

Dietary fiber can also reduce the risk of diabetes, and the iron content of oat-based cereals is good for the prevention of anemia.

Muesli

High in protein with a low glycemic load. Like most cereals, muesli is low in saturated fat and cholesterol, and is a good source of the free-radical-zapping antioxidant vitamin E (alpha tocopherol). B vitamins and iron promote the production of "good" cholesterol, which can help protect against heart disease, and contribute to maintaining good overall health. Muesli is also an excellent source of manganese, providing about 93% of your recommended daily intake. This trace mineral is very important for maintaining the normal functioning of the brain and proper activity of the nervous system, as well as bone health. The only downside is that muesli often has quite a high sugar content.

NUTRIENTS IN 1 CUP OF MUESLI:

Calories, 289
Carbohydrate, 66 g
Dietary fiber, 6 g
Folate, 207 mcg
Niacin, 10.3 mg
Pantothenic acid, 3.9 mg
Protein, 8 g
Riboflavin, 0.9 mg
Sodium, 196 mg
Sugars, 26 g
Thiamin, 0.8 mg
Total fat, 4 g
Vitamin A (RAE), 139.4 mcg
Vitamin B6, 1 mg
Vitamin B12, 3.1 mcg
Vitamin E, 6.1 mg
Vitamin K, 2.5 mcg

Glycemic load: 11
Inflammatory index: Minimally inflammatory

RECOMMENDED FOR HELP WITH:

- Allergies
- Diabetes (type 2)
- Metabolism

HEALTH AND HEALING BENEFITS:

HEART AND BLOOD CIRCULATION:

Riboflavin (vitamin B2), niacin (vitamin B3), along with the iron content ensure the production of "good" cholesterol (HDL), which can help protect against heart disease and aid efficient metabolism of hemoglobin.

MAINTAINING GOOD HEALTH:

Pantothenic acid (vitamin B5) helps to alleviate the symptoms of asthma, hair loss, allergies, stress, respiratory disorders, and heart problems.

KIDNEYS:

The thiamin (vitamin B1) can help prevent kidney disorders in type 2 diabetes.

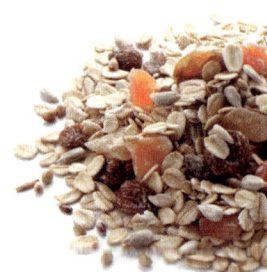

OATS

Some oats are gluten free, and all are high in protein. A steaming bowl of oatmeal for breakfast is packed with minerals, including calcium, potassium, and magnesium. Along with the B-complex vitamins, these are vital for maintaining a healthy nervous system, building strong bones and teeth, and supplying lots of silicon for healthy arterial walls. No wonder oats have been the staple food of some of the hardiest peoples, such as the Scottish Highlanders.

Oat-based cereal

In common with most cereals, oats are low in saturated fat and sodium and contain no cholesterol. They are a good source of dietary fiber, bone-building phosphorus, and the antioxidants selenium and manganese. Oat cereal products can be obtained in many different forms, often with added vitamins (fortified).

NUTRIENTS IN 1 CUP OF REGULAR CEREAL OATS COOKED WITH WATER, WITHOUT SALT:

Calories, 166
Calcium, 21.1 mg
Carbohydrate, 28.1 g
Dietary fiber, 4 g
Iron, 2.1 mg
Magnesium, 63.2 mg
Manganese, 1.4 mg

Glycemic load: 14
Inflammatory index: Moderately inflammatory

Phosphorus, 180 mg
Potassium, 163.8 mg
Protein, 5.9 g
Selenium, 12.6 mcg
Sodium, 9 mg
Sugars, 0.6 g
Total fat, 3.6 g

Oats, whole

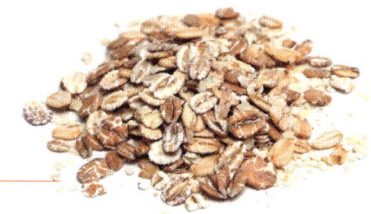

Whole oats, sometimes called old-fashioned or rolled oats, are made when whole oat groats are steamed and then rolled into flakes. The healthy oils are stabilized, they stay fresh longer, and they cook more quickly. The Scots traditionally stone-grind their oats, creating broken bits of varying sizes, resulting in the oats commonly sold in stores.

NUTRIENTS IN ½ CUP OF REGULAR ROLLED OATS, UNFORTIFIED, DRY:

Calories, 153.5
Calcium, 21.1 mg
Carbohydrate, 28 g
Copper, 0.2 mg
Dietary fiber, 4 g
Folate, 13 mcg
Iron, 1.7 mg
Magnesium, 56 mg
Manganese, 1.5 mg
Niacin, 0.5 mcg
Pantothenic acid, 0.5 mg
Phosphorus, 166 mg
Potassium, 146.5 mg
Protein, 5.5 g
Riboflavin, 0.1 mg
Selenium, 11.7 mcg
Sodium, 2.5 mg
Sugars, 0.5 g
Thiamin, 0.2 mcg
Vitamin B6, 0.1 mg
Vitamin K, 0.8 mcg
Zinc, 1.5 mg

Glycemic load: 17
Inflammatory index: Moderately inflammatory

Whole oat groats

A groat is the basic grain kernel with the inedible outer husk removed. They are low in saturated fat and very low in cholesterol and sodium, but lack the manganese and selenium content of rolled oats and cereals.

Rice, black

Black rice contains a high level of antioxidants, which help to combat free radical damage to cells, which if left unchecked can lead to disease. Anthocyanins, the antioxidants also found in blueberries, are responsible for the dark purplish color of black rice. Anthocyanins have been linked to a decreased risk of heart disease and cancer. Black rice is also rich in metabolism-boosting iron and zinc.

NUTRIENTS IN ½ CUP OF BLACK RICE:

Calories, 160
Carbohydrate, 34 g
Calcium, 33 mg
Copper, 0.3 mg
Dietary fiber, 3.4 g
Folate, 20 mcg
Iron, 1.8 mg
Magnesium, 143 mg
Manganese, 3.7 mg
Niacin, 4.3 mg
Pantothenic acid, 1.5 mg
Phosphorus, 264 mg
Potassium, 268 mg
Protein, 7.5 g
Riboflavin, 0.1 mg
Sodium, 4 mg
Thiamin, 0.4 mg
Vitamin B6, 0.5 mg
Zinc, 2 mg

HEALTH AND HEALING BENEFITS:

IMMUNE HEALTH:

Zinc supports immunity and contributes to metabolic balance. Zinc deficiency can lead to a weak immunity (frequent colds and flu, etc.), diarrhea, hair loss, skin lesions, loss of appetite and anorexia, ADHD, hypertension, diabetes, decreased sense of taste, ulcerative colitis, and enlarged prostate.

BLOOD:

Iron helps to prevent anemia, enabling your red blood cells to carry more oxygen around the body in the form of hemoglobin.

ANTIOXIDANT:

Anthocyanins, the antioxidants found in various superfoods, have been linked to a decreased risk of heart disease and cancer.

Glycemic load: 12
Inflammatory index: Moderately inflammatory

RECOMMENDED FOR HELP WITH:

- Immunity
- Heart disease
- Cancer prevention

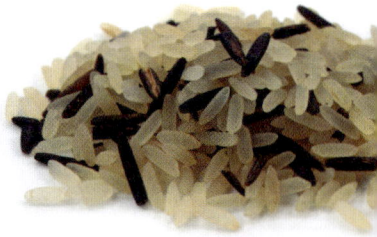

Rice, brown

A better source of protein than white rice. It is gluten free, making it suitable for those on gluten-free diets. Brown rice takes longer to cook than white rice, but the nutritional benefits are worth the wait. The outer bran and germ layers are where the health-boosting vitamins, minerals, and fiber are stored. As a rule of thumb, the longer the grain, the less sticky and starchy the rice. Long-grain rice is ideal for light, fluffy, pilaf-style dishes.

NUTRIENTS IN ½ CUP OF COOKED LONG-GRAIN BROWN RICE:

Calories, 111
Carbohydrate, 23 g
Calcium, 10 mg
Copper, 0.1 mg
Dietary fiber, 1.8 g
Folate, 4 mcg
Iron, 0.4 mg
Magnesium, 43 mg
Manganese, 0.9 mg
Niacin, 1.5 mg
Pantothenic acid, 0.3 mg
Phosphorus, 83 mg
Potassium, 43 g
Protein, 2.6 g
Riboflavin 0.1 mg
Selenium, 9.8 mcg
Sodium, 5 mg
Thiamin, 0.1 mg
Vitamin B6, 0.1 mg
Zinc, 0.6 mg

HEALTH AND HEALING BENEFITS:

ANTIOXIDANT:

A half-cup serving of cooked long-grain brown rice contains almost half the recommended daily value of manganese, a trace mineral that helps protect cells against free radical damage and synthesize fatty acids.

HEART DISEASE:

Brown, red, and black rice contain anthocyanins, the antioxidants found in various superfoods, including blueberries, grapes, and acai, which have been linked to a decreased risk of heart disease and cancer.

CHOLESTEROL:

The oil found in the bran of brown rice has been shown to have cholesterol-lowering benefits.

Glycemic load: 11
Inflammatory index: Moderately inflammatory

RECOMMENDED FOR HELP WITH:

- Lowering cholesterol
- Digestion
- Heart disease

Herbs, spices, and seasonings

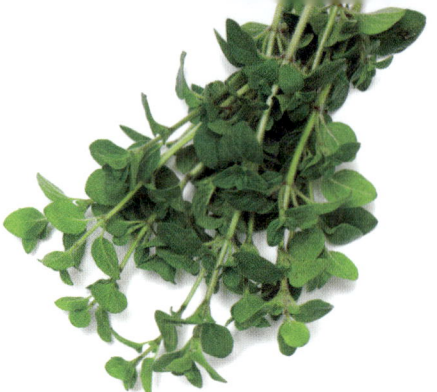

In general, all spices, seasonings, and herbs have much greater concentrations of antioxidants than fruits and vegetables; carbohydrates, fats, and meats tend to be relatively low in antioxidants, and many of these create inflammation.

One of the most interesting reports on the benefits of antioxidants was published in *The Journal of Nutrition* in 2011. The study, from the University of Pennsylvania, demonstrated that two tablespoons of high-oxidant spices lowered oxidative stress and triglyceride levels by 30% after high-fat and high-carbohydrate meals. An article by Monica H. Carlsen, et al., in *Nutrition Journal* (2010, 9:3) listed the total antioxidant content of more than 3,100 foods, beverages, spices, herbs, and supplements. The highest mean antioxidant values of the dried and ground herbs and spices ranged from 44 to 277 mmol/100 g, with the highest in clove, "followed by peppermint, allspice, cinnamon, oregano, thyme, sage, rosemary, saffron, and estragon (tarragon)."

The best way to measure antioxidant capacity is Oxygen Radical Absorbance Capacity (ORAC). The recommended daily intake is 5,000 ORAC, while 10,000 is more ideal. According to Modern Survival Blog's Top 100 High ORAC Value Antioxidant Foods (modernsurvivalblog.com/health/high-orac-value-antioxidant-foods-top-100/), the highest ORAC content foods are: ground cloves, sumac bran, ground cinnamon, raw sorghum bran, oregano, turmeric, freeze-dried acai berry, and cumin seed.

The bottom line is that virtually all herbs and spices are excellent additives and help mitigate the inflammatory aspects of the more inflammatory foods. All of the following are strongly recommended for overall health. Use liberally, except for the Himalayan salt, of which half a teaspoon daily is optimal. In general, a teaspoon or less of most of these will add 5,000 to 10,000 ORAC units to your diet.

Allspice	Dill	Red bell peppers
Black pepper	Echinacea	Rue
Black tea	Fenugreek	Sage
Borage	Ginger	Sarsaparilla
Burdock	Ginseng	Sassafras
Caraway	Green tea	Sorrel
Cardamom	Himalayan salt (far better than other salt sources, as it contains 3% trace minerals)	St. John's wort
Chamomile		Turmeric
Cilantro (coriander)		Willow tea
Cinnamon		
Cloves	Marjoram	
Cohosh	Mint	
Comfrey	Nettle	
Cumin	Nutmeg	
	Oregano	

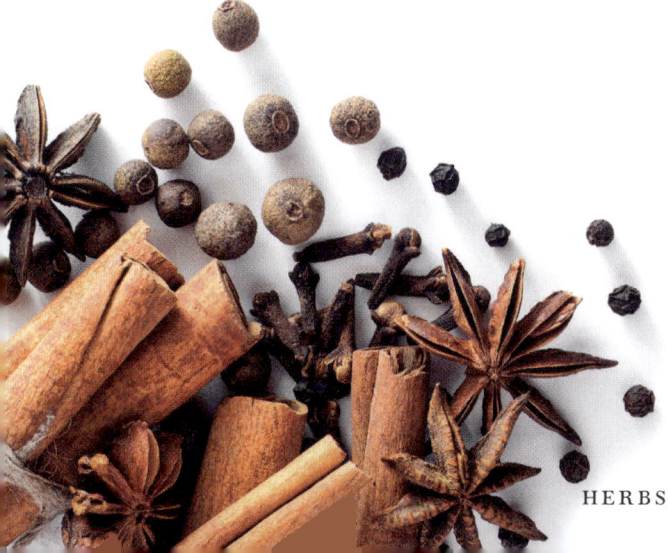

Allspice

Popular in Mexican and Central American cuisine, allspice is warming, soothing, and fragrant. Like black peppercorns, it's thought to aid the motility (or contractions) of the gastrointestinal tract, and promote digestion by boosting the secretions of enzymes in the stomach and intestines. Rich in minerals, a tablespoon of allspice provides 2% of your recommended daily values of iron and potassium, contributing to the healthy function of the blood and heart. It's also high in vitamin C, a powerful natural antioxidant that helps the body combat infection.

NUTRIENTS IN 1 TBSP. OF ALLSPICE:

Calories, 16
Calcium, 39.7 mg
Dietary fiber, 1 g
Iron, 0.4 mg
Magnesium, 8.1 g
Manganese, 0.2 mg
Potassium, 62.6 g
Vitamin A (RAE), 1.6 mcg
Vitamin C, 2.4 mg

HEALTH AND HEALING BENEFITS:

BLOOD AND HEART HEALTH:

Iron is required to produce red blood cells in bone marrow, while potassium helps in the regulation of blood pressure and heart rate.

ANTIOXIDANT/ANTI-INFLAMMATORY:

One tablespoon is packed with 4% of your recommended daily value of nature's own powerful antioxidant, vitamin C, which helps prevent cell damage from free radicals.

ANTIBACTERIAL:

The essential oil eugenol found in allspice has local anesthetic and antiseptic properties. Research shows that preparations of allspice oil mixed with garlic and oregano can help fight E. coli, salmonella, and other bacterial infections.

Glycemic load: 1
Inflammatory index: Anti-inflammatory

RECOMMENDED FOR HELP WITH:

- Rheumatoid arthritis
- Digestion
- Immune health

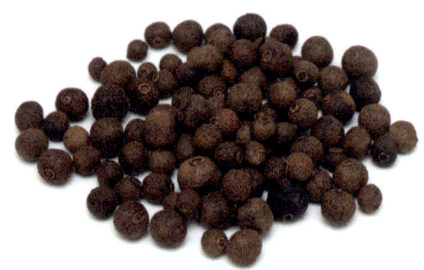

Basil

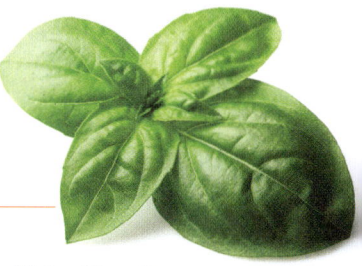

Popular for its fragrant aroma and sweet, punchy flavor, just a handful of basil leaves will transform a bland snack into a delicious treat. Loaded with antioxidants which help prevent cell damage from free radicals, basil offers more than just a flavor boost. Considered one of the healthiest of the herbs, just two tablespoons of chopped fresh basil are packed with over a quarter of your recommended daily value of vitamin K, essential for blood clotting. For a basil-packed flavor hit, try making your own pesto.

NUTRIENTS IN 2 TBSP. OF CHOPPED FRESH BASIL:

Calories, 1
Calcium, 9.3 mg
Dietary fiber, 0.1 g
Folate, 3.6 mcg
Iron, 0.2 mg
Magnesium, 3.4 mg
Manganese, 0.1 mg
Phosphorus, 2.9 mg
Potassium, 15.5 mg
Protein, 0.2 g
Vitamin A (RAE), 14 mcg
Vitamin C, 0.9 mg
Vitamin K, 21.8 mcg

HEALTH AND HEALING BENEFITS:

ANTIBACTERIAL:

Essential oils found in basil, including eugenol, help fight harmful bacteria, restricting the growth of E. coli, salmonella, and other bacterial infections.

CARDIOVASCULAR HEALTH:

A good source of vitamin A through its concentration of carotenoids such as beta-carotene, a powerful antioxidant that protects cells from free radical damage. It also helps prevent free radicals from oxidizing cholesterol in the bloodstream—oxidized cholesterol can build up in blood vessel walls, initiating the development of atherosclerosis, which can result in heart attack or stroke.

ANTI-INFLAMMATORY:

Studies show that eugenol can block the activity of the enzyme cyclooxygenase (COX), contributing to relief from the symptoms of inflammatory health problems such as rheumatoid arthritis and inflammatory bowel conditions.

Glycemic load: 0
Inflammatory index: Moderately inflammatory

RECOMMENDED FOR HELP WITH:

- Rheumatoid arthritis
- Atherosclerosis
- Inflammatory bowel conditions

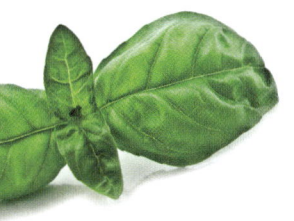

Cinnamon

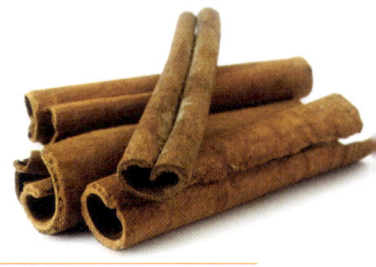

A powerhouse of the spices, with higher antioxidant properties than almost any other food. The brown bark of the cinnamon tree native to Sri Lanka is popular for its warm, woody flavor and sweet, fragrant aroma. For centuries, it's been prized as a spice, a trading commodity, and for its medicinal properties. There are two types of cinnamon. Cassia cinnamon comes mainly from China, Vietnam, and Indonesia, while Ceylon cinnamon, which is slightly sweeter, is produced in Sri Lanka, India, Madagascar, Brazil, and the Caribbean. Cinnamon is available as dried quills or ground powder.

NUTRIENTS IN 1 TBSP. GROUND CINNAMON:

Calories, 19
Calcium, 77.7 mg
Dietary fiber, 4 g
Iron, 0.6 mg
Magnesium, 4.7 mg
Manganese, 1.4 mg
Potassium, 33.4 mg
Protein, 0.3 g
Vitamin K, 2.4 mcg

HEALTH AND HEALING BENEFITS:

ANTIOXIDANT:

Antioxidants are essential for health. These compounds help decrease free radicals, which damage cells and lead to every known disease.

BLOOD/ANTI-INFLAMMATORY:

Cinnamaldehyde, an oil found in cinnamon bark, has been shown to prevent unwanted coagulation of blood and clumping of blood platelets. It does this by inhibiting the release of inflammatory fatty acid, making it helpful as an anti-inflammatory.

BRAIN ACTIVITY:

Studies have shown that even the smell of cinnamon can boost brain activity. Tests showed improvement in memory, visual recognition, and motor speed in individuals who smelled cinnamon, compared to individuals who smelled jasmine, peppermint, or no fragrance at all.

Glycemic load: 1
Inflammatory index: Mildly inflammatory

RECOMMENDED FOR HELP WITH:

- Diabetes
- Atherosclerosis
- Heart disease
- Irritable bowel syndrome

Cloves

Native to the rainforests of Indonesia, cloves are the unopened flower buds of the evergreen clove tree. The manganese content in cloves is higher than in almost any other food. Just a couple of teaspoons of cloves provides in excess of your daily recommended value of this trace element, a potent antioxidant that helps protect cells against free radical damage and contributes to healthy skin. For millennia, cloves have been prized for their warm, sweet flavor and medicinal properties.

NUTRIENTS IN 1 TBSP. OF GROUND CLOVES:

Calories, 18
Calcium, 41.1 g
Dietary fiber, 2.2 g
Folate, 1.6 mcg
Iron, 0.8 mg
Magnesium, 16.8 mg
Manganese, 3.9 mg
Vitamin A (RAE), 0.5 mcg
Vitamin C, 0 mg
Vitamin E, 0.6 mg
Vitamin K, 9.2 mcg

HEALTH AND HEALING BENEFITS:

ANTIOXIDANT:

Manganese produces a potent antioxidant. Antioxidants are essential for optimal health. These compounds help decrease free radical molecules, which damage cells and lead to every known disease. Diets low in manganese have been linked to conditions marked by increased oxidative stress, including skin problems and asthma.

ANTI-INFLAMMATORY:

The essential oil eugenol found in cloves is an anti-inflammatory. Eugenol may help lower the risk of digestive-tract cancers and reduce joint inflammation. Cloves also contain a variety of flavonoids, including kaempferol and rhamnetin, which contribute to clove's anti-inflammatory properties.

DIGESTION:

Aids the motility (or contractions) of the gastrointestinal tract, and promotes digestion by boosting the secretions of enzymes in the stomach and intestines, helping to relieve indigestion and constipation.

Glycemic load: 1
Inflammatory index: Anti-inflammatory

RECOMMENDED FOR HELP WITH:

- Indigestion
- Joint inflammation
- Dental care

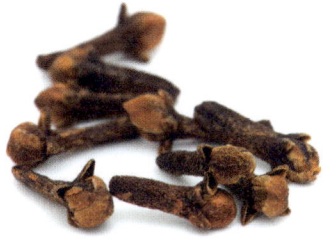

HERBS, SPICES AND SEASONINGS

Cumin

Packed with energy-boosting iron, cumin is an ordinary-looking little seed with extraordinary health benefits. One teaspoon contains almost a quarter (22%) of your recommended daily value of iron. An integral component of hemoglobin, which transports oxygen from the lungs to the cells around the body, iron is particularly important for menstruating women, who lose iron each month during menses. Growing children and adolescents have an increased need for iron, as do women who are pregnant or lactating. As well as packing a healthy punch, cumin is popular for its nutty, peppery taste, and adds a distinctive flavor to Mexican, Middle Eastern, and Indian cuisine.

NUTRIENTS IN 1 TBSP. OF WHOLE CUMIN SEEDS:

Calories, 22.5
Calcium, 55.9 mg
Copper, 0.1 mg
Dietary fiber, 0.6 g
Iron, 4 mg
Magnesium, 22 mg
Manganese, 0.2 mg
Phosphorus, 29.9 mg
Potassium, 107 mg
Protein, 1.1 g
Vitamin A (RAE), 3.8 mcg
Vitamin C, 0.5 mg

HEALTH AND HEALING BENEFITS:

BLOOD AND HEART HEALTH:

Iron is required to produce red blood cells in bone marrow, while potassium helps in the regulation of blood pressure and heart rate.

DIGESTIVE SYSTEM:

Cumin may stimulate the secretion of pancreatic enzymes, compounds necessary for proper digestion and nutrient assimilation.

IMMUNE HEALTH:

Iron is a part of key enzyme systems for metabolism and is instrumental in keeping your immune system healthy.

LIVER HEALTH:

Cumin seeds boost the liver's detoxification enzymes and may also have anticarcinogenic properties. In one study, cumin was shown to protect animals from developing stomach or liver tumors.

Glycemic load: 1
Inflammatory index: Anti-inflammatory

RECOMMENDED FOR HELP WITH:

- Metabolism
- Digestion
- Immune health
- Cancer prevention for stomach and liver

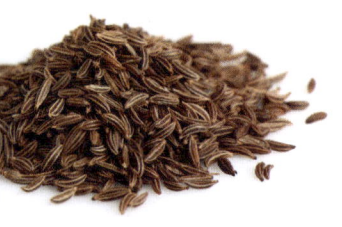

Dill

Dill takes its name from a Saxon word meaning "to lull," which is apt given its soothing effect on the digestive tract. Rich in antioxidants, both the feathery leaves and the seeds have been used in healing remedies since ancient Greek and Roman times. Just one tablespoon of dill seeds contains 10% of your recommended daily value of calcium, an integral ingredient in maintaining healthy bones.

NUTRIENTS IN 1 TBSP. OF DILL SEEDS:

Calories, 20
Calcium, 98.5 mg
Copper, 0.3 mg
Dietary fiber, 1.4 g
Iron, 1.1 mg
Magnesium, 16.6 mg
Manganese, 0.1 mg
Potassium, 77.1 mg
Vitamin C, 1.4 mg
Zinc, 0.3 mg

HEALTH AND HEALING BENEFITS:

ANTIOXIDANT:

Antioxidants are essential for optimal health. These compounds help decrease free radical molecules, which damage cells and lead to every known disease.

BONE HEALTH:

A very good source of calcium, which plays an important role in reducing the bone loss that occurs after menopause, and in conditions such as rheumatoid arthritis.

COMBATING CARCINOGENS:

Dill's essential oils make it a "chemoprotective" food that may help neutralize particular carcinogens, such as benzopyrenes found in cigarette smoke.

Glycemic load: 1
Inflammatory index: Mildly inflammatory

RECOMMENDED FOR HELP WITH:

- Digestion
- Cancer prevention
- Rheumatoid arthritis

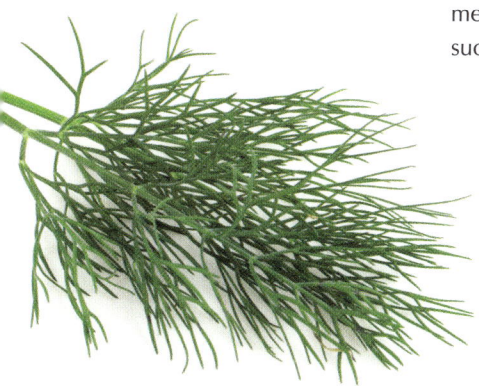

HERBS, SPICES AND SEASONINGS

Fennel

Loaded with antioxidants and fiber, fennel has long been used in folk remedies to aid digestion and combat a variety of ailments, from congestion to conjunctivitis. A storehouse of many vital vitamins and minerals, it was used by the ancient Chinese to stimulate appetite, soothe sore throats, and increase the flow of breast milk in lactating mothers. Native to southern Europe, fennel is sought after for its distinctive anise flavor, and is a favorite in many Mediterranean dishes.

NUTRIENTS IN 1 TBSP. OF WHOLE FENNEL SEEDS:

Calories, 20
Calcium, 68.8 mg
Copper, 0.1 mg
Dietary fiber, 2.3 g
Iron, 1.1 mg
Magnesium, 22.1 mg
Manganese, 0.4 mg
Niacin, 0.3 mg
Phosphorus, 28 mg
Potassium, 97.4 mg
Protein, 0.9 g
Vitamin C, 1.2 mg

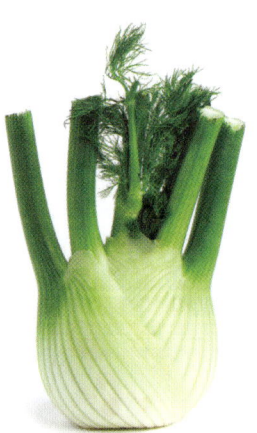

HEALTH AND HEALING BENEFITS:

ANTIOXIDANT/ANTI-INFLAMMATORY:

The essential oil anethole found in fennel is an anti-inflammatory. Anethole may help lower the risk of liver cancer and reduce joint inflammation. Fennel also contains a variety of flavonoids, including kaempferol and quercetin, which contribute to its antioxidant and anti-inflammatory properties.

IMMUNE HEALTH:

A good source of vitamin C, which neutralizes free radicals. Left unchecked, free radicals cause cellular damage that results in the pain and joint deterioration that occurs in conditions such as osteoarthritis and rheumatoid arthritis.

DIGESTION:

Supported by manganese, calcium, iron, magnesium, phosphorus, and copper, the dietary fiber in fennel limits cholesterol buildup, absorbs water in the digestive system, and helps eliminate carcinogens from the colon, possibly preventing colon cancer.

Glycemic load: 0
Inflammatory Index:
Anti-inflammatory

RECOMMENDED FOR HELP WITH:

- Digestion
- Prevention of colon cancer
- Rheumatoid arthritis

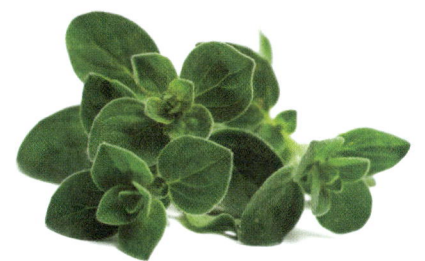

Oregano

Oregano takes its name from the Greek *oros* and *ganos*, meaning "mountain joy." It has long been prized in Europe and is a staple of Italian cuisine. So much more than a tasty pizza topping, oregano is packed with fiber to aid digestion, and vitamins A and K to boost the immune system, provide antioxidant power to protect against cell damage from free radicals, and prevent unwanted blood clotting.

NUTRIENTS IN 1 TSP. OF DRIED OREGANO LEAVES:

Calories, 3
Calcium, 15.8 mg
Dietary fiber, 0.4 g
Folate, 2.4 mcg
Iron, 0.4 mg
Magnesium, 2.7 mg
Manganese, 0.1 mg
Potassium, 12.6 mg
Vitamin A (RAE), 0.9 mcg
Vitamin E, 0.2 mg
Vitamin K, 6.2 mcg

HEALTH AND HEALING BENEFITS:

ANTIOXIDANT:

A good source of antioxidants, found in vitamins C and E. Antioxidants are essential for optimal health. These compounds help decrease free radical molecules, which damage cells and lead to every known disease.

IMMUNITY:

Vitamin A is key in maintaining a healthy immune system and helps boost vision, too.

DIGESTION:

A good source of fiber, which binds bile salts and cancer-causing toxins in the colon and removes them from the body, forcing the body to break down cholesterol to make more bile salts. Diets high in fiber have been shown to lower high cholesterol levels and reduce the risk of colon cancer.

Glycemic load: 0
Inflammatory index: Anti-inflammatory

RECOMMENDED FOR HELP WITH:

- Digestion
- Immunity
- Lowering cholesterol

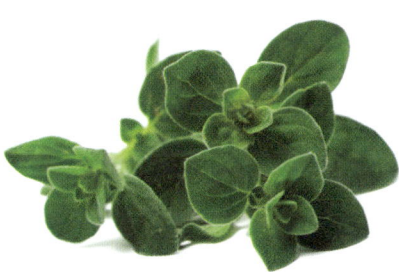

Parsley

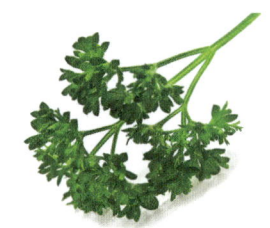
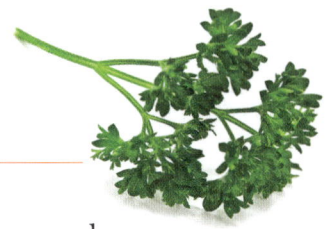

An excellent source of vitamins A, C, and K. Just one cup of fresh raw parsley contains in excess of your recommended daily value of vitamins A and C, and a huge 1,230% of your recommended daily value of vitamin K. Vitamin C is one of the most critical vitamins supporting immune health, while vitamin A also boosts immune health as well as vision. Vitamin K prevents unwanted clotting of the blood and promotes bone health. Add to that twice the amount of iron as in spinach, and it's easy to see why parsley is so much more than just a garnish.

NUTRIENTS IN 1 CUP OF FRESH PARSLEY:

Calories, 22
Calcium, 82.8 mg
Copper, 0.1 mg
Dietary fiber, 2 g
Folate, 91.2 mcg
Iron, 3.7 mg
Magnesium, 30 mg
Manganese, 0.1 mg
Niacin, 0.8 mg
Pantothenic acid, 0.2 mg
Potassium, 332 mg
Protein, 1.8 g
Riboflavin, 0.1 mg
Thiamin, 0.1 mg
Vitamin A (RAE), 253 mcg
Vitamin B6, 0.1 mg
Vitamin C, 79.8 mg
Vitamin E, 0.4 mg
Vitamin K, 984 mcg
Zinc, 0.6 mg

HEALTH AND HEALING BENEFITS:

BLOOD, BONES, AND BRAIN:

Vitamin K prevents unwanted clotting of the blood, promotes bone strength, and also has a part to play in the treatment and possible prevention of Alzheimer's disease by limiting neuronal damage in the brain.

EYES:

The vitamin A content helps maintain healthy eyes and vision and prevents diseases such as macular degeneration and cataracts.

ANTIOXIDANT/IMMUNE HEALTH:

Parsley is an excellent source of immune-boosting vitamin C, containing three times that of oranges. Antioxidants are essential for optimal health, helping to decrease free radical molecules, which damage cells and lead to every known disease.

Glycemic load: 2
Inflammatory index: Strongly anti-inflammatory

RECOMMENDED FOR HELP WITH:

- Macular degeneration
- Alzheimer's disease
- Immunity

Peppermint

Popular for its cool, fresh flavor, peppermint has long been prized for its distinctive taste and medicinal properties. The essential oil menthol is what gives peppermint its distinctive aroma, taste, and cooling sensation. Menthol is also thought to be responsible for the calming effect of peppermint on the digestive system and bowels, alleviating the symptoms of irritable bowel syndrome. It is also beneficial for respiratory function and heart health.

NUTRIENTS IN 2 TBSP. OF FRESH PEPPERMINT:

Calories, 2
Calcium, 7.8 mg
Dietary fiber, 0.3 g
Folate, 3.7 mcg
Iron, 0.2 mg
Magnesium, 2.6 mg
Niacin, 0.1 mg
Phosphorus, 2.3 mg
Potassium, 18.2 mg
Vitamin A (RAE), 6.8 mcg
Vitamin C, 1 mg

HEALTH AND HEALING BENEFITS:

HEART HEALTH:

A good source of minerals, including potassium, one of the critical electrolytes for healthy cell function, which helps regulate blood pressure, heart rate, and nerve conduction.

DIGESTIVE HEALTH:

Peppermint has been shown to have a calming effect on the symptoms of irritable bowel syndrome, including indigestion, dyspepsia, and colonic muscle spasms. The essential oil menthol in peppermint may play a key role in this bowel-comforting effect.

RESPIRATORY HEALTH:

Rosmarinic acid found in peppermint has been shown to be beneficial in alleviating the symptoms of asthma. In addition to its antioxidant abilities to neutralize free radicals, rosmarinic acid has been shown to inhibit production of inflammatory chemicals and promote the production of prostacyclins that keep the airways open for easy breathing.

Glycemic load: 0
Inflammatory index: Anti-inflammatory

RECOMMENDED FOR HELP WITH:

- Irritable bowel syndrome
- Blood pressure
- Asthma

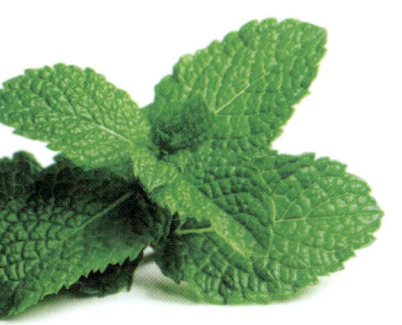

Rosemary

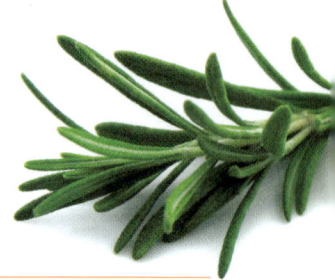

The piney flavor of rosemary is a favorite accompaniment to lamb, pork, chicken, and salmon dishes. Not only is rosemary a tasty addition to many recipes, it is associated with numerous health benefits and has long been used in folk remedies for boosting circulation, improving blood flow to the heart and brain to enhance concentration and memory, stimulating the immune system, and aiding digestion. What's more, it's hardy and easy to grow, making it a perfect herb for your kitchen garden.

NUTRIENTS IN 1 TBSP. OF FRESH ROSEMARY:

Calories, 2
Calcium, 5.4 mg
Dietary fiber, 0.2 g
Folate, 1.9 mcg
Iron, 0.1 mg
Magnesium, 1.6 mg
Potassium, 11.4 mg
Vitamin A (RAE), 2.5 mcg
Vitamin C, 0.4 mg

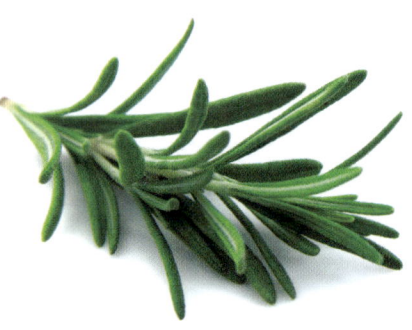

HEALTH AND HEALING BENEFITS:

ANTIOXIDANT:

A good source of the trace mineral manganese, a potent antioxidant that helps protect cells against free radical damage and contributes to healthy skin.

RESPIRATORY HEALTH:

Rosmarinic acid found in rosemary has been shown to be beneficial in alleviating the symptoms of asthma. In addition to its antioxidant abilities to neutralize free radicals, rosmarinic acid has been shown to inhibit production of inflammatory chemicals and promote the production of prostacyclins that keep the airways open for easy breathing.

EYES:

The vitamin A content helps maintain healthy eyes and vision and prevents diseases such as macular degeneration and cataracts.

Glycemic load: 0
Inflammatory index: Anti-inflammatory

RECOMMENDED FOR HELP WITH:

- Asthma
- Digestion
- Immune health

Saffron

Saffron has long been highly prized for its distinctive, vibrant yellow color and unique flavor. The spice is made from the dried stigmas of the crocus flower. It takes around 4,500 crocus flowers to produce one ounce of saffron spice. This labor-intensive process, which is carried out by hand, means saffron comes with the highest price tag of any of the common spices. However, its many health benefits—as an antioxidant, immune booster, and blood sugar regulator—coupled with its distinctive flavor and hue means it remains a popular commodity.

NUTRIENTS IN 1 TBSP. OF SAFFRON:

Calories, 6
Iron, 0.2 mg
Magnesium, 5.3 mg
Manganese, 0.6 mg
Potassium, 34.5 mg
Vitamin B6, 0.1 mg
Vitamin C, 1.6 mg

HEALTH AND HEALING BENEFITS:

ANTIOXIDANT/SKIN AND BONES:

A good source of the trace mineral manganese, a potent antioxidant that helps protect cells against free radical damage, contributes to healthy skin, helps regulate blood sugar, metabolize carbohydrates, and absorb calcium, which contributes to maintaining healthy bones. The high magnesium content also benefits bone health.

IMMUNITY:

A good source of carotenoids—the family of yellow, orange, and red compounds, which includes beta-carotene, astaxanthin, and lycopene. Vitamin C, beta-carotene, and vitamin E work synergistically, and all three are essential for a healthy immune system. Saffron is also a good source of vitamin C.

BLOOD AND NERVOUS SYSTEM:

A good source of vitamin B6, which helps nerve cells to communicate and helps to maintain blood sugars within the normal range.

Glycemic load: 0
Inflammatory index: Anti-inflammatory

RECOMMENDED FOR HELP WITH:

- Immune health
- Skin
- Maintaining blood sugar levels

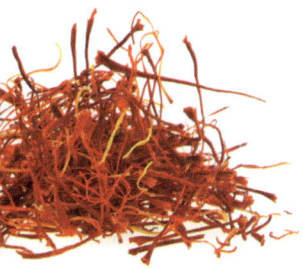

Sage

For centuries, sage has been revered for its culinary and medicinal uses and was considered sacred by the Romans. Like its sister herb, rosemary, sage contains a potent blend of essential oils, flavonoids, and phenolic acids, including rosmarinic acid, with powerful antioxidant and anti-inflammatory properties. It's also packed with vitamin K, with just one tablespoon containing 43% of your recommended daily value, helping to prevent unwanted clotting of the blood and maintain healthy bones. Sage has been used as a folk remedy for millennia to treat ailments from excessive perspiration to sore throats.

NUTRIENTS IN 1 TBSP. OF GROUND SAGE:

Calories, 6
Calcium, 33 mg
Copper, 0.1 mg
Dietary fiber, 0.8 g
Folate, 5.5 mcg
Iron, 0.6 mg
Magnesium, 8.6 mg
Manganese, 0.1 mg
Thiamin, 0.1 mg
Vitamin A (RAE), 5.9 mcg
Vitamin B6, 0.1 mg
Vitamin C, 0.6 mg
Vitamin E, 0.1 mg
Vitamin K, 34.3 mcg

HEALTH AND HEALING BENEFITS:

RESPIRATORY HEALTH:

Rosmarinic acid found in sage has been shown to be beneficial in alleviating the symptoms of asthma. In addition to its antioxidant abilities to neutralize free radicals, it has been shown to inhibit production of inflammatory chemicals and promote the production of prostacyclins that keep the airways open for easy breathing.

ANTI-INFLAMMATORY/ ANTIOXIDANT:

The blend of flavonoids, phenolic acids, and enzymes found in sage contain powerful antioxidant powers for neutralizing harmful free radicals, as well as compounds that fight inflammation, bronchial asthma, and atherosclerosis.

BRAIN FUNCTION:

Tests have shown sage to significantly boost memory recall. In other studies, sage has also been shown to inhibit acetylcholinesterase (AChE), an increase in which accompanies the memory loss characteristic of Alzheimer's disease.

Glycemic load: 0
Inflammatory index: Strongly anti-inflammatory

RECOMMENDED FOR HELP WITH:

- Rheumatoid arthritis
- Bronchial asthma
- Atherosclerosis
- Alzheimer's disease

Sorghum bran

Native to Africa, sorghum is said to be the fifth most important cereal crop grown in the world. It is very low in saturated fat, cholesterol, and sodium, and is gluten free, making it a good alternative to wheat bran for celiacs or those on a gluten-free diet. Sorghum bran also packs a healthy antioxidant punch, helping to protect cells against free radical damage. A good source of fiber, a 3½ oz. serving of sorghum bran contains a quarter of your recommended daily value of fiber. Sorghum bran is also rich in iron and niacin, fueling healthy metabolism and immune function.

NUTRIENTS IN 3.5 OZ. OF SORGHUM BRAN:

Calories, 339
Calcium, 28 mg
Dietary fiber, 6.3 g
Iron, 4.4 mg
Niacin, 2.9 mg
Phosphorus, 287 mg
Potassium, 350 mg
Protein, 11.3 g
Riboflavin, 0.1 mg
Thiamin, 0.2 mg

HEALTH AND HEALING BENEFITS:

DIGESTION:

Fiber helps move food through your digestive system. Additionally, getting more fiber in your diet lowers blood cholesterol levels, prevents constipation, and helps you feel full faster.

METABOLISM:

Iron aids in fuel production, and niacin helps you break down and metabolize nutrients into energy. Niacin and iron also support healthy circulation, and iron plays a role in immune function.

BLOOD AND HEART HEALTH:

Iron is required to produce red blood cells in bone marrow, while potassium helps in the regulation of blood pressure and heart rate.

Glycemic load: 47
Inflammatory index: Anti-inflammatory

RECOMMENDED FOR HELP WITH:

- Digestion
- Metabolism
- Immune health

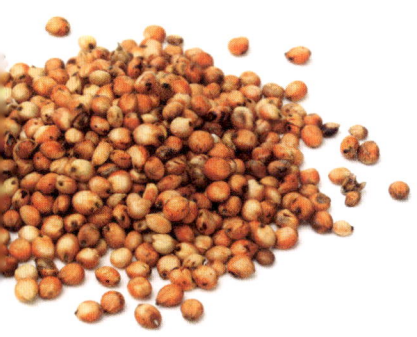

HERBS, SPICES AND SEASONINGS

Soy sauce

Very low in saturated fat and cholesterol, soy sauce is a good substitute for salt. Research suggests that soy sauce may not carry the same cardiovascular health risks linked to other high-sodium foods, including high blood pressure. However, those on a salt-restricted diet or at risk of excessive salt intake should still consult with a health-care provider before including more soy sauce in a meal plan than would otherwise be allowed based on sodium content. Look for products that do not contain artificial colors or flavors. Wheat-free varieties are also available—"tamari" soy sauces are made using less or no wheat.

NUTRIENTS IN 1 TBSP. OF SOY SAUCE:

Calories, 11
Carbohydrate, 1 g
Copper, 0.1 mg
Iron, 0.4 mg
Magnesium, 7.2 mg
Manganese, 0.1 mg
Niacin, 0.7 mg
Phosphorus, 23.4 mg
Protein, 1.9 g
Riboflavin, 0.1 mg
Vitamin B6, 0.1 mg

HEALTH AND HEALING BENEFITS:

DIGESTIVE HEALTH:

Studies suggest that oligosaccharides, carbohydrates created in the fermentation process of soy sauce, promote the growth of "friendly" bacteria in our large intestine.

BLOOD PRESSURE:

Studies also suggest that peptides produced from protein during the fermentation process may inhibit the activity of angiotensin I-converting enzyme (ACE) that is needed to constrict our blood vessels. Our blood pressure tends to go up when our blood vessels constrict because there is less room for our blood to flow through. By decreasing ACE activity, peptides in soy sauce may be able to help prevent this process from happening.

ANTIOXIDANT:

A good source of the trace element manganese, a potent antioxidant that helps protect cells against free radical damage and contributes to healthy skin.

> **Glycemic load:** 1
> **Inflammatory index:** Mildly inflammatory
>
> **RECOMMENDED FOR HELP WITH:**
>
> - Immunity
> - Digestive health
> - Blood pressure

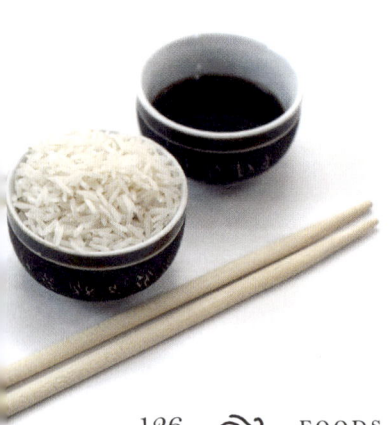

Tarragon

Tarragon is rich in immune-boosting antioxidants, and minerals such as calcium, iron, and manganese, contributing to healthy bones, blood, and skin. Also known as dragon wort, in folk traditions tarragon's cooling properties make it a popular remedy for menopausal hot flashes, as well as for a variety of ailments from stimulating the appetite to hiccups. Different varieties include French, Russian, and Spanish tarragon, French being the most popular and widely used as a tasty addition to a range of dishes, from roast chicken to omelets.

NUTRIENTS IN 1 TBSP. OF DRIED TARRAGON:

Calories, 5
Calcium, 20.5 mg
Folate, 4.9 mcg
Iron, 0.6 mg
Magnesium, 6.3 mg
Manganese, 0.1 mg
Niacin, 0.2 mg
Phosphorus, 5.6 mg
Potassium, 54.4 mg
Vitamin A (RAE), 3.8 mcg
Vitamin B6 0.1. mg
Vitamin C, 0.9 mg

HEALTH AND HEALING BENEFITS:

ANTIOXIDANT:

A good source of the trace element manganese, a potent antioxidant that helps protect cells against free radical damage and contributes to healthy skin.

NERVOUS AND IMMUNE HEALTH:

Pyridoxine, also known as vitamin B6, is a water-soluble vitamin needed by the nervous and immune systems. Vitamin B6 helps nerve cells to communicate. It is involved in making hormones, insulin, antibodies, and cell membranes, and is needed for the normal breakdown of protein, carbohydrate, and fat. Vitamin B6 helps to maintain blood sugar within the normal range.

BLOOD AND HEART HEALTH:

Iron is required to produce red blood cells in bone marrow, while potassium helps in the regulation of blood pressure and heart rate.

Glycemic load: 0
Inflammatory index: Anti-inflammatory

RECOMMENDED FOR HELP WITH:

- Carpal tunnel syndrome
- Premenstrual syndrome
- Atherosclerosis

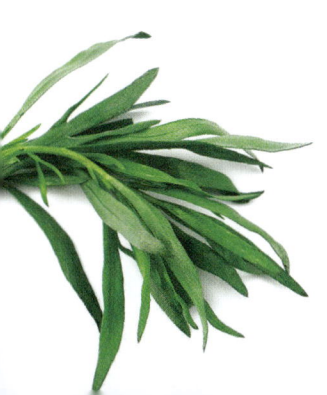

Thyme

This delicate-looking herb packs a healthy antioxidant punch—it's loaded with immune-boosting vitamin C, antimicrobial thymol, and free-radical-zapping manganese. Thyme has long been used in natural remedies for chest and respiratory complaints, including coughs, bronchitis, and chest congestion, and as an antiseptic mouthwash. The ancient Greeks prized thyme for its aromatic qualities, burning it as incense in sacred temples. It is one of the herbs in the French bouquet garni, used to season soups, stocks, and stews. Enjoy its distinctive flavor in a bean, beef, or lamb stew on a cold winter's day for an immune system boost.

NUTRIENTS IN 1 TSP. OF FRESH THYME:

Calories, 1
Calcium, 3.2 mg
Dietary fiber, 0.1 g
Folate, 0.4 mcg
Iron, 0.1 mg
Magnesium, 1.3 mg
Phosphorus, 0.8 mg
Potassium, 4.9 mg
Vitamin A (RAE), 1.9 mcg
Vitamin C, 1.3 mg

HEALTH AND HEALING BENEFITS:

ANTIOXIDANT:

The flavonoids in thyme—including apigenin, naringenin, luteolin, and thymonin—increase its antioxidant capacity, and combined with its status as a good source of manganese, put it high on the list of antioxidant foods.

ANTISEPTIC/ANTI-FUNGAL:

Thymol, one of the most important essential oils in thyme, has been shown to have antiseptic and antifungal characteristics, combating various microbial diseases such as E. coli.

IMMUNITY:

A good source of vitamin C, a powerful natural antioxidant that helps the body fight infection.

Glycemic load: 0
Inflammatory index: Anti-inflammatory

RECOMMENDED FOR HELP WITH:

- Immune health
- Bronchitis
- Digestion

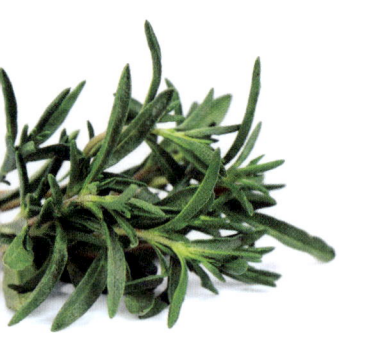

Turmeric

Turmeric is made from the bright orange root of the *Curcuma longa* plant, native to the sub-Himalayan mountain region. A powerhouse of the spices, it has long been used in Indian and Chinese medicine for its anti-inflammatory, pain-killing, and antioxidant properties. Just one tablespoon of turmeric contains over a quarter of your recommended daily value of manganese, a potent antioxidant that helps protect cells against free radical damage and contributes to healthy skin. Use it to add a unique, warm, peppery kick to curry dishes—even small amounts can have a beneficial health impact.

NUTRIENTS IN 1 TBSP. OF GROUND TURMERIC:

Calories, 24
Calcium, 12.4 mg
Dietary fiber, 1.4 g
Iron, 2.8 mg
Magnesium, 13 mg
Manganese, 0.5 mg
Potassium, 170 mg
Vitamin B6, 0.1 mg
Vitamin C, 1.7 mg

HEALTH AND HEALING BENEFITS:

ANTI-INFLAMMATORY/ANTIOXIDANT:

Curcumin, the main active ingredient in turmeric, is a potent anti-inflammatory and antioxidant with the power to zap free radicals, which damage cells and lead to every known disease.

DIGESTIVE HEALTH:

Its potent anti-inflammatory properties mean that even small amounts of turmeric can help alleviate the symptoms of inflammatory bowel conditions, such as Crohn's disease and ulcerative colitis.

HEART HEALTH:

Curcumin has a cholesterol-lowering effect, and it may help to prevent the oxidation of cholesterol, which can have protective effects in those with coronary artery disease and atherosclerosis.

Glycemic load: 0
Inflammatory index: Strongly anti-inflammatory

RECOMMENDED FOR HELP WITH:

- Inflammatory bowel syndrome
- Rheumatoid arthritis
- Coronary artery disease
- Atherosclerosis

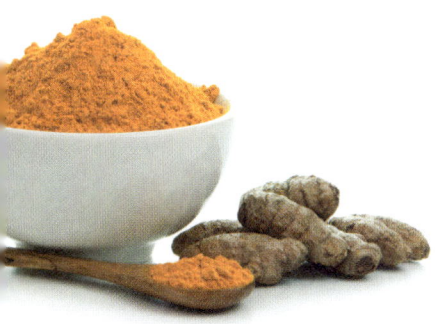

Legumes

In general, legumes—including peas, beans, and lentils—are high in fiber and protein; however, they are "incomplete" proteins, lacking some essential amino acids. They need to be eaten alongside milk, meat, or egg protein to be complete. Legumes are also high in carbohydrates, which is where most of their calorific content comes from.

Alfalfa seeds, sprouted

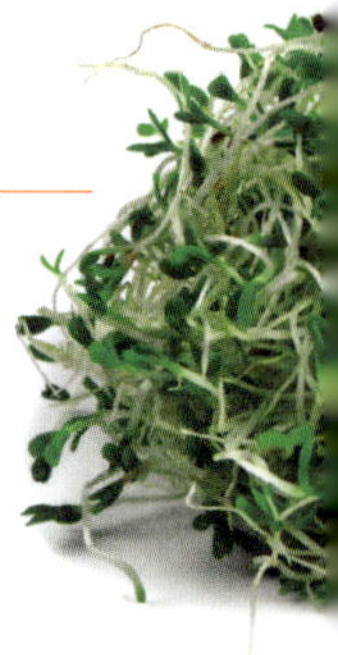

Low in saturated fat, sodium, and cholesterol, sprouted alfalfa seeds are the shoots of the plant harvested before they are fully grown. They're packed with concentrated amounts of essential vitamins and minerals, including vitamin K, essential for blood clotting, immune-boosting vitamin C, and bone-strengthening calcium. Wash thoroughly before eating and add to salads for a tasty nutritional boost.

NUTRIENTS IN 1 CUP OF RAW SPROUTED ALFALFA SEEDS:

Calories, 8
Carbohydrate, 1 g
Calcium, 10.6 mg
Copper, 0.1 mg
Dietary fiber, 1 g
Folate, 11.9 mcg
Iron, 0.3 mg
Manganese, 0.1 mg
Niacin, 0.2 mg
Pantothenic acid, 0.2 mg
Phosphorus, 23.1 mg
Potassium, 26.1 mg
Protein, 1 g
Riboflavin, 0.1 mg
Sodium, 2 mg
Thiamin, 0.1 mg
Vitamin A (RAE), 2.6 mcg
Vitamin C, 2.7 mg
Vitamin K, 10.1 mcg
Zinc, 0.3 mg

Glycemic load: 0
Inflammatory index: Mildly anti-inflammatory

RECOMMENDED FOR HELP WITH:

- Lowering cholesterol
- Healthy blood
- Immunity

HEALTH AND HEALING BENEFITS:

BLOOD CLOTTING:

Vitamin K is valuable in helping blood to clot, while the iron content keeps the red corpuscles healthy.

CHOLESTEROL:

The dietary fiber contained in alfalfa helps to lower LDL, or "bad cholesterol", and raise levels of HDL, or "good cholesterol."

GENERAL HEALTH:

The wide variety of essential vitamins and minerals are beneficial to maintaining good all-around levels of health.

Garbanzo beans (chickpeas)

Like other beans, garbanzo beans are rich in soluble and insoluble fiber. Soluble fiber helps with the removal of cholesterol, and insoluble fiber prevents constipation. Garbanzo beans are low in saturated fat and sodium, and a very good source of anemia-busting folate and the free-radical-zapping antioxidant manganese. These beans produce less intestinal gas than many legumes.

NUTRIENTS IN 1 CUP OF GARBANZO BEANS, BOILED, WITHOUT SALT:

Calories, 269
Carbohydrate, 45 g
Calcium, 80.4 mg
Copper, 0.6 mg
Dietary fiber, 12 g
Fat, 4 g
Folate, 282 mcg
Iron, 4.7 mg
Manganese, 1.7 mg
Protein, 15 g
Sodium, 11 mg
Sugars, 8 g
Vitamin A (RAE), 1.6 mcg
Vitamin B6, 0.2 mg
Vitamin C, 2.1 mg

Glycemic load: 5
Inflammatory index: Mildly inflammatory

RECOMMENDED FOR HELP WITH:

- Constipation
- Blood circulation
- Cholesterol reduction

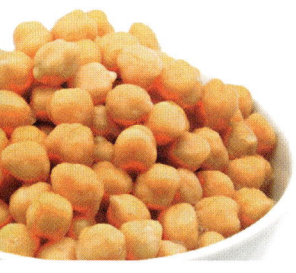

LEGUMES 131

HEALTH AND HEALING BENEFITS:

DIGESTION:

Fiber helps move food through your digestive system. Additionally, getting more fiber in your diet lowers blood cholesterol levels, prevents constipation, and helps you feel full faster.

WEIGHT LOSS:

On their own or mixed with other foods, garbanzo beans will keep you feeling full for longer.

OXYGENATION OF THE BLOOD:

Iron improves the ability of the red blood cells to carry oxygen from the lungs to the cells around the body in the form of hemoglobin. It is particularly important for menstruating women, who lose iron each month during menses. Growing children and adolescents have an increased need for iron, as do women who are pregnant or lactating.

Haricot beans

Also known as navy beans, as they were a staple of the United States Navy in the early twentieth century. They are low in saturated fat, cholesterol, and sodium. Haricot beans are packed with fiber and anemia-busting folate. They are also a good source of energy-boosting thiamin (B1). All animals require vitamin B1, which is made in bacteria, fungi, and plants, but a big portion of the nutritional B1 content of foods is often lost due to modern food processing.

NUTRIENTS IN 1 CUP OF HARICOT BEANS, BOILED, WITHOUT SALT:

Calories, 255
Calcium, 126 mg
Carbohydrate, 48 g
Dietary fiber, 19.1 g
Fat, 1 g
Folate, 255 mcg
Manganese, 1 mg
Phosphorus, 262 mg
Protein, 15 g
Thiamin, 0.4 mg

Glycemic load: 17
Inflammatory index: Minimally inflammatory

RECOMMENDED FOR HELP WITH:

- Diabetes
- Constipation
- Good general health

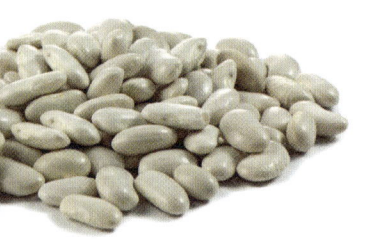

HEALTH AND HEALING BENEFITS:

METABOLISM:

Vitamin B1 plays a key role in energy metabolism. Deficiency of vitamin B1 can lead to beriberi, optic nerve damage, Korsakoff's syndrome, peripheral neuropathy, and heart failure.

CHOLESTEROL AND BLOOD SUGAR:

Like most beans, haricot beans are an excellent source of cholesterol-lowering fiber. In addition, the high fiber content prevents blood sugar levels from rising too rapidly after a meal, making these beans an especially good choice for individuals with diabetes, insulin resistance, or hypoglycemia.

DIGESTION:

As with all legumes, the high dietary fiber content helps to move food through your digestive system and prevent constipation. Additionally, getting more fiber in your diet lowers blood cholesterol levels and helps you feel full faster.

Kidney beans

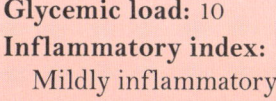

Low in saturated fat, cholesterol, and sodium, kidney beans are packed with protein and digestion-boosting soluble and insoluble fiber. One cup of boiled kidney beans contains more than half (58%) of your recommended daily value of anemia-busting folate, which contributes to healthy heart and brain function. In common with most legumes, cooking red kidney beans by boiling will considerably reduce the sodium content, which is high in the raw product.

NUTRIENTS IN 1 CUP OF BOILED KIDNEY BEANS, WITHOUT SALT:

Calories, 255
Carbohydrate, 40 g
Calcium, 62 mg
Dietary fiber, 11 g
Fat, 1 g
Folate, 230 mcg
Manganese, 0.8 mg
Phosphorus, 244 mg
Protein, 15 g
Sodium, 2 mg
Sugars, 1 g

Glycemic load: 10
Inflammatory index: Mildly inflammatory

RECOMMENDED FOR HELP WITH:

- Heart health
- Digestion
- Brain function

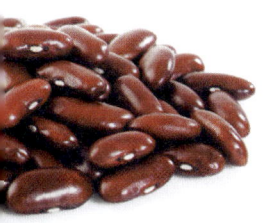

HEALTH AND HEALING BENEFITS:

DIGESTION:

Dietary fiber, especially the insoluble fiber, speeds the digestive process through the intestinal tract, thereby reducing the risk of constipation. Soluble fiber helps reduce cholesterol.

CORONARY DISEASE:

Folic acid works with other B vitamins to control homocysteine levels. An excess of homocysteine has been linked to an increased risk of coronary disease, stroke, and other diseases such as osteoporosis and Alzheimer's.

BRAIN FUNCTION:

A good source of folate, one of the most critical vitamins, especially during pregnancy, where deficiencies increase the risk of spinal defects and mental retardation in the fetus. In the general population, folate is particularly important in all aspects of brain function and in cholesterol metabolism.

PEANUTS

Low in cholesterol but high in sodium and calories, peanuts are one of the anti-inflammatory and alkalizing legumes. They're a good source of free-radical-zapping manganese and niacin (vitamin B3). Nutritional properties vary according to variety: for example, Virginia peanuts are much more anti-inflammatory than Valencia peanuts. It's worth noting that although they are called "nuts," peanuts are actually legumes and therefore not harmful to nut-allergy sufferers. However, some people do have a specific allergy to peanuts.

NUTRIENTS IN 1 CUP OF CHOPPED OIL-ROASTED PEANUTS WITH SALT:

Calories, 862
Carbohydrate, 22 g
Dietary fiber, 14 g
Fat, 76 g
Manganese, 2.7 mg
Niacin, 19.9 mg
Protein, 40 g
Saturated fat, 13 g
Sodium, 460 mg
Sugars, 6 g

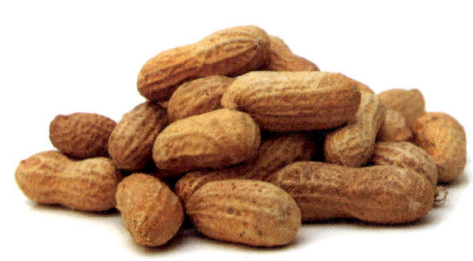

Peanut butter

One cup of peanut butter contains in excess of your recommended daily values of the antioxidants manganese and niacin, making peanut butter an even richer source of these nutrients than peanuts.

NUTRIENTS IN 2 TBSP. OF SMOOTH PEANUT BUTTER:

Calories 188
Carbohydrate, 7.7 g
Dietary fiber, 1.8 g
Fat, 15.8 g
Manganese, 0.4 mg
Niacin, 4.2 mg
Protein, 7 g
Saturated fat, 3 g
Sodium, 152 mg
Sugars, 2.1 g

HEALTH AND HEALING BENEFITS:

BONE BUILDING:

Manganese works with calcium to help in the formation of skeletal tissue.

ANTIOXIDANT:

Niacin (vitamin B3) is also involved in energy metabolism and in protecting the body against excessive tissue damage from free radicals.

CHOLESTEROL:

Niacin (vitamin B3) contributes to the formation of HDL (high-density lipoproteins), or "good" cholesterol. This lowers blood pressure and improves blood flow.

Glycemic load: 1
Inflammatory index: Mildly anti-inflammatory

RECOMMENDED FOR HELP WITH:

- Lowering cholesterol
- Bone formation

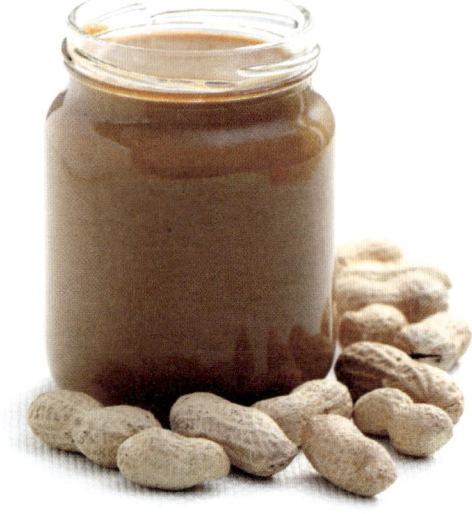

Green beans (French beans)

Also known as snap beans or string beans. Low in sodium and very low in saturated fats and cholesterol, green beans are packed with dietary fiber, vision-boosting vitamin A, immune-boosting vitamin C, and vitamin K, essential for blood clotting. They are also a good source of the antioxidants folate and manganese, which help to protect cells from free radical damage.

NUTRIENTS IN 1 CUP OF RAW GREEN BEANS:

Calories, 31
Carbohydrate, 7 g
Calcium, 37 mg
Copper, 0.1 mg
Dietary fiber, 2.7 g
Folate, 33 mcg
Iron, 1 mg
Magnesium, 25 mg
Manganese, 0.2 mg
Niacin, 0.7 mg
Phosphorus, 38 mg
Potassium, 211 mg
Protein, 1.8 g
Riboflavin, 0.1 mg
Sodium, 6 mg
Sugars, 3.3 g
Thiamin, 0.1 mg
Vitamin A (RAE), 35 mcg
Vitamin B6, 0.1 mg
Vitamin C, 12.2 mg
Vitamin K, 43 mcg

HEALTH AND HEALING BENEFITS:

VISION:

Vitamin A improves vision and helps with eye disorders including age-related macular degeneration (AMD), glaucoma, and cataracts.

BLOOD CLOTTING:

Vitamin K is essential for the blood clotting process, and also contributes to the strength and maintenance of bones.

STORING ENERGY:

Pyridoxine or vitamin B6 is essential in the using and storing of energy from proteins and carbohydrates.

Glycemic load: 2
Inflammatory index: Mildly anti-inflammatory

RECOMMENDED FOR HELP WITH:

- Age-related macular degeneration
- Blood clotting
- Storing energy

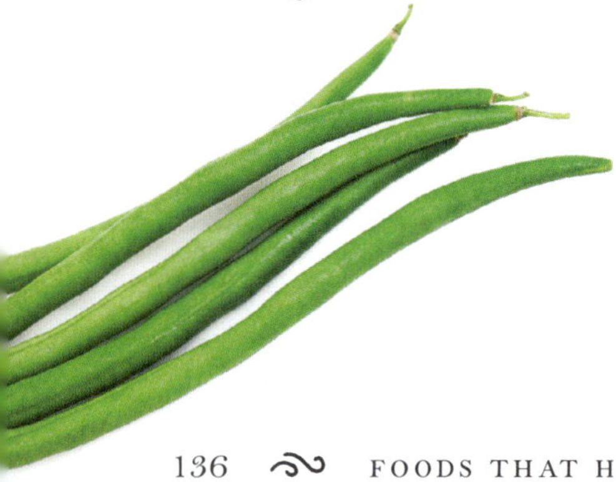

Snow peas, sugar snap peas

Snow peas are flatter than round garden peas, while sugar snap peas are a cross between the garden pea and the snow pea. Both snow peas and sugar snap peas have edible pods and are sweeter than garden peas. Eat them raw in salads for a healthy crunch or enjoy them sautéed in a range of dishes. They're loaded with antioxidants, including vitamins C and E, and zinc, as well as anti-inflammatory nutrients associated with a lowered risk of conditions such as type 2 diabetes.

NUTRIENTS IN 1 CUP OF RAW WHOLE SNOW PEAS OR SUGAR SNAP PEAS:

Calories, 27
Carbohydrate, 4.8 g
Dietary fiber, 1.6 g
Folate, 26.5 mcg
Iron, 1.3 mg
Magnesium, 15.1 mg
Manganese, 0.2 mg
Pantothenic acid, 0.5 mg
Phosphorus, 33.4 mg
Potassium, 126 mg
Protein, 1.8 g
Riboflavin, 0.1 mg
Thiamin, 0.1 mg
Vitamin A (RAE), 34 mcg
Vitamin B6, 0.1 mg
Vitamin C, 37.8 mg
Vitamin K, 15.8 mcg

HEALTH AND HEALING BENEFITS:

ANTIOXIDANT:

Packed with antioxidants, including vitamins C and E, and zinc. Antioxidants are essential for optimal health. These compounds help decrease free radical molecules, which damage cells and lead to every known disease.

HEART HEALTH:

Packed with omega-3 fats, antioxidants, and anti-inflammatory nutrients that contribute to cardiovascular health.

BLOOD SUGAR REGULATION:

Rich in protein and dietary fiber, which help to regulate the pace at which we digest our food, helping to control the breakdown of starches into sugars and the general passage of carbohydrates through our digestive tract. Better regulation of carbohydrates can help to maintain steadier blood sugar levels.

Glycemic load: 1
Inflammatory index: Mildly anti-inflammatory

RECOMMENDED FOR HELP WITH:

- Cardiovascular health
- Maintaining healthy blood sugar levels
- Immunity

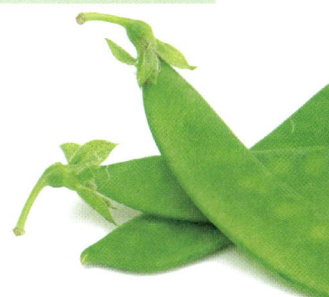

Meats

All meats have optimal essential amino acids, including taurine, which is vital for many biological functions in humans. Meats are also one of the best sources of vitamin B12. No plant food contains either taurine or vitamin B12. Including a couple of servings of red meat in your weekly meal plan as part of a healthy diet can provide your body with many vital nutrients.

BEEF

Depending on the cut and the preparation method, beef tends to be low in sodium and is a good source of many vital nutrients. However, it is relatively high in saturated fat, which can lead to a buildup of cholesterol in the arteries and a higher risk of heart disease, so should be included in your diet in moderation. As a rule of thumb, the leaner the beef, the lower the levels of saturated fat. Choose lower-fat cuts such as top round, bottom round, eye round, flank, and strip for healthier options. Higher-fat cuts such as tenderloin, porterhouse steak, or ribeye contain higher levels of total fat, saturated fat, and calories, which can be difficult for the body to process. Cooking methods impact the level of fat as well as cut. Grilling, baking, poaching, or steaming are healthier options, while frying or roasting increase the fat content.

Note: The entries below allow quick comparison between calories, cholesterol, protein, sodium, saturated fat, and total fat for many cuts of beef and various cooking methods, as well as highlighting beneficial nutrients associated with each particular beef product.

Beef, ground, grass-fed

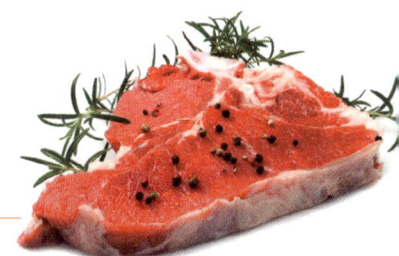

Research has shown that grass-fed beef contains more than double the carotenoid content of conventionally fed beef. Carotenoids are the family of yellow, orange, and red compounds, essential for a healthy immune system. Grass-fed beef contains significantly lower levels of cholesterol than conventionally fed beef. Labeling on beef products can be confusing or misleading—even products that state "pasture-fed" or "grass-fed" do not guarantee that cows have spent a significant amount of time in an outdoor pasture setting. Look for labels that state "100% grass-fed beef."

NUTRIENTS IN 4 OZ. OF GROUND GRASS-FED BEEF:

Calories, 216
Cholesterol, 68 mg
Protein, 20 g
Saturated fat, 4 g
Sodium, 76 mg
Total fat, 14 g
Niacin, selenium, vitamin B12, zinc

Glycemic load: 0
Inflammatory index: Mildly anti-inflammatory

Kidney, beef

Beef kidneys are protein-rich, with a 4-ounce serving containing nearly half of your recommended daily value of protein. They're a good source of iron and B vitamins. However, they are also high in cholesterol and trans fat.

NUTRIENTS IN 4 OZ. OF COOKED, SIMMERED BEEF KIDNEYS:

Calories, 178.6
Cholesterol, 811.8 mg
Protein, 30.7 g
Saturated fat, 1.3 g
Sodium, 106.6 mg
Total fat, 5.3 g
Calcium, copper, folate, iron, niacin, phosphorus, riboflavin, selenium, vitamins B6 and B12, zinc

Glycemic load: 0
Inflammatory index: Moderately inflammatory

Liver, beef

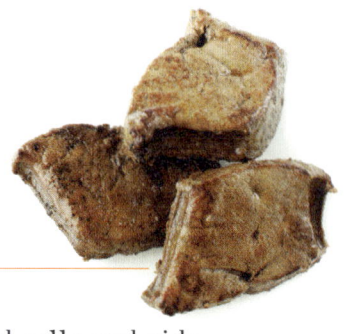

Rich in vitamin B12, which helps maintain healthy red blood cells and aids neurological health. Vitamin B12 deficiency leads to pernicious anemia, and damage to the spinal cord and brain. However, liver is high in cholesterol and trans fat. Pan-frying compared to braising increases the glycemic load. Calves' liver tends to be more tender and milder in flavor than meat from older animals.

NUTRIENTS IN 4 OZ. OF COOKED BEEF LIVER, BRAISED:

Calories, 208
Carbohydrate, 4.8 g
Cholesterol, 430.4 mg
Protein, 32 g
Saturated fat, 1.6 g
Sodium, 86.4 mg
Total fat, 6.4 g
Copper, folate, iron, niacin, pantothenic acid, phosphorus, riboflavin, selenium, vitamin A (very high), vitamins B6 and B12, vitamin C, zinc

Glycemic load: 2
Inflammatory index: Mildly inflammatory

Round steak

Round steak comes from the rear leg of the cow. It's a lean cut, making it a healthier option than cuts such as porterhouse steak. However, it is high in cholesterol. The lack of fat and marbling means it can dry out when cooking, so slow, moist heat methods of cooking such as braising help retain the moisture.

NUTRIENTS IN 4 OZ. BEEF ROUND, TRIMMED OF FAT, ROASTED:

Calories, 215.1
Cholesterol, 97 mg
Protein, 31.5 g
Saturated fat, 26.8 g
Sodium, 41 mg
Total fat, 9 g
Calcium, iron, niacin, selenium, vitamin B12, zinc

Glycemic load: 0
Inflammatory index: Mildly anti-inflammatory

Tongue

Rich in anemia-busting iron and immune-boosting zinc. However, tongue is high in saturated fat and trans fat. Like other organ meats, such as liver, it is high in cholesterol and should be eaten in moderation.

NUTRIENTS IN 4 OZ. OF COOKED, SIMMERED TONGUE:

Calories, 321.3
Cholesterol, 149.3 mg
Protein, 21.3 g
Saturated fat, 9.3 g
Sodium, 73.2 mg
Total fat, 25.3 g
Trans fat, 1.3 g
Iron, vitamin B12, vitamin C

HEALTH AND HEALING BENEFITS OF BEEF:

ENERGY:

Vitamins B6 and B12 work together to use and store energy from proteins and carbohydrates, and also help to control levels of homocysteine, an excess of which has been linked to increased risk of coronary diseases, as well as osteoporosis and Alzheimer's disease.

IMMUNE SYSTEM:

Zinc is important for the maintenance of a healthy immune system, thyroid function, good vision, and overall cell function. The body cannot store zinc, so a daily intake is necessary to maintain healthy levels. Protein in red meat also contains amino acids necessary to build muscle and repair tissue. Muscle mass is essential because it gives you the ability to be physically active, and it also produces enzymes and hormones that help prevent illness.

OXYGENATION OF THE BLOOD:

Iron improves the ability of the red blood cells to carry oxygen from the lungs to the cells around the body in the form of hemoglobin. Iron is particularly important for menstruating women, who lose iron each month during menses. Growing children and adolescents have an increased need for iron, as do women who are pregnant or lactating.

Glycemic load: 0
Inflammatory index: Mildly inflammatory

ANTIOXIDANT:

Rich in the antioxidant minerals selenium and zinc. Antioxidants are essential for optimal health. These compounds help decrease free radical molecules, which damage cells and lead to every known disease.

RECOMMENDED FOR HELP WITH:

- Iron-deficient anemia
- Immune health
- Muscle maintenance

LAMB

Lamb is low in sodium, and a good source of protein, energy-boosting niacin, immune-boosting zinc, and vitamin B12, essential for red blood cell production and nerve function. Most meat products lack dietary fiber, and should be eaten with vegetables to provide this essential nutrient. It is worth noting that most meat is high in saturated fat and cholesterol, though the presence of vitamin B complexes help to control "bad" cholesterol. Lamb is a source of purines, which your body converts into puric acid, which can increase the risk of kidney stones and gout—those susceptible to these conditions should avoid foods high in purines, including lamb.

Note: The entries below allow quick comparison between calories, cholesterol, sodium, total fat, saturated fat, and protein for many cuts of lamb and various cooking methods, as well as highlighting beneficial nutrients associated with each particular lamb product.

Lamb loin, cooked

Along with shank and leg, loin is one of the leaner, healthier cuts of lamb, and is comparable to beef or pork in terms of calories and fat. Lamb is an excellent source of essential amino acids. It is, however, high in saturated fat and cholesterol.

NUTRIENTS IN 4 OZ. LAMB LOIN, TRIMMED TO ⅛ INCH FAT, BROILED:

Calories, 247.4
Cholesterol, 93.1 mg
Protein, 29.3 g
Saturated fat, 6.7 g
Sodium, 87.8 mg
Total fat, 13.3 g
Calcium, iron, niacin, vitamins B6 and B12

Glycemic load: 0
Inflammatory index: Mildly inflammatory

Lamb chops

Grilling is one of the healthiest, most delicious ways to prepare lamb chops. Broiling is another healthy cooking method that maintains the benefits of grilling. Lamb chops are, however, high in saturated fat and cholesterol.

NUTRIENTS IN 4 OZ. OF SIRLOIN CHOPS, BONELESS, TRIMMED TO $1/8$ INCH FAT, BROILED:

Calories, 266
Cholesterol, 95.8 mg
Protein, 29.3 g
Saturated fat, 6.6 g
Sodium, 71.8 mg
Total fat, 16 g
Calcium, iron, niacin, vitamin B12, zinc

Glycemic load: 0
Inflammatory index: Mildly inflammatory

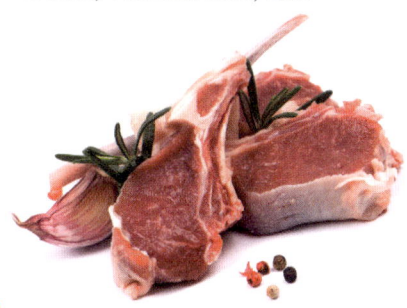

Leg of lamb

Along with shank and loin, leg is one of the leaner, healthier cuts of lamb, and is comparable to beef or pork in terms of calories and fat. However, it is high in saturated fat and cholesterol.

NUTRIENTS IN 4 OZ. OF LAMB LEG, BONE-IN, TRIMMED TO $1/8$ INCH FAT, BROILED:

Calories, 243.4
Cholesterol, 95.8 mg
Protein, 29.3 g
Saturated fat, 6.7 g
Sodium, 73.2 mg
Total fat, 13.3 g
Calcium, iron, niacin, phosphorus, riboflavin, vitamin B12, zinc

Glycemic load: 0
Inflammatory index: Mildly inflammatory

Liver, lamb

Lamb liver is particularly rich in vitamin A, which helps promote healthy skin and hair, and iron, essential to delivering oxygen around the body. However, it is also very high in cholesterol, high levels of which can lead to heart problems.

NUTRIENTS IN 11 OZ. OF PAN-FRIED LAMB LIVER:

Calories, 278.6
Carbohydrate, 4.4 g
Cholesterol, 577.1 mg
Protein, 29.8 g
Saturated fat, 5.8 g
Sodium, 145.1 mg
Total fat, 14.9 g
Very high in vitamin A and iron; also contains vitamins B6, B12, C, calcium, phosphorus, zinc, manganese, riboflavin, niacin, folate, pantothenic acid, copper, selenium.

HEALTH AND HEALING BENEFITS OF LAMB:

OXYGENATION OF THE BLOOD:

Iron is essential in the production of hemoglobin, which carries oxygen from the lungs to cells in all parts of the body. Iron is particularly important for menstruating women, who lose iron each month during menses. Growing children and adolescents have an increased need for iron, as do women who are pregnant or lactating.

PROSTATE CANCER:

Studies suggest that selenium may help reduce the risk of prostate cancer. Selenium also contributes to the healthy function of the immune and reproductive systems.

Glycemic load: 0
Inflammatory index: Strongly inflammatory

BONE FORMATION AND MAINTENANCE:

Calcium and manganese are both important in the building and maintenance of skeletal tissue.

RECOMMENDED FOR HELP WITH:

- Immune health
- Bone building
- Hair and skin health

MIXED MEATS

While not considered health foods, even mixed meats such as sausages can provide the body with essential nutrients that contribute to body maintenance and muscle building. These include choline for cell membrane construction and relieving pain and depression. The iron available assists in healthy red blood cells, and protein is vital for building and maintaining muscle.

Pork

Like most meats, pork is a good source of protein, iron, energy-boosting niacin and thiamin, bone-building calcium, and selenium, which has been linked to combating cancer. However, pork is also high in saturated fat, cholesterol, and, depending on the cut and preparation method, can be high in sodium. Most meat products lack dietary fiber, and should be eaten with vegetables to provide this essential nutrient. Including a couple of servings of pork in your weekly meal plan as part of a healthy diet can provide your body with many vital nutrients.

Note: The entries below provide a quick look at the calories, cholesterol, sodium, total fat, saturated fat, and protein for many cuts of pork and various cooking methods, as well as highlighting beneficial nutrients associated with each particular pork product.

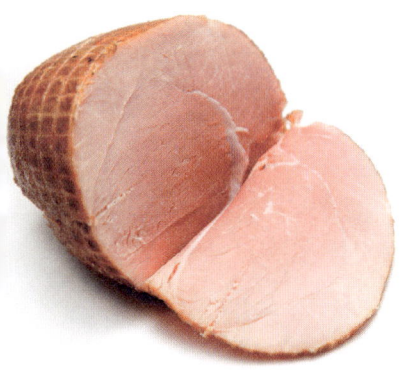

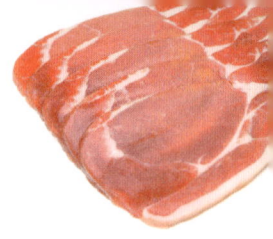

Bacon, Canadian

Two slices of Canadian-style bacon provide just over a quarter (26%) of your recommended daily value of energy-boosting thiamin. However, this food is also high in cholesterol and sodium. Two slices contain 30% of your recommended daily value of sodium, so should be avoided by those on a sodium-restricted diet.

NUTRIENTS IN 1 SLICE OF CANADIAN BACON, PAN-FRIED:

Calories, 20
Cholesterol, 9.3 mg
Protein, 3.9 g
Saturated fat, 0.1 g
Sodium, 137 mg
Total fat, 0.4 g
Niacin, phosphorus, selenium, thiamin, vitamin B6

Glycemic load: 2
Inflammatory index: Mildly anti-inflammatory

Bacon, cured

Bacon contains protein, niacin, and selenium. However, it is high in sodium, so should be avoided by those on a sodium-restricted diet. Low-sodium bacon is a good alternative for those who want to avoid excess sodium.

NUTRIENTS IN 1 SLICE OF BACON, PAN-FRIED:

Calories, 54
Cholesterol, 11.4 mg
Protein, 3.9 g
Saturated fat, 1.4 g
Sodium, 193 mg
Total fat, 4 g
Niacin, selenium

Glycemic load: 0
Inflammatory index: Mildly inflammatory

Pork chops, center loin

The loin runs along the back of the pig from the legs to the shoulder and includes the upper portion of the pig's body. Blade chops come from near the shoulder, sirloin chops from near the rump, with center between the two. Center is the leanest choice. All provide an energy-enhancing vitamin B boost.

NUTRIENTS IN 3 OZ. CENTER LOIN PORK CHOPS, BONE-IN, PAN-FRIED:

Calories, 235
Cholesterol, 78 mg
Protein, 25 g
Saturated fat, 5 g
Sodium, 68 mg
Total fat, 14 g
Selenium, thiamin

Glycemic load: 0
Inflammatory index:
  Mildly anti-inflammatory

Ground pork

Three ounces of ground pork contain over 40% of your recommended daily value of thiamin, which helps to maintain the healthy function of your heart, muscles, and central nervous system. All animals require vitamin B1, which is made in bacteria, fungi, and plants, but a big portion of the nutritional B1 content of foods is often lost due to modern food processing.

NUTRIENTS IN 3 OZ. OF GROUND PORK, COOKED:

Calories, 252
Cholesterol, 80 mg
Protein, 22 g
Saturated fat, 7 g
Sodium, 62 mg
Total fat, 18 g
Calcium, iron, selenium, thiamin, vitamin C

Glycemic load: 0
Inflammatory index:
  Moderately inflammatory

Ham, rump

Ham rump is a very good source of copper, which helps to boost the body's antioxidant defenses, protecting against free radical damage to cells. It also plays an important role in energy production and contributes to bone and blood vessel health. However, rump is high in cholesterol and very high in sodium (30% recommended daily value in 3 ounces), so should be eaten in moderation.

NUTRIENTS IN 3 OZ. OF CURED RUMP HAM, BONE-IN, LEAN ONLY, ROASTED:

Calories, 112
Cholesterol, 60 mg
Saturated fat, 82 g
Sodium, 719 mg
Total fat, 3 g
Trans fat, 0 g
Calcium, copper, iron, niacin, phosphorus, riboflavin, selenium, thiamin, vitamin B6, zinc

Glycemic load: 0
Inflammatory index: Mildly inflammatory

Ham, whole leg

Whole leg of ham is lower in sodium than cured cuts of ham. Three ounces of roasted whole leg of ham contains just 2% of your recommended daily value of sodium. It's also a very good source of protein—contains half your recommended daily value. However, it is high in cholesterol.

NUTRIENTS IN 3 OZ. OF WHOLE LEG HAM, LEAN ONLY, ROASTED:

Calories, 179
Cholesterol, 80 mg
Protein, 25 g
Saturated fat, 3 g
Sodium, 54 mg
Total fat, 8 g
Niacin, phosphorus, selenium, thiamin, vitamin B6, zinc

Glycemic load: 0
Inflammatory index: Mildly inflammatory

Liver cheese, pork

Liver cheese is an outstanding source of vision-boosting vitamin A and vitamin B12, which maintains healthy red blood cells and contributes to neurological health. Three ounces contains 133% of your recommended daily value of vitamin A, and 155% of vitamin B12. However, it is high in saturated fat, cholesterol, and sodium, so should be eaten in moderation.

NUTRIENTS IN 1.5 OZ. OF PORK LIVER CHEESE:

Calories, 116
Cholesterol, 66 mg
Protein, 6 g
Saturated fat, 3 g
Sodium, 465 mg
Total fat, 10 g
Iron, niacin, pantothenic acid, riboflavin, selenium, vitamin A and vitamin B12

Glycemic load: 0
Inflammatory index: Mildly anti-inflammatory

Pork tenderloin

Low in sodium and rich in energy-enhancing B vitamins, pork tenderloin is a lean cut, providing a lower-fat alternative to other cuts, such as chops or bacon. It is also a good source of metabolism-regulating selenium and bone-tissue-strengthening phosphorus.

NUTRIENTS IN 3 OZ. OF FRESH PORK TENDERLOIN, LEAN ONLY, ROASTED:

Calories, 122
Cholesterol, 62 mg
Saturated fat, 3 g
Sodium, 48 mg
Total fat, 3 g
Niacin, phosphorus, potassium, riboflavin, selenium, thiamin, vitamin B6, zinc

Glycemic load: 0
Inflammatory index: Mildly inflammatory

HEALTH AND HEALING BENEFITS OF PORK:

ENERGY RELEASE:

Thiamin is essential for carbohydrate metabolism, releasing energy for growth, nerve function, and muscle tone. All animals require thiamin, made in bacteria, fungi, and plants, but a big portion of its nutritional content in foods is often lost in processing.

MUSCLE HEALTH:

Pork is a good source of protein, which is vital for repairing and maintaining body tissue and muscle mass, among other functions.

IMMUNE HEALTH:

Zinc is important for the maintenance of a healthy immune system, thyroid function, good vision, and overall cell function. The body cannot store zinc, so a daily intake is necessary to maintain healthy levels. Protein in red meat also contains amino acids necessary to build muscle and repair tissue. Muscle mass is essential because it gives you the ability to be physically active, and it also produces enzymes and hormones that help prevent illness.

RECOMMENDED FOR HELP WITH:
- Nerve function
- Energy
- Immunity

VEAL

Veal is the meat from young cattle, usually less than twenty weeks old. Like pork, veal tends to be lower in fat than beef. It is also richer in energy-boosting thiamin and niacin. Like other red meats, veal is a good source of protein and can contribute to meeting your daily protein requirement, whether in stir-fries, grilled, stewed, or using ground meat to make burgers or meatloaf. The nutritional value of meats varies according to the type and the cut, while cooking methods impact the level of fat: broiling, baking, poaching, or steaming are healthier options, while frying or roasting increase the fat content.

Note: The entries below allow quick comparison between calories, cholesterol, sodium, total fat, saturated fat, and protein for various cuts of veal and cooking methods, as well as highlighting beneficial nutrients associated with each particular veal product.

Veal breast

Veal breast is a good source of B vitamins, which are necessary for energy systems and metabolism. However, it is high in saturated fat and cholesterol.

NUTRIENTS IN 4 OZ. OF WHOLE VEAL BREAST, BONELESS, BRAISED:

Calories, 301.2
Cholesterol: 128 mg
Protein, 30.4 g
Saturated fat: 7.6 g
Sodium: 73.6 mg
Total fat: 18.8 g
Iron, niacin

Glycemic load: 0
Inflammatory index: Mildly anti-inflammatory

Veal chops, sirloin

Veal chops are very lean. Unlike beef, most cuts of veal are appropriate for broiling; however, veal chops are the most commonly broiled because they are among the thickest and most tender of all the veal cuts.

NUTRIENTS IN 4 OZ. OF SIRLOIN VEAL CHOPS, ROASTED:

Calories, 241.3
Cholesterol, 121.8 mg
Protein, 30.2 g
Saturated fat, 5.3 g
Sodium, 99.1 mg
Total fat, 12.4 g
Iron, niacin, phosphorus, riboflavin, vitamin B6, vitamin B12, zinc

Glycemic load: 0
Inflammatory index: Moderately inflammatory

Liver, veal

Veal liver is very high in vision-boosting vitamin A, which also helps promote healthy skin and hair; and iron, essential to delivering oxygen around the body. However, it is also high in cholesterol.

NUTRIENTS IN 4 OZ. OF VEAL LIVER, PAN-FRIED:

Calories, 258
Cholesterol, 650 mg
Protein, 36 g
Saturated fat, 2 g
Sodium, 114 mg
Total fat, 8 g
Copper, folate, iron, niacin, phosphorus, riboflavin, selenium, vitamin A, vitamin B6, vitamin B12, zinc

Glycemic load: 2
Inflammatory index: Moderately inflammatory

Veal loin

Veal loin is a good source of B vitamins, which are necessary for energy systems and metabolism. However, it is high in saturated fat and cholesterol.

NUTRIENTS IN 4 OZ. OF VEAL LOIN, ROASTED:

Calories, 248.5
Cholesterol, 118 mg
Protein, 28.5 g
Saturated fat, 6 g
Sodium, 106.5 mg
Total fat, 14 g
Niacin, phosphorus, vitamin B6, vitamin B12, zinc

Glycemic load: 0
Inflammatory index: Moderately inflammatory

Veal rump

Veal rump is a good source of selenium; studies have shown a link between consumption of the trace mineral selenium and a reduction in the risk of cancer.

NUTRIENTS IN 4 OZ. OF VEAL RUMP, ROASTED:

Calories, 123.1
Cholesterol, 62.7 g
Protein, 17.8 g
Saturated fat, 1.3 g
Sodium, 262.2 mg
Total fat, 3.6 g
Selenium, vitamin B6, vitamin B12

Glycemic load: 0
Inflammatory index: Mildly inflammatory

Veal shoulder

Veal shoulder is a good source of energy-boosting B vitamins, including niacin, and immune-boosting zinc. However, it is high in cholesterol.

NUTRIENTS IN 4 OZ. OF VEAL SHOULDER, WHOLE (ARM AND BLADE), BRAISED:

Calories, 248.6
Cholesterol, 137.7 mg
Protein, 34.9 g
Saturated fat, 4 g
Sodium, 103.4 mg
Total fat, 10.9 g
Niacin, phosphorus, selenium, vitamin B12, zinc

HEALTH AND HEALING BENEFITS OF VEAL:

OXYGENATION OF THE BLOOD:

Iron improves the ability of the red blood cells to carry oxygen from the lungs to the cells around the body in the form of hemoglobin. Iron is particularly important for menstruating women, who lose iron each month during menses. Growing children and adolescents have an increased need for iron, as do women who are pregnant or lactating.

MUSCLE MAINTENANCE:

The proteins found in animal foods are complete because they provide essential amino acids, the small molecules required to form protein. Your body cannot synthesize these, so the amino acids in veal and other red meats help to maintain the right balance for your body to function healthily.

IMMUNE SYSTEM:

Zinc is important for the maintenance of a healthy immune system, thyroid function, good vision, and overall cell function. The body cannot store zinc, so a daily intake is necessary to maintain healthy levels. Protein in red meat also contains amino acids necessary to build muscle and repair tissue. Muscle mass is essential because it gives you the ability to be physically active, and it also produces enzymes and hormones that help prevent illness.

ENERGY:

Vitamins B6 and B12 work together to use and store energy from proteins and carbohydrates, and also help to control levels of homocysteine, an excess of which has been linked to increased risk of coronary diseases, as well as osteoporosis and Alzheimer's.

Glycemic load: 0
Inflammatory index: Mildly inflammatory

RECOMMENDED FOR HELP WITH:

- Muscle maintenance
- Energy
- Immune health

VENISON

Venison (deer) is high in protein and stacked with vitamins and iron. From a nutrient perspective it is similar in some ways to beef, but different in others. Venison is lower in saturated fat than beef. For example, a 4-ounce serving of beef flank steak has more than 9 grams of total fat, nearly 4 grams of which is saturated. An equivalent serving of venison contains only 3 grams of total fat, 1 gram of which is saturated. Both meats provide many other important nutrients, notably iron and complex B vitamins, which are necessary for maintaining healthy energy systems and metabolism. Including a couple of servings of red meat in your weekly meal plan as part of a healthy diet can provide your body with many vital nutrients.

Note: The entries below allow quick comparison between calories, cholesterol, sodium, total fat, saturated fat, and protein for various cuts of deer and various cooking methods, as well as highlighting beneficial nutrients associated with each particular deer product.

Ground venison

Ground venison can be made into patties or meatloaf. It is a good source of energy-boosting B vitamins, but is high in saturated fat and cholesterol.

NUTRIENTS IN 4 OZ. PAN-BROILED:

Calories, 232
Cholesterol, 121.3 mg
Protein, 33.3 g
Saturated fat, 5.3 g
Sodium, 97.3 mg

Total fat, 10.7 g
Niacin, phosphorus, riboflavin, thiamin, vitamin B6, vitamin B12, zinc

Glycemic load: 0
Inflammatory index: Mildly inflammatory

Venison loin

Venison loin is a healthy, lean choice of cut. It is rich in energy and immune-boosting B vitamins. However, it is high in cholesterol.

NUTRIENTS IN 4 OZ. OF VENISON LOIN, PAN-BROILED:

Calories, 162
Cholesterol, 83 mg
Protein, 32 g
Sodium, 62 mg
Total fat, 2 g
Iron, niacin, phosphorus, riboflavin, selenium, thiamin, vitamin B6, vitamin B12, zinc

HEALTH AND HEALING BENEFITS OF VENISON (DEER):

ANEMIA PREVENTION:

Venison is very iron-rich (more so than beef). Iron prevents anemia and is important in the production of hemoglobin in the blood, which carries oxygen to all parts of the body.

MUSCLE HEALTH:

Venison is higher in protein than other red meats, which is vital for repairing and maintaining body tissue and muscle mass, among other functions. High levels of protein also mean that deer sates the appetite well.

ENERGY:

Vitamins B6 and B12 in venison help to break down protein, carbohydrates, and fat to provide the body with energy. These B vitamins may also lower homocysteine buildup in the blood, thus lowering the risk of heart attacks and strokes.

Glycemic load: 0
Inflammatory index: Mildly anti-inflammatory

IMMUNE SYSTEM:

The body has no means of storing zinc, so a daily intake of this nutrient is necessary to maintain a healthy immune system. Zinc is also good for hair and skin health, and overall cell function.

RECOMMENDED FOR HELP WITH:

- Heart health
- Energy levels
- Immunity
- Iron-deficient anemia

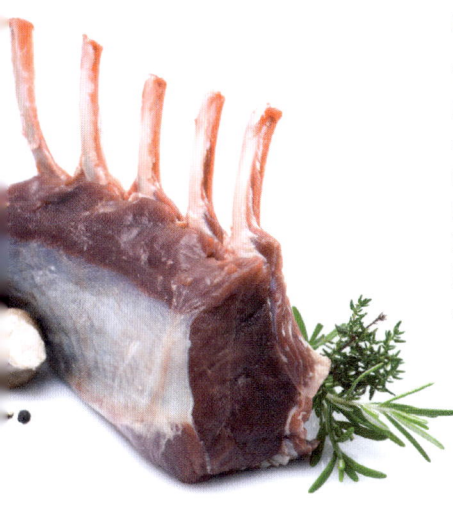

Mushrooms

Mushrooms are widely known for their high levels of nutrition and their many health benefits. Low in calories, saturated fat, cholesterol, and sodium, they also contain many vital nutrients, and are being hailed as one of the "superfoods."

Morel mushroom

A great source of vitamin D, essential for helping your body absorb calcium, thus supporting bone health. The morel has an intense, woodsy flavor. Dried morels are also tasty and less expensive than the fresh variety, ideal for cooking. Morel mushrooms are low in calories and a good source of fiber and iron, supporting healthy digestion and oxygenation of the blood.

NUTRIENTS IN 5 PIECES OF DRIED WILD MOREL MUSHROOMS:

Calories, 30
Calcium, 39 mg
Dietary fiber, 1.8 g
Iron, 7.9 mg
Potassium, 265 mg
Protein, 2 g
Vitamin D, 15 IU

HEALTH AND HEALING BENEFITS:

DIGESTION:

Fiber helps move food through your digestive system. Additionally, getting more fiber in your diet lowers blood cholesterol levels, prevents constipation, and helps you feel full faster.

BLOOD HEALTH:

Iron is essential for blood manufacture and helps the blood cells and muscles to carry and hold oxygen and then release it when needed.

BONES:

Vitamin D contributes to maintaining healthy bones by aiding the body's absorption of calcium.

Glycemic load: 0
Inflammatory index: Anti-inflammatory

RECOMMENDED FOR HELP WITH:

- Digestion
- Immune health
- Bone strength

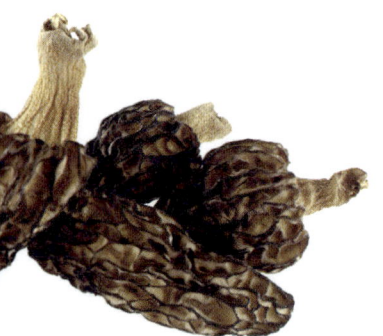

Portobello mushroom

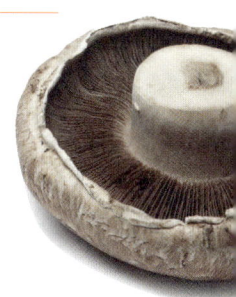

Portobello mushrooms are fat-free, low in calories, and a rich source of antioxidant-boosting copper and selenium, as well as metabolism-enhancing B vitamins. They are instantly recognizable by their large tan brown caps, dark undersides, and thick white stems. Their dense, meaty texture makes them a versatile ingredient in the kitchen, and an ideal meat substitute in many dishes.

NUTRIENTS IN 1 CUP OF DICED RAW PORTOBELLO MUSHROOMS:

Calories, 22
Calcium, 0.5 mg
Copper, 0.3 mg
Dietary fiber, 1.3 g
Folate, 18.9 mcg
Iron, 0.5 g
Magnesium, 9.5 mg
Manganese, 0.1 mg
Niacin, 3.9 mg
Pantothenic acid, 1.3 mg
Phosphorus, 112 mg
Potassium, 416 mg
Protein, 2.2 g
Riboflavin, 0.4 mg
Selenium, 9.5 mcg
Thiamin, 0.1 mg
Vitamin B6, 0.1 mg
Zinc, 0.5 mg

HEALTH AND HEALING BENEFITS:

ANTIOXIDANT:

A rich source of the antioxidants copper and selenium, which help to combat free radicals that damage cells and lead to every known disease. Copper also helps form connective tissue, metabolize iron, and produce energy.

METABOLISM:

One cup of sliced fresh portobello mushrooms contains 19% of your recommended daily value of niacin and 4% of vitamin B6. Your body doesn't contain its own stores of these vitamins, so it's essential to get a regular supply through your diet to help metabolize food into energy and synthesize fatty acids.

IMMUNE HEALTH:

Vitamin B6 supports the immune system, while studies have shown that selenium also helps to regulate the immune system and reduce inflammation.

Glycemic load: 2
Inflammatory index: Mildly anti-inflammatory

RECOMMENDED FOR HELP WITH:

- Immune health
- Digestion
- Metabolism protection

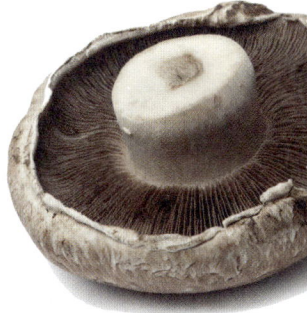

SHIITAKE MUSHROOM

Great for maintaining a healthy immune system, and also thought to lower cholesterol. These meaty and delicious mushrooms contain a substance called eritadenine, which encourages body tissues to absorb cholesterol and lower the amount circulating in the blood. Shiitakes are also thought to have antiviral and anticarcinogenic effects. Widely available fresh or dried, the dried variety have a particularly intense smoky flavor. Sauté for roughly seven minutes to get the best flavor, while keeping maximum nutritional value.

Shiitake mushroom, raw

Raw shiitake mushrooms are a good source of antioxidant-boosting copper and selenium, as well as metabolism-enhancing B vitamins. Wash raw mushrooms to remove dirt—you may want to chop off the bottom of the hard stem, then slice thinly and sprinkle over salads to add a tasty nutritional boost.

NUTRIENTS IN 1 CUP OF RAW SHIITAKE MUSHROOMS:

Calories, 34
Copper, 0.1 mg
Dietary fiber, 2.5 g
Folate, 13 mcg
Magnesium, 20 mg
Manganese, 0.2 mg
Niacin, 3.9 mg
Pantothenic acid, 1.5 mg
Potassium, 304 mg
Riboflavin, 0.2 mg
Selenium, 5.7 mcg
Vitamin B6, 0.3 mg
Zinc, 1 mg

Glycemic load: 7
Inflammatory index: Mildly inflammatory

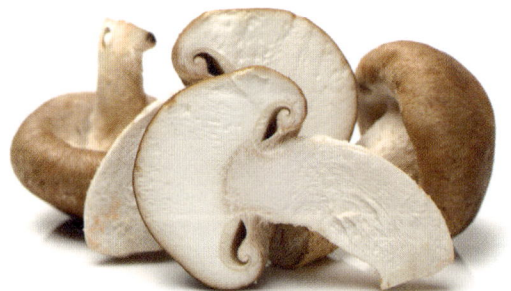

Shiitake mushroom, dried

A one-cup serving of dried shiitake mushrooms provides almost double your recommended daily values of copper and the B vitamin pantothenic acid. Dried shiitake mushrooms also contain even higher levels of niacin, riboflavin, vitamin B6, manganese, selenium, zinc, and dietary fiber than raw. Soak dried shiitake mushrooms in water before using. Chop and use to add depth of flavor to soups, stews, and stir-fries.

NUTRIENTS IN 1 CUP OF DRIED SHIITAKE MUSHROOMS:

Calories, 98.7
Copper, 1.7 mg
Dietary fiber, 3.8 g
Folate, 54.3 mcg
Magnesium, 44 mg
Manganese, 0.4 mg
Niacin, 4.7 mg
Pantothenic acid, 7.3 mg
Potassium, 511.3 mg
Riboflavin, 0.4 mg
Selenium, 15.4 mcg
Vitamin B6, 0.3 mg
Zinc, 2.6 mg

HEALTH AND HEALING BENEFITS (RAW AND DRIED):

IMMUNE SUPPORT:

Many studies have been carried out on the beneficial effects on the immune system of the polysaccharides (large carbohydrate molecules composed of many different sugars arranged in chains and branches) in shiitake mushrooms.

CARDIOVASCULAR HEALTH:

Eritadenine (also called lentinacin, or lentsine, sometimes abbreviated as DEA), one of the most unusual naturally occurring nutrients in shiitake mushrooms, has been shown to help lower total blood cholesterol.

Glycemic load: 35
Inflammatory index: Mildly inflammatory

ANTI-CANCEROUS:

Research has shown that "anti-cancer immunity" may be enhanced by shiitake mushroom intake, by activating macrophage cells, responsible for identifying and clearing potentially cancerous cells from the body.

RECOMMENDED FOR HELP WITH:

- Immune health
- Lowering cholesterol
- Cancer prevention

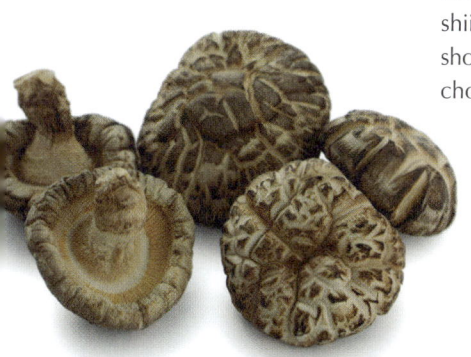

White button mushroom

Low in saturated fat and sodium and very low in cholesterol. A good source of the immune-boosting B-complex vitamins riboflavin, niacin, pantothenic acid, and folate, as well as antioxidant-boosting copper and selenium. White button are the most common and least expensive mushrooms. Their mild taste means they can be used in a wide range of dishes, from salads to sauces, yet their flavor intensifies when cooked, making them ideal for sautéing and grilling.

NUTRIENTS IN 1 CUP OF SLICED RAW WHITE BUTTON MUSHROOMS:

Calories, 15
Copper, 0.2 mg
Dietary fiber, 0.7 g
Niacin, 2.5 mg
Pantothenic acid, 1 mg
Phosphorus, 60.2 mg
Potassium, 223 mg
Riboflavin, 0.3 mg
Selenium, 6.5 mcg
Thiamin, 0.1 mg
Vitamin B6, 0.1 mg
Vitamin C, 1.5 mg
Vitamin D, 12.6 IU

HEALTH AND HEALING BENEFITS:

IMMUNE HEALTH:

Vitamin B6 supports the immune system, while studies have shown that selenium also helps to regulate the immune system and reduce inflammation.

ANTIOXIDANT:

A rich source of the antioxidants copper and selenium, which help to combat free radicals that damage cells and lead to every known disease. Copper also helps form connective tissue, metabolize iron, and produce energy.

DIGESTION:

Fiber helps move food through your digestive system. Additionally, getting more fiber in your diet lowers blood cholesterol levels, prevents constipation, and helps you feel full faster.

Glycemic load: 2
Inflammatory index: Mildly inflammatory

RECOMMENDED FOR HELP WITH:

- Immune health
- Digestion
- Metabolism

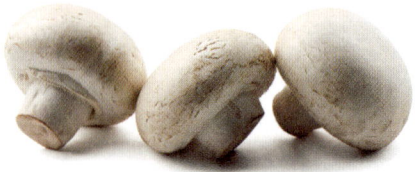

Nuts and seeds

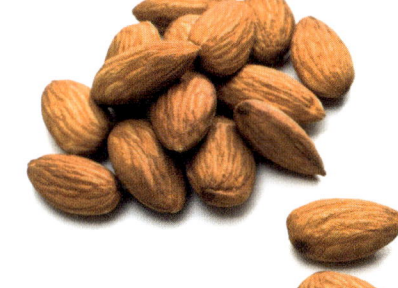

Nuts and seeds are among the nutritional superfoods—packed full of health-giving nutrients, such as proteins healthy fats, and fiber. However, please beware and avoid if you have a nut allergy.

Almonds

Eating almonds five times a week may lower the risk of coronary artery disease by 50%. All nuts are good, but almonds and Brazil nuts are the only two that produce an alkaline reaction in the body. Since most people's bodies are far too acidic, almonds are a welcome addition to any diet. They also have more magnesium than other nuts and are an excellent source of monounsaturated fat. And, of course, its excellent taste means that the almond is an all-time favorite. Additionally, almond butter is terrific, either alone or with any other food.

NUTRIENTS IN 23 ALMONDS (1 OZ.):

Calories, 164
Iron, 1 mg
Magnesium, 76.5 mg
Manganese, 0.6 mg
Potassium, 208 mg
Vitamin E, 7.3 mg
Zinc, 0.9 mg
14 amino acids, including 0.7 mg l-arginine, the nitric oxide enhancer

Glycemic load: 0
Inflammatory index: Strongly anti-inflammatory

Almond butter

Almond butter is an alkalizing food that's low in cholesterol; add a spoonful of almond butter to your breakfast shake for a tasty protein boost. Almond butter provides folate, iron, magnesium, potassium, and zinc.

Almond oil

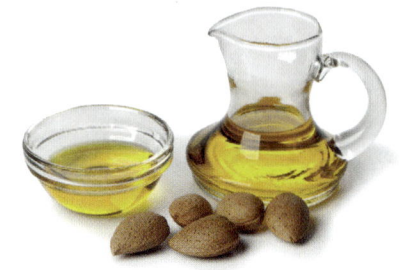

Almond oil is a great substitute for more unhealthy fats and oils. While it lacks the B vitamins of whole almonds or almond butter, just one ounce of almond oil contains over half your recommended daily value of the antioxidant vitamin E, helping to protect cells from free radical damage.

HEALTH AND HEALING BENEFITS OF ALMONDS:

PREVENTING CANCER:

Provides excellent antioxidants, and there is clinical evidence for decreased colon, prostate, and cervical cancers.

HEART HEALTH:

One of the best foods for lowering blood pressure, decreasing cholesterol, and improving blood flow.

DIABETES:

Stabilizes blood sugar and lowers glycemic index. Especially good in lowering rises when eaten with higher glycemic foods.

RECOMMENDED FOR HELP WITH:

- Diabetes
- Coronary artery disease
- Cancer prevention
- Carpal tunnel syndrome

Brazil nuts, dried

Native to the Amazon rainforest, Brazil nuts are one of only two nuts (almond is the second) that produce an alkaline reaction in the body. Since most people's bodies are too acidic, Brazil nuts are a welcome addition to any diet. They are also an excellent source of selenium; just one ounce contains a huge 767% of your recommended daily value, making them the highest natural source of this mineral.

NUTRIENTS IN 6 DRIED BRAZIL NUTS (1 OZ.):

Calories, 187
Copper, 0.5 mg
Magnesium, 107 mg
Phosphorus, 206 mg
Selenium, 544 mcg
Thiamin, 0.2 mg
Vitamin E, 1.6 mg

Glycemic load: 2
Inflammatory index: Mildly anti-inflammatory

RECOMMENDED FOR HELP WITH:

- Lowering cholesterol
- Reducing the risk of heart disease
- Type 2 diabetes

HEALTH AND HEALING BENEFITS:

CHOLESTEROL:

A good source of monounsaturated fatty acids, which help to lower LDL, or "bad cholesterol," and increase HDL, or "good cholestero,l" levels in the blood. Studies suggest that diets rich in monounsaturated fatty acids and omega-3 fatty acids help to prevent coronary artery disease and strokes.

METABOLISM:

B-complex vitamins work with enzymes to promote healthy metabolism.

IMMUNITY:

Selenium has antioxidant properties that help the body prevent cellular damage from free radicals. It also helps to support a strong immune system, while getting adequate selenium into your diet may help prevent coronary artery disease, liver cirrhosis, and cancers.

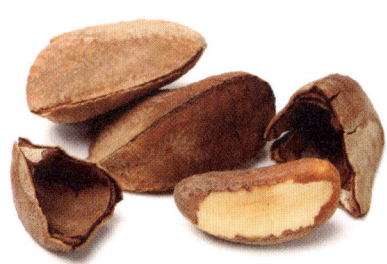

Cashew nuts

Native to the Amazon, these sweet, crunchy nuts are packed with free-radical-zapping antioxidants, energy, vitamins, and minerals—as well as energy-boosting copper and bone-strengthening magnesium. They are low in cholesterol and sodium. Cashews are one of the best legumes, with excellent fat ratios and protein, though with incomplete amino acids. Delicious as a snack, raw, or roasted, and as an addition to salads and stir-fry dishes.

NUTRIENTS IN 18 RAW CASHEW NUTS (1 OZ.):

Calories, 157
Copper, 0.6 mg
Fat, 12 g
Magnesium, 82.8 mg
Manganese, 0.5 mg
Phosphorus, 168 mg
Protein, 5.2 g
Thiamin, 0.1 mg
Vitamin K, 9.7 mcg
Zinc, 1.6 mg

Glycemic load: 3
Inflammatory index: Mildly anti-inflammatory

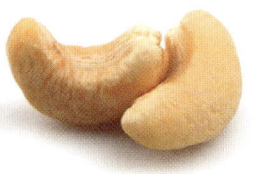

Cashew butter

Cashew butter is low in cholesterol, with good-quality fats. One tablespoon four times a week can help to lower the risk of cardiovascular disease and coronary heart disease. It provides copper, folate, protein, and zinc.

HEALTH AND HEALING BENEFITS OF CASHEWS:

CHOLESTEROL:

Rich in "heart-friendly" monounsaturated fatty acids that help lower harmful LDL-cholesterol while increasing "good" HDL cholesterol. Studies suggest that a diet rich in monounsaturated fatty acids helps to prevent coronary artery disease and strokes.

ANTIOXIDANT:

Copper helps to boost the body's antioxidant defenses, protecting against free radical damage to cells. It also plays an important role in energy production and contributes to bone and blood vessel health.

HEALTHY BONES:

Everyone knows that calcium is needed for strong, healthy bones, but magnesium is also vital for the same function. Insufficient magnesium can also contribute to high blood pressure, muscle spasms, and migraine headaches, as well as muscle cramps, tension, soreness, and fatigue.

Glycemic load: 0
Inflammatory index: Anti-inflammatory

RECOMMENDED FOR HELP WITH:

- Lowering cholesterol
- Reducing the risk of heart disease
- Diabetes

Chestnuts, roasted

Unlike most nuts, chestnuts are rich in complex carbohydrates. They are chiefly composed of starch and have a similar nutritional composition to staple starch foods such as sweet potato. Chestnuts stand out from other edible nuts for being rich in vitamin C, nature's own powerful antioxidant, which helps prevent cell damage from free radicals. One ounce of roasted chestnuts contains 12% of your recommended daily value of immune-boosting vitamin C. Chestnuts are also a good source of energy-boosting copper.

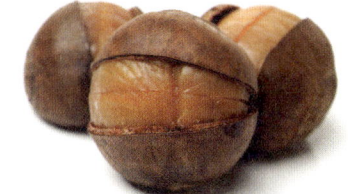

NUTRIENTS IN 3 ROASTED CHESTNUTS (1 OZ.):

Calories, 70
Copper, 0.1 mg
Dietary fiber, 1.5 g
Manganese, 0.3 mg
Vitamin B6, 0.1 mg
Vitamin C, 7.3 mg

HEALTH AND HEALING BENEFITS:

IMMUNITY:

A good source of vitamin C, nature's own powerful antioxidant and one of the most critical vitamins for immune health.

CHOLESTEROL:

Like other nuts, chestnuts are a good source of monounsaturated fatty acids, which help to lower LDL, or "bad cholesterol," and increase HDL, or "good cholesterol," levels in the blood. Studies suggest that diets rich in monounsaturated fatty acids and omega-3 fatty acids help to prevent coronary artery disease and strokes.

ANTIOXIDANT:

Copper helps to boost the body's antioxidant defenses, protecting against free radical damage to cells. It also plays an important role in energy production and contributes to bone and blood vessel health.

Glycemic load: 42
Inflammatory index: Inflammatory

RECOMMENDED FOR HELP WITH:

- Lowering cholesterol
- Reducing the risk of heart disease
- Immunity

Chia seeds

A super-quality protein and source of fiber, chia seeds are also packed with omega-3s. There may be no other food as rich in overall nutrients and health benefits as chia—the "strength" food of the Aztecs. If I had only one food to eat, I would choose chia! No other food has the overall balance of quality protein, fat, and fiber, and these small black or white seeds pack more energy and value than any other known food. Plus, no other plant protein comes close in terms of the quality of the protein/amino mix. Just ¼ cup of chia seeds contains as much quality protein as a glass of milk.

NUTRIENTS IN 2 TBSP. (1 OZ.) OF CHIA SEEDS:

Calories, 138
Carbohydrate, 11.9 g
Boron, trace
Calcium, 179 mg
Fiber, 9.8 g
Magnesium, 95 mg
Niacin, 2.5 mg
Thiamin, 0.2 mg
Omega-3 fats, 5.1 g
Polyunsaturated fat, 6.7 g
Potassium, 115 mg
Protein, 4.7 g
Vitamin E, 0.1 mg
Zinc, 1.3 mg

HEALTH AND HEALING BENEFITS:

ANTI-INFLAMMATORY/ ANTIOXIDANT:

All diseases include some degree of inflammation. Omega-3s are converted to positive prostaglandins. Perhaps the most important benefit of these tiny seeds is that they contain more ORACS than blueberries.

BLOOD SUGAR STABILIZER:

The high fiber content slows carbohydrate metabolism and helps keep blood sugars level—part of chia's excellence in providing energy.

BONE HEALTH:

The perfect ratio of magnesium to calcium, plus boron.

BRAIN POWER:

Omega-3s are critical for nerve function, memory, and, essentially, holding our cells together.

DETOXIFICATION:

Fiber is essential for good digestion and bowel function in general. Many of our natural probiotics are dependent upon adequate fiber.

ENERGY:

Chia means strength. Many claims have been made that Aztecs could function on one tablespoon of chia daily. Today, it is widely used by marathon runners.

DIGESTION:

The amount of fiber in chia is ideal as a percentage of calories. Soothes the lining of the bowel.

HEART SUPPORT:

Lowers blood pressure and cholesterol—far better than any drug.

WEIGHT BALANCE:

Provides bulk, decreases hunger, helps slow the digestive process, and boosts metabolism overall, while supplying all essential amino acids for muscle building.

Glycemic load: 4
Inflammatory index: Mildly anti-inflammatory

RECOMMENDED FOR HELP WITH:

- Irritable bowel syndrome
- Diabetes
- Hypertension
- Weight loss

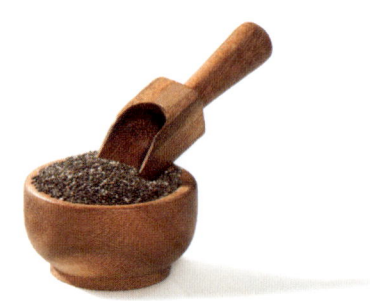

Flaxseeds

A powerhouse of the seed kingdom, flaxseeds are a great source of fiber, omega-3s, and antioxidants. They make a nutritious addition to everything from muffins, cookies, and breads, to pizza crusts and casseroles. And the good news is that studies suggest that the cooking process doesn't impact the effectiveness of the omega-3 fatty acids, which help to lower LDL, or "bad cholesterol," and increase HDL, or "good cholesterol," levels in the blood. Flaxseeds are also ranked as the number one source of lignans—phytonutrients that provide both antioxidant and fiber-like benefits to the body. They contain a whopping seven times the amount of lignans as sesame seeds, the closest runner-up in the lignan-rich food stakes.

NUTRIENTS IN 1 TBSP. OF FLAXSEEDS:

Calories, 37
Copper, 0.1 mg
Dietary fiber, 1.9 g
Magnesium, 27.4 mg
Manganese, 0.2 mg
Phosphorus, 44.9 mg
Thiamin, 0.1 mg

Glycemic load: 0
Inflammatory index: Strongly anti-inflammatory

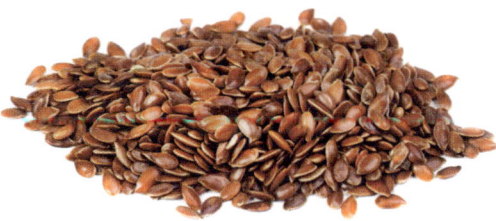

Flaxseed oil

One of the best sources of essential fatty acids, which help to lower LDL, or "bad cholesterol," and increase HDL, or "good cholesterol," levels in the blood. One ounce provides 5 milligrams of vitamin E.

HEALTH AND HEALING BENEFITS OF FLAXSEEDS:

ANTIOXIDANT:

Lignans provide free-radical-zapping antioxidant benefits, protecting cells from free radical damage.

HEART HEALTH:

The antioxidant benefits of flaxseeds have long been associated with the prevention of cardiovascular diseases and have also been linked to decreased insulin resistance.

DIGESTION:

Lignans also provide fiber-like benefits to the body. Fiber helps move food through your digestive system. Additionally, getting more fiber in your diet lowers blood cholesterol levels, prevents constipation, and helps you feel full faster.

RECOMMENDED FOR HELP WITH:

- Reducing the risk of heart disease and diabetes
- Lowering cholesterol
- Colon health
- Immunity

Ginkgo nuts

Traditionally used in Chinese medicine in a range of contexts, from easing asthma to improved memory and concentration. Ginkgo nuts decrease the ability of the blood to clot, and should be discontinued a week before elective surgery. Despite the health benefits of ginkgo nuts, it's recommended to limit consumption to no more than ten a day as ginkgotoxin can cause poisoning by interfering with vitamin B6, causing symptoms from stomachache to vomiting, and can even prove fatal.

NUTRIENTS IN 1 OZ. OF RAW GINKGO NUTS:

Calories, 51
Copper, 0.1 mg
Niacin, 1.7 mg
Vitamin C, 4.2 mg

Glycemic load: 6
Inflammatory index: Anti-inflammatory

RECOMMENDED FOR HELP WITH:

- Boosting memory
- Immunity

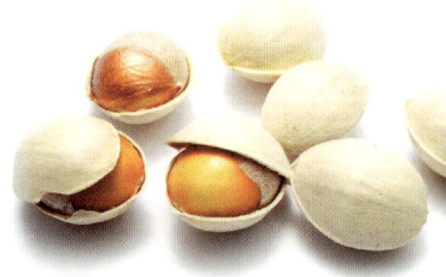

HEALTH AND HEALING BENEFITS:

ANTIOXIDANT:

High in free-radical-zapping antioxidants. One ounce contains 7% of your daily recommended value of vitamin C, nature's own powerful antioxidant, which helps prevent cell damage from free radicals.

MEMORY BOOST:

Minerals such as copper are required for healthy functioning of neurotransmission.

ENERGY:

Like the other B complex vitamins, niacin (vitamin B3) is important in energy production. It plays an essential role in converting dietary proteins, fats, and carbohydrates into usable energy.

Hazelnuts

These sweet, nutritious nuts are a good source of "healthy" fats, which help to lower cholesterol, and of free-radical-zapping vitamin E, which also contributes to healthy skin. Hazelnuts are packed with the antioxidant manganese and energy-boosting copper. One ounce of hazelnuts contains nearly a quarter (24%) of your recommended daily value of copper, which plays an important role in keeping your energy levels well stoked.

NUTRIENTS IN 21 HAZELNUTS (1 OZ.):

Calories, 178
Copper, 0.5 mg
Manganese, 1.8 mg
Thiamin, 0.2 mg
Vitamin E, 4.3 mg

HEALTH AND HEALING BENEFITS:

ENERGY:

Not only does copper help to boost the body's antioxidant defenses, protecting against free radical damage to cells, it also plays an important role in energy production and contributes to bone and blood vessel health.

Glycemic load: 0
Inflammatory index: Strongly anti-inflammatory

RECOMMENDED FOR HELP WITH:

- Reducing the risk of heart disease and diabetes
- Weight loss
- Lowering cholesterol

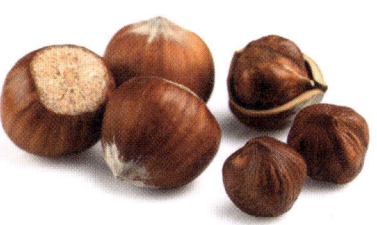

CHOLESTEROL:

The essential fatty acid linoleic acid helps lower LDL, or "bad cholesterol," and increase HDL, or "good cholesterol." Studies suggest that a diet that is plentiful in monounsaturated fatty acids helps to prevent coronary artery disease and strokes.

ANTIOXIDANT:

Manganese and vitamin E are powerful antioxidants. Antioxidants are essential for optimal health. These compounds help decrease free radical molecules, which damage cells and lead to every known disease. Diets low in manganese have been linked to conditions marked by increased oxidative stress, including skin problems and asthma.

Macadamia nuts, raw

Native to the rainforests of Australia, macadamia nuts are packed with energy and contain high levels of monounsaturated fats, which may help to lower cholesterol. They're also rich in antioxidants, which protect cells from free radical damage. One ounce of macadamia nuts contains over half (58%) of your recommended daily value of free-radical-zapping manganese.

NUTRIENTS IN 10–12 RAW RAW MACADAMIA NUTS (1 OZ.):

Calories, 204
Copper, 0.2 mg
Manganese, 1.2 mg
Thiamin, 0.3 mg

HEALTH AND HEALING BENEFITS:

ANTIOXIDANT:

A good source of the trace element manganese, a powerful antioxidant. Antioxidants are essential for optimal health. These compounds help decrease free radical molecules, which damage cells and lead to every known disease. Diets low in manganese have been linked to conditions marked by increased oxidative stress, including skin problems and asthma.

CHOLESTEROL:

Rich in "heart-friendly" monounsaturated fatty acids that help lower harmful LDL cholesterol while increasing "good" HDL cholesterol. Studies suggest that a diet rich in monounsaturated fatty acids helps to prevent coronary artery disease and strokes.

Glycemic load: 0
Inflammatory index: Strongly anti-inflammatory

RECOMMENDED FOR HELP WITH:

- Reducing the risk of heart disease and diabetes

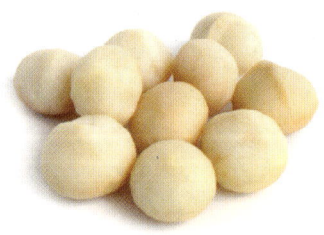

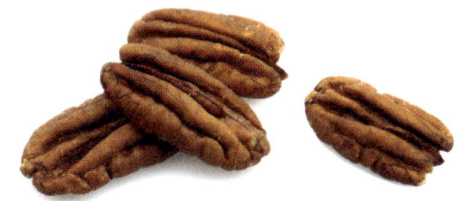

Pecan nut

These rich, buttery nuts are the most antioxidant-rich tree nut, protecting cells against damage from free radicals. They're also packed with energy, and rich in omega-6 fatty acids, which can help lower the risk of heart disease. They're popular in sweet desserts such as pecan pie, but can also be enjoyed as a healthy snack raw or roasted (with or without salt), or as a healthy addition to a range of dishes.

NUTRIENTS IN 19 HALVES OF PEACAN NUTS (1 OZ.):

Calories, 196
Copper, 0.3 mg
Manganese, 1.3 mg
Thiamin, 0.2 mg
Vitamin E, 0.4 mg

HEALTH AND HEALING BENEFITS:

ANTIOXIDANT:

Rich in the antioxidant ellagic acid. Antioxidants are essential for optimal health. These compounds help decrease free radical molecules, which damage cells and lead to every known disease.

CHOLESTEROL:

Rich in "heart-friendly" monounsaturated fatty acids, such as oleic acid, that help lower harmful LDL cholesterol while increasing "good" HDL cholesterol. Studies suggest that a diet rich in monounsaturated fatty acids helps to prevent coronary artery disease and strokes.

Glycemic load: 0
Inflammatory index: Moderately anti-inflammatory

RECOMMENDED FOR HELP WITH:

- Reducing the risk of heart disease and diabetes
- Lowering cholesterol

Pine nuts, dried

The sweet, crunchy, edible seeds of the pine tree are a good source of protein and dietary fiber. Low in cholesterol and sodium, they're packed with cardiovascular-system-boosting vitamins E and K, and the antioxidant manganese to help protect cells from free radical damage. One ounce of pine nuts contains in excess (123%) of your recommended daily value of manganese.

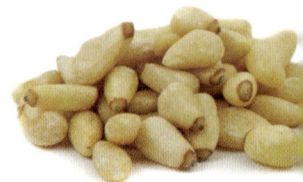

NUTRIENTS IN APPROX. 167 PINE NUTS (1 OZ.):

Calories, 191
Copper, 0.4 mg
Dietary fiber, 1 g
Magnesium, 71.2 mg
Manganese, 2.5 mg
Protein, 3.9 g
Vitamin E, 2.6 mg
Vitamin K, 15.3 mcg
Zinc, 1.8 mg

HEALTH AND HEALING BENEFITS:

CARDIOVASCULAR HEALTH:

Vitamins E and K both contribute to the healthy function of the cardiovascular system. Vitamin E helps to produce red blood cells vital to transporting oxygen around the body, while vitamin K allows blood to clot properly.

CHOLESTEROL:

Rich in "heart-friendly" monounsaturated fatty acids, such as oleic acid, that help lower harmful LDL cholesterol while increasing good HDL cholesterol. Studies suggest that a diet rich in monounsaturated fatty acids helps to prevent coronary artery disease and strokes.

WEIGHT LOSS:

The essential fatty acid pinolenic acid found in pine nuts has been shown to curb the appetite by triggering a release of hunger-suppressant enzymes in the gut, making it potentially beneficial for weight loss.

Glycemic load: 0
Inflammatory index: Moderately anti-inflammatory

RECOMMENDED FOR HELP WITH:

- Reducing the risk of heart disease and diabetes
- Weight loss
- Maintaining healthy levels of cholesterol

Pistachio nuts

One of the healthiest, low-calorie nuts. Pistachios are a good source of "heart-friendly" monounsaturated fats, which help to lower cholesterol. They're packed with antioxidant minerals, such as free-radical-busting manganese and copper, to help protect cells from free radical damage, and crammed with vitamins too—just one ounce of pistachios contains almost a quarter (24%) of your recommended daily value of nervous-system-boosting vitamin B6.

NUTRIENTS IN 49 RAW PISTACHIO NUTS (1 OZ.):

Calories, 159
Copper, 0.4 mg
Dietary fiber, 3 g
Manganese, 0.3 mg
Protein, 5.7 g
Thiamin, 0.2 mg
Vitamin B6, 0.5 mg
Vitamin E, 0.8 mg

HEALTH AND HEALING BENEFITS:

ANTIOXIDANT:

Copper and manganese help to boost the body's antioxidant defenses, protecting against free radical damage to cells. Copper also plays an important role in energy production and contributes to bone and blood vessel health.

BLOOD AND NERVOUS SYSTEM:

A good source of vitamin B6, which helps nerve cells to communicate. Deficiency is found especially in patients with heart disease, atherosclerosis, premenstrual syndrome, and carpal tunnel syndrome.

CHOLESTEROL:

Rich in "heart-friendly" monounsaturated fatty acids, such as oleic acid, that help lower harmful LDL cholesterol while increasing "good" HDL cholesterol. Studies suggest that a diet rich in monounsaturated fatty acids helps to prevent coronary artery disease and strokes.

Glycemic load: 1
Inflammatory index: Mildly anti-inflammatory

RECOMMENDED FOR HELP WITH:

- Reducing the risk of heart disease and diabetes
- Lowering cholesterol

Pumpkin seeds

A great source of magnesium and zinc. Eating the entire seed, including the shell, will maximize your intake of zinc. They can also be enjoyed roasted, though it's worth noting that roasted seeds have a significantly higher glycemic load (10) compared to dried seeds (0). It's recommended to roast pumpkin seeds for no more than 15–20 minutes, as after this time unwanted changes occur in the fat structure, altering their nutrient content.

NUTRIENTS IN APPROX. 142 DRIED PUMPKIN SEED KERNELS (1 OZ.):

Calories, 158
Copper, 0.4 mg
Iron, 2.5 mg
Magnesium, 168 mg
Manganese, 1.3 mg
Phosphorus, 349 mg
Protein, 8.6 g
Vitamin K, 2.1 mcg
Zinc, 2.2 g

Glycemic load: 0
Inflammatory index: Moderately anti-inflammatory

NUTRIENTS IN 85 WHOLE ROASTED PUMPKIN SEEDS (1 OZ.):

Calories, 126
Copper, 0.2 mg
Iron, 0.9 mg
Magnesium, 74.3 mg
Manganese, 0.1 mg
Phosphorus, 26.1 mg
Protein, 5.3 g
Zinc, 2.9 mg

HEALTH AND HEALING BENEFITS:

ANTIOXIDANT:

While pumpkin seeds aren't exceptionally high in vitamin E, they contain a diverse range of forms of this vitamin, which are thought to carry a variety of health benefits, including free-radical-zapping antioxidant power to help protect cells against damage from free radicals.

IMMUNE HEALTH:

Zinc plays an important role in the activity of more than 300 enzymes, and has far-reaching effects on immunity, reproduction, skin health, and vision. Diets low in zinc can lead to decreased activity of the immune system.

METABOLISM:

Magnesium is a key mineral in healthy metabolism. It plays a role in maintaining healthy bones, energy production, and controlling inflammation and blood sugar levels. Ongoing magnesium deficiency can lead to a significant amount of bone loss.

Glycemic load: 10
Inflammatory index: Moderately anti-inflammatory

RECOMMENDED FOR HELP WITH:

- Reducing the risk of heart disease and diabetes
- Prostate health
- Immunity

Sesame seeds

An excellent source of copper and other minerals, sesame seeds are packed with a rich mix of nutrients to maintain healthy bones and muscles, and contribute to good overall health. Sesamin and sesamoli are a type of lignan—phytonutrients with antioxidant and anti-inflammatory properties that have been shown to help lower cholesterol. Sesame seeds add a delicate nutty crunch and a nutritional boost to a range of foods, from breads to desserts, and salads to cereals. Sesame seed butter paste is a healthy, nut-free alternative to peanut butter, containing large amounts of omega fatty acids, as well as calcium, copper, and iron.

NUTRIENTS IN 1 TBSP. OF WHOLE, DRIED SESAME SEEDS:

Calories, 52
Calcium, 87.8 mg
Copper, 0.4 mg
Dietary fiber, 1.1 g
Iron, 1.3 mg
Magnesium, 31.6 mg
Manganese, 0.2 mg
Phosphorus, 56.6 mg
Thiamin, 0.1 mg
Vitamin B6, 0.1 mg
Zinc, 0.7 mg

HEALTH AND HEALING BENEFITS:

LIVER HEALTH:

Sesamin has also been found to protect the liver from oxidative damage.

CHOLESTEROL:

Sesamin and sesamoli are unique substances found in sesame seeds. They are a type of lignan—phytonutrients with antioxidant and anti-inflammatory properties that have been shown to help lower cholesterol.

ANTIOXIDANT/ ANTI-INFLAMMATORY:

A very good source of the trace element manganese, a potent antioxidant that helps protect cells against free radical damage and contributes to healthy skin. Copper also has antioxidant properties, as well as being an anti-inflammatory that can ease symptoms in conditions such as rheumatoid arthritis.

Glycemic load: 0
Inflammatory index: Mildly anti-inflammatory

Glycemic load: 0
Inflammatory index: Mildly anti-inflammatory

RECOMMENDED FOR HELP WITH:

- Reducing the risk of heart disease and diabetes
- Prostate health
- Liver health

Sunflower seeds

A rich source of vitamin E and the B-complex group of vitamins. A handful of these mildly nutty seeds provides a tasty, nutritious, health-boosting snack. Not only do they stave off hunger, sunflower seeds are also packed with vitamin E and magnesium, which help keep your heart and bones healthy. Upping your intake of vitamin E can significantly reduce the risk of developing atherosclerosis and boost heart health. B-complex vitamins also provide a boost to the metabolism, ensuring energy levels are well stocked.

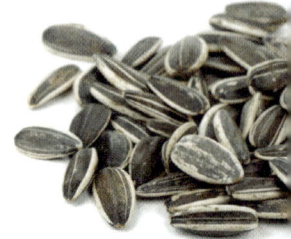

NUTRIENTS IN ¼ CUP (1 OZ.) OF SUNFLOWER SEEDS, ROASTED WITH SALT:

Calories, 165
Copper, 0.5 mg
Manganese, 0.6 mg
Pantothenic acid, 2 mg
Phosphorus, 329 mg
Selenium, 22.5 mcg
Vitamin B6, 0.2 mg
Vitamin E, 7.4 mg

HEALTH AND HEALING BENEFITS:

CARDIOVASCULAR HEALTH:

The antioxidant vitamin E helps prevent free radicals from oxidizing cholesterol. Only after it has been oxidized is cholesterol able to stick to blood vessel walls and start the process of atherosclerosis, which can lead to blocked arteries, heart attack, or stroke.

CANCER PREVENTION:

Studies have shown a link between consumption of the trace mineral selenium and a reduction in the risk of cancer. It is thought that selenium combats cancer by promoting DNA repair in damaged cells and inhibiting the proliferation of cancer cells.

METABOLISM:

Magnesium is a key mineral in healthy metabolism. It plays a role in maintaining healthy bones, energy production, and controlling inflammation and blood sugar levels. Ongoing magnesium deficiency can lead to a significant amount of bone loss.

Glycemic load: 0
Inflammatory index: Moderately anti-inflammatory

RECOMMENDED FOR HELP WITH:

- Reducing the risk of heart disease and diabetes
- Cancer prevention

WALNUTS

Walnuts contain valuable and rare nutrients not found in many other food sources, including the tannin tellimagrandin and the flavonol morin. These antioxidant and anti-inflammatory phytonutrients have been linked with a decreased risk of breast cancer and prostate cancer related to walnut consumption. It's thought that walnut skin—the whitish outermost part of the nut—contains many of the key nutrients, so eating the skin is encouraged to gain the full nutritional benefit of these marvelous nuts.

Black walnuts, dried

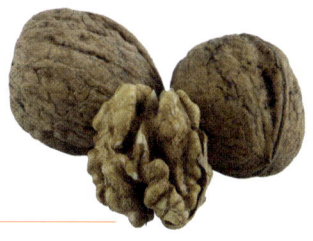

Black walnuts contain more protein than English walnuts, and are a great source of essential fatty acids, which help to lower cholesterol.

English walnuts

A great source of omega-3 fatty acids, they contain slightly higher levels of energy-boosting thiamin, and can help with weight loss.

NUTRIENTS IN 14 HALVES OF ENGLISH WALNUTS (1 OZ.):

Calories, 185
Copper, 0.5 mg
Magnesium, 44.8 mg
Manganese, 1 mg
Pantothenic acid, 0.2 mg
Phosphorus, 98.1 mg
Protein, 4.3 g
Thiamin, 0.1 mg
Vitamin B6, 0.2 mg

HEALTH AND HEALING BENEFITS OF WALNUTS:

CARDIOVASCULAR HEALTH:

The type of vitamin E present in walnuts is called gamma-tocopherol, which is more unusual than the alpha-tocopherol form of vitamin E. Studies have shown it provides significant protection against heart problems.

CHOLESTEROL:

An important source of omega-3 essential fatty acids, which help to lower LDL, or "bad cholesterol," and increase HDL, or "good cholesterol," levels in the blood. Studies suggest that diets rich in monounsaturated fatty acids and omega-3 fatty acids help to prevent coronary artery disease and strokes.

ANTIOXIDANT/ ANTI-INFLAMMATORY:

Walnuts contain valuable and rare antioxidant and anti-inflammatory phytonutrients, such as the tannin tellimagrandin and the flavonol morin, which have been linked with a decreased risk of breast cancer and prostate cancer.

Glycemic load: 0
Inflammatory index: Moderately anti-inflammatory

Glycemic load: 0
Inflammatory index: Moderately anti-inflammatory

RECOMMENDED FOR HELP WITH:

- Reducing the risk of heart disease
- Type 2 diabetes
- Lowering cholesterol
- Boosting memory

Poultry

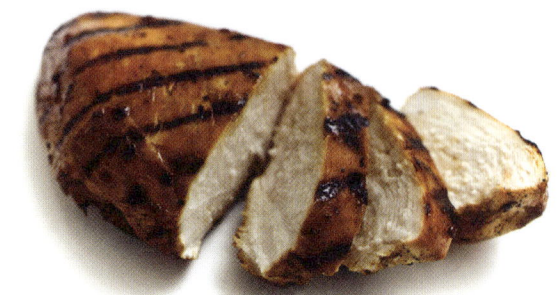

"Poultry" includes chicken, turkey, duck, goose, pheasant, and quail. In general, poultry meat is low in fat and high in protein. The white meat found in most poultry is healthier than the dark meat, so consider this when choosing your cut. Additionally, baking and broiling are healthier means of cooking poultry than frying. All poultry is even healthier if it is grass-fed and/or pasture-fed, rather than restricted to only being fed grains. Grass-fed poultry meat is also considered tastier and more tender.

CHICKEN

Chicken is one of the best sources of complete protein, featuring all essential amino acids. Protein is a building block of bones, muscles, and most components of the body. The human body requires a large amount of protein, so chicken is a good part of any meat-eater's well-balanced diet. Amino acids are required for cell and muscle development, and chicken also has a healthy ratio of fats. White meat is healthier than dark meat, while breast meat is particularly low in fat; gizzards and giblets are especially high in protein, and liver contains high levels of iron and vitamin B12.

Chicken, breast meat

Breast meat has a lower fat content than other pieces of chicken.

NUTRIENTS IN 4 OZ. OF CHICKEN, BREAST MEAT:

Calories, 160
Niacin, 9 mg
Phosphorus, 175 mg
Protein, 31 g
Selenium, 22 mcg
Vitamin B6, 0.4 mg

Glycemic load: 0
Inflammatory index: Mildly inflammatory

Chicken, dark meat (and thigh)

Thigh meat provides roughly the same nutrients as below.

NUTRIENTS IN 4 OZ. OF CHICKEN, DARK MEAT:

Calories, 200
Niacin, 4.5 mg
Phosphorus, 140 mg
Protein, 27 g
Selenium, 19 mcg
Vitamin B6, 0.26 mg
Zinc, 1.9 mg

Glycemic load: 0
Inflammatory index: Moderately inflammatory

Chicken, drumstick

NUTRIENTS IN 4 OZ.* OF CHICKEN, DRUMSTICK:

Calories, 170
Niacin, 4.5 mg
Phosphorus, 140 mg
Protein, 28 g
Selenium, 19 mcg
Vitamin B6, 0.26 mg
Zinc, 1.9 mg

*Roughly 2 chicken drumsticks

Glycemic load: 0
Inflammatory index: Moderately inflammatory

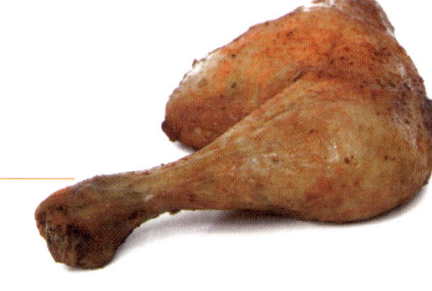

Chicken, giblets

Chicken giblets are particularly high in protein.

NUTRIENTS IN 4 OZ. OF CHICKEN GIBLETS (FOR ROASTING):

Calories, 144
Folate, 312 mcg
Iron, 6.1 mg
Niacin, 7 mg
Phosphorus, 208 mg
Protein, 20.5 g
Riboflavin, 0.9 mg
Selenium, 61.1 mcg
Vitamin A (RAE), 3,250 mcg
Vitamin B12, 10.6 mcg
Zinc, 3.8 mg

Glycemic load: 1
Inflammatory index: Strongly inflammatory

Chicken, liver

Chicken livers also contain high levels of iron and vitamin B12.

NUTRIENTS IN 4 OZ. OF CHICKEN LIVERS:

Calories, 134
Folate, 664 mcg
Iron, 10.2 mg
Niacin, 11 mg
Phosphorus, 336 mg
Protein, 19.1 g
Riboflavin, 2 mg
Selenium, 61.7 mcg
Vitamin A (RAE), 3,730 mcg
Vitamin B6, 1 mg
Vitamin B12, 18.8 mcg
Vitamin C, 20.2 mg
Zinc, 3 mg

Glycemic load: 0
Inflammatory index: Mildly inflammatory

HEALTH AND HEALING BENEFITS OF CHICKEN:

STRONG MUSCLES AND BONES:

A great source of complete protein, a building block of bones, muscles, blood, skin, nails, and hair. Protein helps build and repair tissues, hormones, and body chemicals. Amino acids help form muscle tissue and increase fat metabolism. This can help keep the body strong, and increases athletic performance. Phosphorus assists healthy bone formation.

INTERNAL HEALTH:

Amino acids work to keep organs healthy and functioning properly, including the heart, brain, and liver.

ENERGY:

Niacin is important in energy production, playing an important role in converting fats, proteins, and carbohydrates into usable energy.

BLOOD HEALTH:

Iron and vitamin B12 maintain healthy red blood cells.

CANCER PROTECTION:

Studies have shown a link between consumption of selenium and a reduction in the risk of cancer.

Glycemic load: 0
Inflammatory index: Moderately inflammatory

RECOMMENDED FOR HELP WITH:

- Muscle maintenance
- Increased energy
- Oxygenation of the blood
- Cancer prevention
- Iron-deficient anemia

DUCK

Duck is an excellent protein, with all essential amino acids and a good ratio of fats. While less common in the United States, duck is a prevalent and delicious protein source in Asia and Europe. There are three main varieties of duck for cooking. In the United States, mild Pekin or Long Island duck is the most common, while the stronger Muscovy is popular in France. Duck has the reputation of being fatty, but in small portions duck is nutritious and protein-packed. The dark color of the meat of this bird of flight comes from high levels of oxygen-storing protein, creating the richer, meatier flavor. Duck has a thick layer of fat under the skin; either remove the skin or score it before cooking to allow the fat to escape.

NUTRIENTS IN 4 OZ. OF DUCK, ROASTED:

Calories, 190
Iron, 2.7 mg
Niacin, 3.7 mg
Phosphorus, 140 mg
Protein, 23 g
Riboflavin, 0.3 mg
Selenium, 22.4 mcg

HEALTH AND HEALING BENEFITS:

BLOOD HEALTH:

Iron maintains healthy red blood cells and improves their ability to carry oxygen to cells around the body. Growing children and adolescents, as well as menstruating, pregnant, or lactating women, have an increased need for iron. Low levels of vitamin B12 lead to anemia and potential damage to the spinal cord and brain.

STRONG MUSCLES AND BONES:

Protein helps build and repair tissues, hormones, and body chemicals. Amino acids help form muscle tissue and increase fat metabolism. Phosphorus assists healthy bone formation.

ENERGY:

Niacin is important for energy, playing an important role in converting fats, proteins, and carbohydrates into energy.

CANCER PROTECTION:

Studies have shown a link between consumption of selenium and a reduction in the risk of cancer. It is thought that selenium promotes DNA repair in damaged cells and inhibits the increase of cancer cells.

INTERNAL HEALTH:

Amino acids aid organ function, including the heart, brain, and liver.

Glycemic load: 0
Inflammatory index: Mildly inflammatory

RECOMMENDED FOR HELP WITH:

- Muscle maintenance
- Increased energy
- Iron-deficient anemia
- Cancer prevention
- Oxygenation of the blood

Goose

Goose is an excellent-quality protein, with all essential amino acids and a good ratio of fats. Goose has a higher total fat content than chicken or turkey, but lower than beef and slightly lower than duck. Like duck, goose meat is rare in the United States but is a Christmas dinner staple in the UK. Goose provides similar nutrients to duck and can also be a tasty and nutritious meal when carefully prepared and served in modest amounts. As it is also a bird of flight, goose meat is red, due to the high levels of the oxygen-storing protein. Employ the same methods of preparation as duck to reduce the amount of fat when cooking.

NUTRIENTS IN 4 OZ. OF GOOSE, ROASTED:

Calories, 230
Niacin, 3 mg
Phosphorus, 210 mg
Protein, 29 g
Riboflavin, 0.3 mg
Selenium, 25.5 mcg
Vitamin B6, 0.3 mg
Zinc, 1.9 mg

HEALTH AND HEALING BENEFITS:

MUSCLES AND BONES:

An excellent quality protein, a building block of bones, muscles, blood, skin, nails, and hair. Protein helps build and repair tissues, hormones, and body chemicals. Amino acids help form muscle tissue and increase fat metabolism. Phosphorus assists healthy bone formation.

STRONG BONES AND TEETH:

The mineral phosphorus is an important part of bones and teeth. It helps in healthy bone formation, hormonal balance, and cellular repair.

STRENGTHENS IMMUNITY:

Zinc has far-reaching effects on immunity, and decreased levels can lower immune activity and the chance of fighting illness. Selenium also works to boost the immune system.

CANCER PROTECTION:

Studies have shown a link between consumption of selenium and a reduction in the risk of cancer. It is thought that selenium promotes DNA repair in damaged cells and inhibits the increase of cancer cells.

INTERNAL HEALTH:

Amino acids aid organ function, including the heart, brain, and liver.

Glycemic load: 0
Inflammatory index: Mildly anti-inflammatory

RECOMMENDED FOR HELP WITH:

- Muscle maintenance
- Enhanced immune health
- Strong bones and teeth
- Cancer prevention

Pheasant

Pheasant is a good-quality protein, with all essential amino acids and a good ratio of fats. Pheasant is more common in the UK and Europe than in the United States. As with duck and goose, pheasant has a higher fat content than chicken and turkey, but about half the amount of fat as beef. Pheasant provides a high level of protein, as well as significant amounts of niacin, potassium, selenium, and vitamin B12, and is one of the best dietary sources of vitamin B6. Pheasant is often roasted, and can be purchased either fresh or frozen from specialty food stores; the fat is reduced by removing the skin.

NUTRIENTS IN 4 OZ. OF PHEASANT, ROASTED:

Calories, 140
Niacin, 6.7 mg
Phosphorus, 240 mg
Potassium, 118 mg
Protein, 26 mg
Selenium, 20 mcg
Vitamin B6, 0.5 mg
Vitamin B12, 0.4 mcg

HEALTH AND HEALING BENEFITS:

INTERNAL HEALTH:

Amino acids work to keep organs healthy and functioning properly, including the heart, brain, and liver. Potassium keeps the organs, brain, and tissues in good condition and strengthens against stroke, kidney disorders, and muscle dysfunction.

STRONG BONES:

Protein helps build and repair tissues, hormones, and body chemicals. Amino acids help form muscle tissue and increase fat metabolism. Phosphorus assists healthy bone formation.

ENERGY:

Niacin is important for energy.

STRONG IMMUNE SYSTEM:

Selenium boosts immunity.

IMPROVED CIRCULATION AND NERVOUS SYSTEM:

Vitamin B6 helps nerves communicate and strengthens blood. Vitamin B6 deficiency is found in people with heart disease and premenstrual syndrome. Vitamin B12 helps maintain red blood cells.

CANCER PROTECTION:

Studies have shown a link between selenium and a reduced risk of cancer. It is thought selenium promotes DNA repair and inhibits cancer cells.

Glycemic load: 0
Inflammatory index: Mildly anti-inflammatory

RECOMMENDED FOR HELP WITH:

- Muscle maintenance
- Strong bones and teeth
- Improved circulation
- Immune health
- Stroke prevention
- Cancer prevention

Quail

Quail is an excellent-quality protein, with all essential amino acids and a good ratio of fats. Quail is another less-common game bird, but one that can be found in dishes served in European restaurants. Why not consider preparing quail at home as part of a delicious, well-balanced meal? A small quail is usually served per person; where quails are larger in size, consider serving the breast meat. Search online or try specialty food stores to find quail.

NUTRIENTS IN 4 OZ. OF QUAIL, ROASTED:

Calories, 130
Iron, 3.3 mg
Niacin, 6 mg
Phosphorus, 210 mg
Protein, 22 g
Selenium, 17.4 mcg
Thiamin, 0.22 mg
Vitamin B6, 0.3 mg
Zinc, 1.9 mg

HEALTH AND HEALING BENEFITS:

STRONG MUSCLES AND BONES:

A great source of complete protein, a building block of bones, muscles, blood, skin, nails, and hair. Protein helps build and repair tissues, hormones, and body chemicals. Amino acids help form muscle tissue and increase fat metabolism. This can help keep a body strong, and also increases athletic performance. Phosphorus assists healthy bone formation.

GOOD INTERNAL HEALTH:

Amino acids also work to keep organs healthy and functioning properly, including the heart, brain, and liver.

BLOOD HEALTH:

Iron maintains healthy red blood cells and improves their ability to carry oxygen to cells around the body. Growing children and adolescents, as well as menstruating, pregnant, or lactating women, have an increased need for iron.

ENERGY:

Niacin is important in energy production, playing a vital role in converting fats, proteins, and carbohydrates into usable energy.

CANCER PROTECTION:

Studies have shown a link between consumption of selenium and a reduction in the risk of cancer. It is thought that selenium promotes DNA repair in damaged cells and inhibits the increase of cancer cells.

Glycemic load: 0
Inflammatory index: Mildly inflammatory

RECOMMENDED FOR HELP WITH:

- Muscle maintenance
- Increased energy
- Oxygenation of the blood
- Cancer prevention
- Iron-deficient anemia

TURKEY

Turkey is a lean white meat that can be purchased in many forms. In the United States, turkey is most commonly served roasted whole for Thanksgiving, but turkey can be used in many dishes and is available in a variety of cuts. Turkey is a quality protein, with all essential amino acids. Turkey also has a good ratio of fats, and is a great source of tryptophan, which, as a precursor to serotonin, can help with mood and relaxation. Turkey is a versatile and inexpensive meat and has more protein and less fat and cholesterol than other meats.

Turkey bacon

NUTRIENTS IN 4 OZ. OF TURKEY BACON:

Calories, 382
Iron, 2.1 mg
Phosphorus, 460 mg
Protein, 29 g
Selenium, 25.8 mcg
Vitamin B6, 0.3 mg
Zinc, 3 mg

Glycemic load: 2
Inflammatory index: Moderately inflammatory

Turkey, breast

NUTRIENTS IN 4 OZ. OF TURKEY BREAST:

Calories, 150
Niacin, 4.5 mg
Phosphorus, 140 mg
Protein, 28 g
Selenium, 31 mcg
Vitamin B6, 0.3 mg

Glycemic load: 0
Inflammatory index: Moderately inflammatory

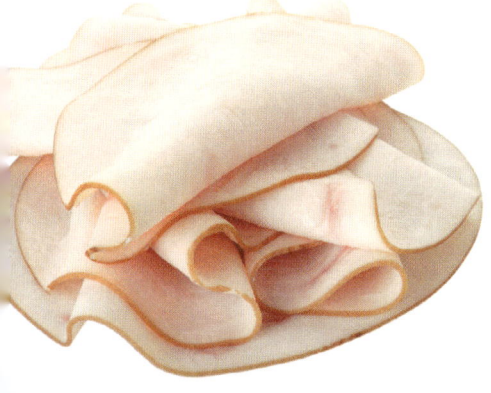

Turkey, dark meat (and thigh)

Thigh meat provides roughly the same nutrients as below.

NUTRIENTS IN 4 OZ. OF TURKEY, DARK MEAT:

Calories, 210
Niacin, 3 mg
Phosphorus, 140 mg
Protein, 27 g
Selenium, 31 mcg
Zinc, 2.9 mg

Glycemic load: 0
Inflammatory index: Moderately inflammatory

Turkey, drumstick

NUTRIENTS 4 OZ. OF TURKEY DRUMSTICKS:

Calories, 200
Niacin, 3 mg
Phosphorus, 140 mg
Protein, 28 g
Selenium, 31 mcg
Zinc, 2.9 mg

Glycemic load: 0
Inflammatory index: Mildly inflammatory

Turkey, giblets

NUTRIENTS 4 OZ. OF TURKEY GIBLETS:

Calories, 140
Folate, 374 mcg
Iron, 6.7 mg
Niacin, 9.8 mg
Phosphorus, 252 mg
Protein, 20.6 g
Riboflavin, 1.6 mg
Selenium, 55.7 mcg
Vitamin A (RAE), 4,450 mcg
Vitamin B12, 14.8 mcg
Zinc, 3.7 mg

Glycemic load: 1
Inflammatory index: Moderately inflammatory

Turkey, ground

NUTRIENTS IN 4 OZ. PATTY:

Calories, 187
Iron, 1.6 mg
Niacin, 4 mg
Protein, 23 g
Selenium, 30.5 mcg
Vitamin B6, 0.3 mg

Glycemic load: 0
Inflammatory index: Mildly inflammatory

Turkey, liver

Turkey livers are a particularly good source of vitamin B12.

NUTRIENTS IN 4 OZ. OF TURKEY LIVERS:

Calories, 145
Folate, 765 mcg
Iron, 10.1 mg
Niacin, 12.7 mg
Phosphorus, 315 mg
Protein, 20.7 g
Riboflavin, 2.5 mg
Selenium, 77.6 mcg
Vitamin A, 9,110 mcg
Vitamin B6, 1.2 mg
Vitamin B12, 22.3 mcg
Zinc, 3.8 mg

HEALTH AND HEALING BENEFITS OF TURKEY:

STRONG IMMUNE SYSTEM:

Selenium works to boost the thyroid and immune system. Zinc has far-reaching effects on immunity, and low zinc levels lead to decreased immune system levels.

STRONG BONES:

An excellent-quality protein, a building block of bones, muscles, blood, skin, nails, and hair. Protein also helps build and repair tissues, hormones, and body chemicals. Amino acids help form muscle tissue and increase fat metabolism. Phosphorous assists healthy bone formation.

IMPROVED CIRCULATION AND NERVOUS SYSTEM:

Vitamin B6 helps nerve cells communicate and strengthens blood. Vitamin B6 deficiency is found in people with heart disease and premenstrual syndrome. Vitamin B12 helps maintain healthy red blood cells. Iron also improves red blood cells' ability to carry oxygen to the body's cells.

CANCER PROTECTION:

Studies have shown a link between consumption of selenium and a reduction in the risk of cancer. It is thought that selenium promotes DNA repair in damaged cells and inhibits the increase of cancer cells.

ENERGY:

Niacin is important in energy production, playing a role in converting fats, proteins, and carbohydrates into usable energy.

Glycemic load: 1
Inflammatory index: Moderately inflammatory

RECOMMENDED FOR HELP WITH:

- Muscle maintenance
- Strong bones and teeth
- Improved circulation and blood oxygenation
- Enhanced immune health
- Cancer prevention

Seafood and fish

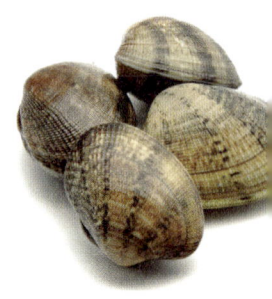

Seafood is among the most health-enhancing of all foods. The quality of the protein, with all essential amino acids, is crucial for building antibodies to strengthen the immune system, and building muscle for strength and endurance. The high quantity and quality of omega-3 fatty acids found in seafood enhance heart and brain health as well as memory. It contains minimal carbohydrate, and helps maintain low blood sugar and normal body fat. Many freshwater fish also have significant levels of omega-3s. The American Heart Association recommends eating two servings of fish per week to promote heart health. Seafood and fish can have high levels of mercury and other toxins, which can be of concern to pregnant women in particular. Each country has its own recommendations regarding the consumption of fish and seafood during pregnancy; these should be referred to. Additionally, allergy to shellfish (including lobster and scallops) is relatively common; if you suffer from any symptoms, get treatment immediately.

Abalone, raw

Abalone is the name for a group of sea mollusks or snails. Abalone contain essential amino acids and are very low in saturated fat. They are a good source of protein, selenium, and vitamin K, as well as providing high levels of vitamin E and iron. However, abalone are also high in sodium and cholesterol, so eat in moderation. Abalone have a special place in many Asian cultures due to their far-reaching health benefits.

NUTRIENTS IN 3 OZ. OF ABALONE, RAW:

Calories, 89
Calcium, 26.4 mg
Copper, 0.2 mg
Iron, 2.7 mg
Magnesium, 40.8 mg
Niacin, 1.3 mg
Pantothenic acid, 2.6 mg
Phosphorus, 162 mg
Potassium, 212 mg
Protein, 15 g
Riboflavin, 0.1 mg
Selenium, 38.1 mcg
Sodium, 256 mg
Thiamin, 0.2 mg
Total omega-3 fatty acids, 76.5 mg
Total omega-6 fatty acids, 6 mg
Vitamin B6, 0.1 mg
Vitamin B12, 0.6 mcg
Vitamin C, 1.7 mg
Vitamin E, 3.4 mg
Vitamin K, 19.6 mcg
Zinc, 0.7 mg

HEALTH AND HEALING BENEFITS:

HEART AND BLOOD HEALTH:

Omega-3 and -6 help protect against stroke, heart disease, and diabetes, as well as regulating blood pressure. Iron and vitamin B12 maintain healthy red blood cells and improve their ability to carry oxygen to the body's cells. Growing children and adolescents, plus menstruating, pregnant, or lactating women, have an increased need for iron. Low levels of B12 lead to anemia and potential damage to the spinal cord and brain.

IMMUNITY:

Selenium, zinc, and omega-6 improve immunity.

MUSCLES AND BONES:

Protein helps build and repair bones, tissues, hormones, and body chemicals. Amino acids help form muscle tissue and increase fat metabolism. This can help keep the body strong, increasing athletic performance. Phosphorus assists healthy bone formation.

INTERNAL HEALTH:

Amino acids aid organ function, including the heart, brain, and liver.

CANCER PROTECTION:

Studies have shown a link between consumption of selenium and a reduction in the risk of cancer. It is thought that selenium promotes DNA repair in damaged cells and inhibits the increase of cancer cells.

ENHANCED BRAIN FUNCTION:

Omega-3 improves brain function, and is believed to aid memory.

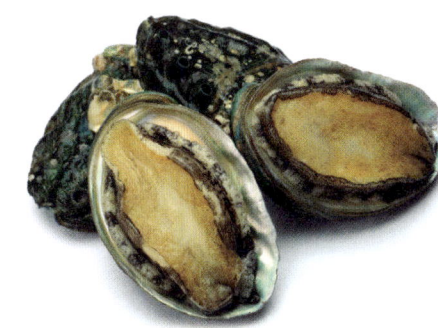

Glycemic load: 3
Inflammatory index: Anti-inflammatory

RECOMMENDED FOR HELP WITH:

- Reducing cardiovascular disease
- Oxygenation of the blood
- Cancer prevention
- Enhanced brain function and memory
- Immunity

SEAFOOD AND FISH

ANCHOVY

Anchovies are small, oily ocean fish. They are very nutritious, if eaten in moderation. They contain essential amino acids and are high in selenium, calcium, iron, and potassium, great for healthy eyes, bones, and muscle. Canned or raw, anchovies are high in cholesterol—canned, they are also high in sodium. Anchovies are a great source of omega-3s. If you suffer from gout, watch your consumption. Low in mercury, they can be eaten during pregnancy.

Anchovy, canned in oil

NUTRIENTS IN 2 OZ. (ROUGHLY 1 CAN) OF ANCHOVY, CANNED IN OIL:

Calories, 94
Calcium, 104 mg
Copper, 0.2 mg
Iron, 2.1 mg
Magnesium, 31.1 mg
Niacin, 9 mg
Phosphorus, 113 mg
Potassium, 245 mg
Protein, 13 g
Riboflavin, 0.2 mg
Selenium, 30.6 mcg
Sodium, 1,650 mg
Total omega-3 fatty acids, 951 mg
Total omega-6 fatty acids, 163 mg
Vitamin B6, 0.1 mg
Vitamin B12, 0.4 mcg
Vitamin E, 1.5 mg
Vitamin K, 5.4 mcg
Zinc, 1.1 mg

Glycemic load: 0
Inflammatory index: Strongly anti-inflammatory

Anchovy, raw

NUTRIENTS IN 1 OZ. OF ANCHOVY, RAW:

Calories, 37
Calcium, 41.2 mg
Copper, 0.1 mg
Iron, 0.9 mg
Magnesium, 11.5 mg
Niacin, 3.9 mg
Phosphorus, 48.7 mg
Potassium, 107 mg
Protein, 6 g
Riboflavin, 0.1 mg
Selenium, 10.2 mcg
Total omega-3 fatty acids, 414 mg
Total omega-6 fatty acids, 27.2 mg
Vitamin B12, 0.2 mcg
Zinc, 0.5 mg

Glycemic load: 0
Inflammatory index: Strongly inflammatory

HEALTH AND HEALING BENEFITS OF ANCHOVY:

HEART AND BLOOD HEALTH:

The omega fatty acids and vitamin E protect against cardiovascular disease, reducing cholesterol. Iron maintains healthy red blood cells and improves their ability to carry oxygen to the body's cells. Growing children and adolescents, plus menstruating, pregnant, or lactating women, have an increased need for iron.

IMPROVED METABOLISM:

Amino acids and vitamin E help form muscle tissue and increase fat metabolism. This can help keep the body strong, increasing athletic performance.

INTERNAL HEALTH:

Amino acids work to keep organs healthy and functioning properly, including the heart, brain, and liver. Potassium maintains the good working order of organs.

STRONG BONES:

Calcium ensures strong bones.

ENERGY:

Niacin is important in energy production, converting fats, proteins, and carbohydrates into usable energy.

EYE HEALTH:

Vitamin E reduces the risk of cataracts.

ENERGY:

Copper and vitamin E boost stamina and energy levels.

CANCER PROTECTION:

Studies have shown a link between consumption of selenium and a reduction in the risk of cancer. It is thought that selenium promotes DNA repair in damaged cells and inhibits the increase of cancer cells.

RECOMMENDED FOR HELP WITH:

- Metabolism
- Stamina
- Eye health
- Heart and blood health
- Cancer prevention

BASS

Bass is low in calories and an excellent source of protein. Whether freshwater bass or sea bass, this fish is high in cholesterol, so maintain portion control and eat in moderation. Freshwater bass in particular is high in manganese and vitamin B12, promoting a strong heart and blood cells and healthy skin. Sea bass is high in selenium and phosphorus, assisting in cellular repair and a reduction in inflammation. It is recommended that bass be avoided or limited during pregnancy due to possible exposure to mercury.

Bass (freshwater)

NUTRIENTS IN 3 OZ.* OF BASS, COOKED:

Calories, 124
Calcium, 87.6 mg
Copper, 0.1 mg
Iron, 1.6 mg
Magnesium, 32.3 mg
Manganese, 1 mg
Niacin, 1.3 mg
Phosphorus, 218 mg
Potassium, 388 mg
Protein, 21 g
Selenium, 13.8 mcg
Thiamin, 0.1 mg
Total omega-3 fatty acids, 861 mg
Total omega-6 fatty acids, 95.2 mg
Vitamin B6, 0.1 mg
Vitamin B12, 1 mcg

*Freshwater bass fillets are on average 2½ oz.

Glycemic load: 0
Inflammatory index: Moderately anti-inflammatory

Bass (sea)

NUTRIENTS IN 3 OZ.* OF SEA BASS, COOKED:

Calories, 105
Magnesium, 45 mg
Niacin, 1.6 mg
Pantothenic acid, 0.7 mg
Phosphorous, 211 mg
Potassium, 279 mg
Protein, 20 g
Riboflavin, 0.1 mg
Selenium, 39.8 mcg
Thiamin, 0.1 mg
Total omega-3 fatty acids, 730 mg
Total omega-6 fatty acids, 26.4 mg
Vitamin B6, 0.4 mg
Vitamin B12, 0.3 mcg

*Sea bass fillets are on average 4 oz.

Glycemic load: 0
Inflammatory index: Strongly inflammatory

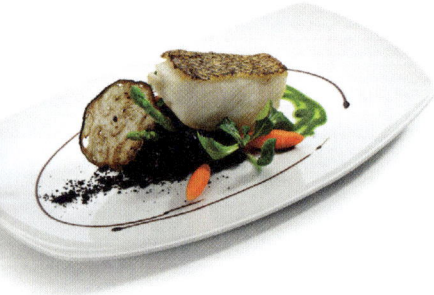

HEALTH AND HEALING BENEFITS OF BASS:

HEALTHY SKIN:

Manganese keeps skin healthy.

STRONG BONES AND TEETH:

Calcium and phosphorus assist in healthy bone and teeth formation.

JOINT HEALTH:

Omega-6 and selenium reduce joint inflammation.

HEART AND BLOOD HEALTH:

Omega-3 and -6 protect against stroke, heart disease, and diabetes, and reduce cholesterol. Vitamin B12 and iron maintain and oxygenate healthy red blood cells.

IMMUNITY:

Selenium and omega-6 boost immunity.

ENHANCED BRAIN FUNCTION:

Omega-3 and -6 enhance brain function and may aid memory.

RECOMMENDED FOR HELP WITH:

- Heart health
- Reducing cardiovascular disease and diabetes
- Strong bones
- Joint health
- Immunity
- Enhanced brain function

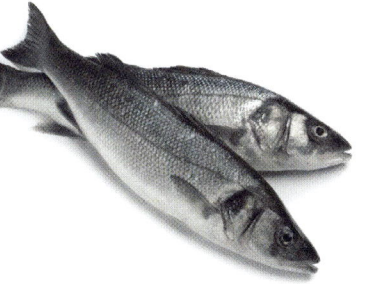

Bream (sea)

Sea bream, also known as porgy, include numerous sea and freshwater species around the world. Sea bream recommendations for pregnant women vary considerably from country to country, and the toxins in sea bream are considered too high for safety by many during this time. However, for non-pregnant people, sea bream is delicious and low in calories. It is also high in omega-3s and seen to lower blood pressure and promote good eye health.

NUTRIENTS IN 4 OZ. BLACK SEA BREAM:

Calories, 194
Magnesium, 36 mg
Niacin, 5.5 mg
Pantothenic acid, 0.6 mg
Phosphorus, 250 mg
Potassium, 400 mg
Protein, 22 g
Sodium, 27 mg
Total omega-3 fatty acids, 890 mg
Total omega-6 fatty acids, 150 mg
Vitamin B2, 0.3 mg
Vitamin B6, 0.4 mg
Vitamin B12, 3.8 mcg
Vitamin D, 4 mcg
Vitamin E, 1.4 mg
Zinc, 0.8 mg

HEALTH AND HEALING BENEFITS:

IMMUNITY:

Zinc and omega-6 improve immune system function.

HEART AND BLOOD HEALTH:

Omega-3 and -6 help protect against stroke, heart disease, and diabetes, as well as regulating blood pressure. Potassium protects against stroke. Vitamin B12 maintains healthy red blood cells. Vitamin B12 maintains healthy red blood cells and improves their ability to carry oxygen to the body's cells. Low levels of B12 lead to anemia and potential damage to the spinal cord and brain.

STRONG MUSCLES AND BONES:

Protein and potassium help build and repair bones, tissues, hormones, and body chemicals. Phosphorus and vitamin D assist healthy bone formation.

EYE HEALTH:

Vitamin E can reduce the risk of cataracts and macular degeneration.

ENHANCED BRAIN FUNCTION:

Omega-3 improves brain function, and is believed to aid memory.

ENERGY:

Niacin and vitamin E are essential for energy production.

Glycemic load: 0
Inflammatory index: Anti-inflammatory

RECOMMENDED FOR HELP WITH:

- Reducing risk of cardiovascular disease
- Heart health
- Immunity
- Energy boost
- Eye health
- Anemia deficiency

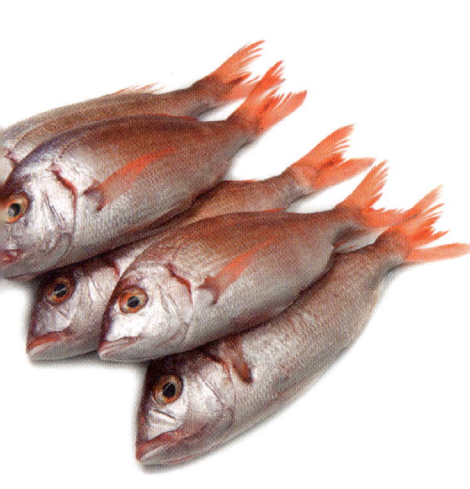

Carp

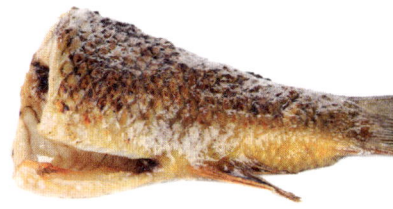

Carp are large, oily freshwater fish. They contain essential fatty acids and are low in sodium but high in cholesterol. Carp are a good source of phosphorus, vitamin B12, selenium, and zinc. Good for promoting heart health, carp consumption also supports the immune system and assists in cellular repair. Due to higher levels of mercury, the American Pregnancy Association recommends limiting carp during pregnancy.

NUTRIENTS IN 3 OZ.* CARP, COOKED:

Calories, 194
Magnesium, 36 mg
Niacin, 5.5 mg
Pantothenic acid, 0.6 mg
Phosphorus, 250 mg
Potassium, 400 mg
Protein, 22 g
Sodium, 27 mg
Total omega-3 fatty acids, 890 mg
Total omega-6 fatty acids, 150 mg
Vitamin B2, 0.3 mg
Vitamin B6, 0.4 mg
Vitamin B12, 3.8 mcg
Vitamin D, 4 mcg
Vitamin E, 1.4 mg
Zinc, 0.8 mg

*Carp fillets are on average 7 oz.

HEALTH AND HEALING BENEFITS:

HEART AND BLOOD HEALTH:

Omega-3 and -6 and potassium protect against stroke, heart disease, and diabetes, and lower blood pressure. Vitamins B6 and B12 maintain and oxygenate healthy red blood cells.

STRONG MUSCLES AND BONES:

Phosphorus assists healthy bone formation and cellular repair. Protein and potassium help build and repair bones, tissues, hormones, and body chemicals.

JOINT HEALTH:

Omega-6 and selenium reduce joint inflammation.

HEALTHY SKIN:

Zinc promotes healthy skin.

IMMUNITY:

Zinc, selenium, and omega-6 improve immune function.

ENHANCED BRAIN FUNCTION:

Omega-3 improves brain function and may aid memory.

Glycemic load: 0
Inflammatory index: Mildly anti-inflammatory

RECOMMENDED FOR HELP WITH:

- Strong bones
- Reducing risk of cardiovascular disease
- Heart health
- Immunity
- Enhanced brain function
- Reducing joint inflammation

Catfish

Catfish is a popular dish in the American South, but a less well-known food source elsewhere. If catfish is prepared correctly and carefully, it can be a delicious and nutritious meal. However, catfish poisoning does result from lack of careful preparation, so ensure you purchase from reputable sources and cook it thoroughly. Catfish contains essential amino acids and is a great source of vitamin B12, phosphorus, and selenium. It is also high in omega-6, which is especially high in farmed catfish. But due to its high cholesterol, it should be eaten in moderation. Due to the low purine content, catfish is considered safe in moderation for those suffering from gout, and because of low mercury, it is deemed safe to eat during pregnancy by the American Pregnancy Association. The same amount of wild catfish provides similar levels of nutrients, but with 89 calories and lower omega fatty acids.

NUTRIENTS IN 3 OZ.* OF FARMED CATFISH, COOKED:

Calories, 129
Copper, 0.5 mg
Iron, 0.7 mg
Magnesium, 22.1 mg
Niacin, 2.1 mg
Pantothenic acid, 0.5 mg
Phosphorus, 208 mg
Potassium, 273 mg
Protein, 16 g
Riboflavin, 0.1 mg
Selenium, 12.3 mcg
Thiamin, 0.4 mg
Total omega-3 fatty acids, 220 mg
Total omega-6 fatty acids, 875 mg
Vitamin B6, 0.1 mg
Vitamin B12, 2.4 mcg
Zinc, 0.9 mg

*Catfish fillets are on average 6 oz.

Glycemic load: 0
Inflammatory index: Mildly anti-inflammatory

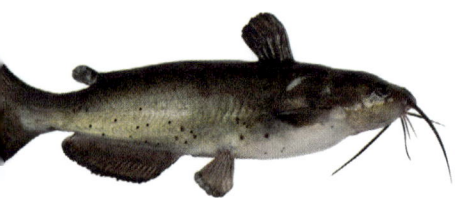

HEALTH AND HEALING BENEFITS:

ENHANCED BRAIN FUNCTION:

Omega-6 is integral to brain function, while omega-3 improves function and is believed to aid memory.

HEART AND BLOOD HEALTH:

Omega-3 and -6 help protect against stroke, heart disease, and diabetes, as well as regulating blood pressure. Potassium protects against stroke. Vitamins B12 and B6 maintain healthy red blood cells and improve their ability to carry oxygen to the body's cells. Low levels of B12 lead to anemia and potential damage to the spinal cord and brain.

STRONG MUSCLES AND BONES:

Phosphorus assists healthy bone formation and cellular repair. Protein and potassium help build and repair bones, tissues, hormones, and body chemicals.

JOINT HEALTH:

Omega-6 and selenium reduce joint inflammation.

HEALTHY SKIN:

Zinc promotes healthy skin.

IMMUNITY:

Omega-6, zinc, and selenium improve immune system function and help combat illness.

RECOMMENDED FOR HELP WITH:

- Enhanced brain function
- Heart health
- Reduced cardiovascular disease
- Immunity
- Reduced joint inflammation
- Strong bones
- Anemia deficiency

Caviar

Caviar is a delicacy in many parts of the world. It is simply fish eggs (notably from the beluga sturgeon), but these little bundles are actually nutritional sources for unborn fish, providing a rich source of nutrients for humans, too. Caviar is very high in cholesterol and sodium, so consume it only as a rare treat—which is just as well, due to the cost. Caviar is extremely high in omega-3 and vitamin B12 (93% of your daily value), as well as vitamins D and A, and selenium. Avoid eating uncooked fish eggs during pregnancy.

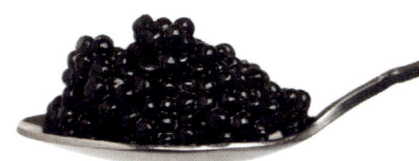

NUTRIENTS IN 1 TBSP. OF CAVIAR:

Calories, 42
Calcium, 44 mg
Iron, 1.9 mg
Magnesium, 48 mg
Pantothenic acid, 0.6 mg
Phosphorus, 57 mg
Protein, 3.9 g
Riboflavin, 0.1 mg
Selenium, 10.5 mcg
Sodium, 240 mg
Thiamin, 0 mg
Total omega-3 fatty acids, 1,088 mg
Total omega-6 fatty acids, 13 mg
Vitamin A (RAE), 43.4 mcg
Vitamin B6, 0.1 mg
Vitamin B12, 3.2 mcg
Vitamin D, 18.7 IU

HEALTH AND HEALING BENEFITS:

HEART AND BLOOD HEALTH:

Omega-3 and -6 and vitamin A protect against stroke, heart disease, and diabetes and lower cholesterol and blood pressure. Vitamin B12 and iron maintain and oxygenate healthy red blood cells.

ENHANCED BRAIN FUNCTION:

Omega-3 improves brain function and may aid memory.

STRONG BONES:

Vitamin D and magnesium maintain strong bones.

IMMUNITY:

Selenium and omega-6 boost immunity.

HEALTHY SKIN:

Vitamin A prevents acne.

Glycemic load: 1
Inflammatory index: Strongly anti-inflammatory

RECOMMENDED FOR HELP WITH:

- Immunity
- Heart health
- Reduced cardiovascular disease
- Anemia deficiency
- Enhanced brain function
- Strong bones
- Healthy skin

Clams

Clams are a type of bivalve mollusk that live in the water. They are eaten all over the world, from Italian shellfish pastas to American clam chowder and Indian curries. Clams contain the highest natural source of the amino acid taurine, believed to lower blood pressure and help fat digestion. They are very low in saturated fat but they are high in cholesterol. Clams are protein-rich and have astoundingly high levels of vitamin B12, plus very high levels of iron and selenium. Clams are low in mercury and can be eaten in moderation during pregnancy.

NUTRIENTS IN 3 OZ. (ROUGHLY 10 SMALL) CLAMS, COOKED:

Calories, 126
Calcium, 78.2 mg
Copper, 0.6 mg
Folate, 24.6 mcg
Iron, 23.8 mg
Manganese, 0.9 mg
Niacin, 2.9 mg
Pantothenic acid, 0.6 mg
Phosphorus, 287 mg
Potassium, 534 mg
Protein, 22 g
Riboflavin, 0.4 mg
Selenium, 54.4 mcg
Thiamin, 0.1 mg
Total omega-3 fatty acids, 337 mg
Total omega-6 fatty acids, 27.2 mg
Vitamin A (RAE), 145 mcg
Vitamin B6, 0.1 mg
Vitamin B12, 84.1 mcg
Vitamin C, 18.8 mg
Zinc, 2.3 mg

HEALTH AND HEALING BENEFITS:

HEART AND BLOOD HEALTH:

Omega-3 and -6 help protect against stroke, heart disease, and diabetes, as well as regulating blood pressure. Taurine is believed to lower blood pressure. Vitamin B12 and iron maintain healthy red blood cells and improve their ability to carry oxygen to the body's cells. Growing children and adolescents, plus menstruating, pregnant, or lactating women have an increased need for iron. Low levels of B12 lead to anemia and potential damage to the spinal cord and brain.

ENHANCED BRAIN FUNCTION:

Omega-3 helps with brain function and may aid memory.

IMMUNITY:

Selenium, vitamin C, omega-6, and zinc boost immunity.

HEALTHY SKIN:

Manganese, vitamin A, and zinc help promote healthy skin.

CANCER PROTECTION:

Studies have shown a link between consumption of selenium and a reduction in the risk of cancer.

> **Glycemic load:** 3
> **Inflammatory index:** Moderately anti-inflammatory
>
> **RECOMMENDED FOR HELP WITH:**
>
> - Lowering blood pressure
> - Anemia deficiency
> - Enhanced brain function
> - Immunity
> - Healthy skin
> - Possible cancer prevention

COD

Atlantic cod, also called scrod, is a distinctively different type of fish from Pacific cod, with varying nutritional contents. Both Atlantic and Pacific cod have incredibly high levels of protein per calorie. There is occasional concern of overfishing of cod, so it is best to monitor this. Atlantic cod is one of the least mercuric fish, and safer to eat during pregnancy.

Cod (Atlantic)

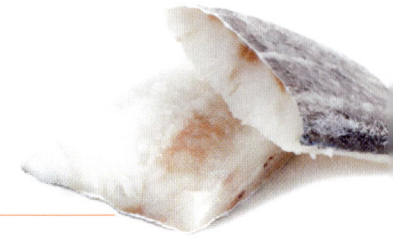

Atlantic cod contains essential fatty acids and is high in selenium, vitamin B12, and vitamin B6 and low in mercury. However, it is high in cholesterol.

NUTRIENTS IN 3 OZ.* OF ATLANTIC COD, COOKED:

Calories, 89
Magnesium, 35.7 mg
Niacin, 2.1 mg
Phosphorus, 117 mg
Potassium, 207 mg
Protein, 19 g
Riboflavin, 0.1 mg
Selenium, 32 mcg
Thiamin, 0.1 mg
Total omega-3 fatty acids, 146 mg
Total omega-6 fatty acids, 5.1 mg
Vitamin B6, 0.2 mg
Vitamin B12, 0.9 mcg

*Atlantic cod fillets are on average 7 oz.

Glycemic load: 0
Inflammatory index: Moderately anti-inflammatory

Cod (Pacific)

Pacific cod contains essential fatty acids and is very low in saturated fat. It is a good source of selenium, vitamin B6, and phosphorus, but is high in cholesterol.

NUTRIENTS IN 3 OZ.* OF PACIFIC COD, COOKED:

Calories, 89
Magnesium, 26.4 mg
Niacin, 2.1 mg
Phosphorus, 190 mg
Potassium, 439 mg
Protein, 20 g
Selenium, 39.8 mcg
Total omega-3 fatty acids, 241 mg
Total omega-6 fatty acids, 6.8 mg
Vitamin B6, 0.4 mg
Vitamin B12, 0.9 mcg
Vitamin C, 2.6 mg

*Pacific cod fillets are on average 4 oz.

Glycemic load: 0
Inflammatory index: Moderately anti-inflammatory

HEALTH AND HEALING BENEFITS OF COD:

STRONG BONES:

Protein is the building block of bones, muscles, blood, skin, nails, and hair. Phosphorus assists healthy bone formation.

IMMUNITY:

Selenium promotes a healthy immune system, as does vitamin C.

CANCER PROTECTION:

Studies have shown a link between consumption of selenium and a reduction in the risk of cancer. It is thought that selenium promotes DNA repair in damaged cells.

HEART AND BLOOD HEALTH:

Omega-6 works with omega-3 to decrease the risk of heart disease and high blood pressure. Vitamins B6 and B12 maintain healthy red blood cells and improve their ability to carry oxygen to the body's cells. Low levels of B12 lead to anemia and potential damage to the spinal cord and brain. Vitamin B6 deficiency is found in people with heart disease, premenstrual syndrome, atherosclerosis, and carpal tunnel syndrome.

RECOMMENDED FOR HELP WITH:

- Strong bones
- Immunity
- Lowering blood pressure
- Anemia deficiency
- Blood health
- Reduced risk of cardiovascular disease
- Possible cancer prevention

Crab (Alaska king), cooked

Crab is a low-calorie food that is very low in saturated fat and high in protein. Crabs come from the sea, so they are very high in sodium, and they are also very high in cholesterol. As a result, ensure you do not add extra salt or butter when preparing crab and limit your intake of this meat. However, crab meat is very high in vitamin B12 (almost twice the recommended daily value) and also has high levels of copper, selenium, and zinc. Crab meat is low in mercury and can be eaten in moderation during pregnancy.

NUTRIENTS IN 3 OZ. OF CRAB, COOKED:

Calories, 82
Calcium, 50.1 mg
Copper, 1 mg
Folate, 43.4 mcg
Iron, 0.6 mg
Magnesium, 53.5 mg
Niacin, 1.1 mg
Phosphorus, 238 mg
Potassium, 223 mg
Protein, 16 g
Selenium, 34 mcg
Sodium, 911 mg
Total omega-3 fatty acids, 389 mg
Total omega-6 fatty acids, 17 mg
Vitamin B6, 0.2 mg
Vitamin B12, 9.8 mcg
Vitamin C, 6.5 mg
Zinc, 6.5 mg

HEALTH AND HEALING BENEFITS:

HEART AND BLOOD HEALTH:

Omega-3 protects against stroke, heart disease, and diabetes, and folate reduces the risk of hypertension. Vitamins B12 and B6 maintain and oxygenate healthy red blood cells. Copper improves blood vessel health.

IMMUNITY:

Selenium, zinc, and omega-6 improve immune system function, as does vitamin C.

STRONG MUSCLES AND BONES:

Protein helps build and repair bones, tissues, hormones, and body chemicals. Phosphorus assists healthy bone formation, and copper contributes to bone health.

Enhanced brain function: Omega-3 improves brain function and may aid memory. Folate is important for brain function, and is especially important during pregnancy for reducing the risk of spinal and mental defects in the fetus. It may also help protect against Alzheimer's.

CANCER PROTECTION:

Studies have shown a link between consumption of selenium and a reduction in the risk of cancer.

ENERGY:

Copper plays an important role in energy production.

HEALTHY SKIN:

Copper and zinc keep the skin healthy.

Glycemic load: 0
Inflammatory index: Moderately anti-inflammatory

RECOMMENDED FOR HELP WITH:

- Reducing cardiovascular disease
- Immunity
- Strong bones
- Energy
- Enhanced brain function
- Developing fetus during pregnancy
- Healthy skin
- Blood health
- Cancer protection

Crappie (wild)

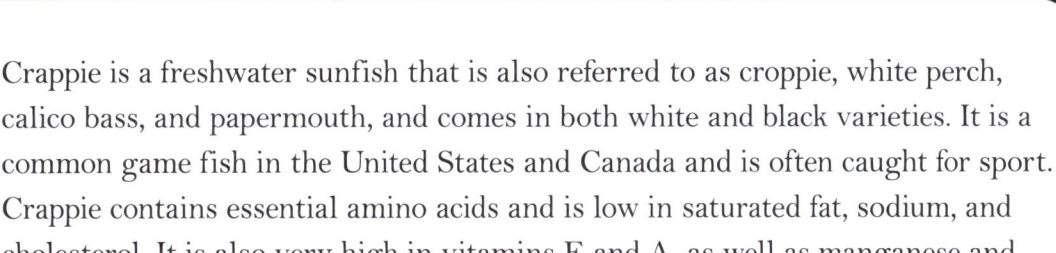

Crappie is a freshwater sunfish that is also referred to as croppie, white perch, calico bass, and papermouth, and comes in both white and black varieties. It is a common game fish in the United States and Canada and is often caught for sport. Crappie contains essential amino acids and is low in saturated fat, sodium, and cholesterol. It is also very high in vitamins E and A, as well as manganese and iron. As a result, crappie is useful in the prevention of cardiovascular disease.

NUTRIENTS IN 3 OZ. OF WILD CRAPPIE:

Calories, 85
Iron, 0.4 mg
Manganese, 6 mg
Protein, 17 g
Vitamin A, 150 IU
Vitamin E, 4.38 IU

HEALTH AND HEALING BENEFITS:

EYE HEALTH:

Vitamin E reduces the risk of cataracts and macular degeneration.

HEALTHY SKIN:

Vitamin A and manganese promote healthy skin.

ENERGY:

Vitamin A boosts stamina.

HEART AND BLOOD HEALTH:

Vitamins A and E help protect the body against cardiovascular disease and lower cholesterol. Iron maintains healthy red blood cells and improves their ability to carry oxygen to the body's cells. Growing children and adolescents, plus menstruating, pregnant, or lactating women have an increased need for iron.

Glycemic load: 0
Inflammatory index: Neutral

RECOMMENDED FOR HELP WITH:

- Blood health
- Vision and eye health
- Reduces risk of cardiovascular disease
- Boosts stamina
- Healthy skin

Eel

While eel may not sound delectable to everyone, it is a delicacy in many cuisines, including jellied eel in the UK and the healthier grilled eel in Korea. Eel is low in sodium and high in omega-3, omega-6, zinc, phosphorus, and vitamins A and B12. However, it is also high in calories and cholesterol, so this meat should be eaten sparingly. With these nutrients, eel can reduce the risk of type-2 diabetes, arthritis, and cardiovascular disease. In Korea, it is believed to improve stamina, but research has so far proved inconclusive.

NUTRIENTS IN 3 OZ.* OF EEL, COOKED:

Calories, 201
Magnesium, 22.1 mg
Niacin, 3.8 mg
Phosphorus, 235 mg
Potassium, 297 mg
Protein, 20 g
Selenium, 7.1 mcg
Thiamin, 0.2 mg
Total omega-3 fatty acids, 712 mg
Total omega-6 fatty acids, 213 mg
Vitamin A (RAE), 969 mcg
Vitamin B12, 2.5 mcg
Zinc, 1.8 mg

*Eel fillets are on average 6 oz.

HEALTH AND HEALING BENEFITS:

HEART AND BLOOD HEALTH:

Omega-3 and -6 and vitamin A protect against stroke, heart disease, and diabetes, and lower cholesterol and high blood pressure. Vitamin B12 maintains healthy red blood cells.

STRONG MUSCLES AND BONES:

Protein helps build and repair bones, tissues, hormones, and body chemicals. Phosphorus assists healthy bone formation.

ENHANCED BRAIN FUNCTION:

Omega-3 improves brain function and may aid memory.

HEALTHY SKIN:

Vitamin A can help prevent acne.

IMMUNITY:

Selenium, zinc, and omega-6 improve immune system function.

Glycemic load: 1
Inflammatory index: Mildly anti-inflammatory

RECOMMENDED FOR HELP WITH:

- Anemia deficiency
- Reduces risk of cardiovascular disease
- Strong bones
- Protection against diabetes
- Brain function
- Healthy skin
- Immunity

Flounder

Flounder is a flat ocean fish that is considered low in calories and protein compared to the density of the meat, meaning you feel fuller quicker. Flounder is low in saturated fat and contains all essential amino acids. Flounder is very high in omega-3 and selenium, as well as vitamin B12, which lead to blood and heart health and a stronger immune system. Due to the low purine content, flounder is considered safe in moderation for those suffering from gout, and because of low mercury is considered safe to eat while pregnant by the American Pregnancy Association.

NUTRIENTS IN 3 OZ.* OF FLOUNDER, COOKED:

Calories, 99
Magnesium, 49.3 mg
Niacin, 1.9 mg
Pantothenic acid, 0.5 mg
Phosphorus, 246 mg
Potassium, 292 mg
Protein, 21 g
Riboflavin, 0.1 mg
Selenium, 49.5 mcg
Thiamin, 0.1 mg
Total omega-3 fatty acids, 478 mg
Total omega-6 fatty acids, 11.9 mg
Vitamin B6, 0.2 mg
Vitamin B12, 2.1 mcg

*Flounder fillets are on average 5 oz.

HEALTH AND HEALING BENEFITS:

JOINT HEALTH:

Selenium and magnesium reduce joint inflammation.

WEIGHT LOSS:

Flounder helps you feel fuller quicker and is low in saturated fat. Magnesium is key to healthy metabolism.

STRONG MUSCLES AND BONES:

Protein helps build and repair bones, tissues, hormones, and body chemicals. Phosphorus and magnesium assist healthy bone formation.

CANCER PROTECTION:

Studies have shown a link between consumption of selenium and a reduction in the risk of cancer.

HEART AND BLOOD HEALTH:

Omega-3 helps protect against stroke, heart disease, and diabetes, and lowers cholesterol. Vitamin B12 maintains healthy red blood cells and improves their ability to carry oxygen to the body's cells. Low levels of B12 lead to anemia and potential damage to the spinal cord and brain.

ENHANCED BRAIN FUNCTION:

Omega-3 improves brain function and is believed to aid memory.

Glycemic load: 0
Inflammatory index: Strongly anti-inflammatory

RECOMMENDED FOR HELP WITH:

- Weight loss
- Reduces risk of cardiovascular disease
- Strong bones
- Heart health
- Joint health
- Cancer protection

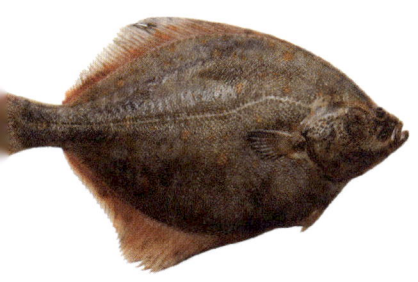

Grouper

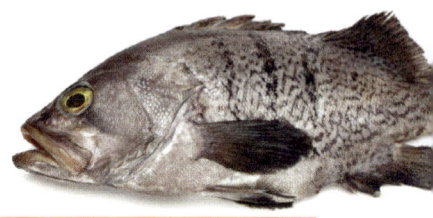

Grouper have large mouths, and some types can grow to a great size. However, as long as you eat small fillets of this meat, the health benefits are sizable. Grouper contains essential amino acids and is low in sodium, calories, and saturated fat, and very high in selenium, protein, and iron. Because of the low calorie content, grouper is excellent for those watching their weight. Both the high protein and selenium are important for repairing new body tissue, and the iron for maintaining healthy red blood cells. Due to high levels of mercury, the American Pregnancy Association recommends limiting grouper consumption during pregnancy.

NUTRIENTS IN 3 OZ.* GROUPER, COOKED:

Calories, 100
Iron, 1 mg
Magnesium, 31.5 mg
Pantothenic acid, 0.7 mg
Phosphorus, 122 mg
Potassium, 104 mg
Protein, 21 g
Selenium, 39.8 mcg
Thiamin, 0.1 mg
Total omega-3 fatty acids, 225 mg
Total omega-6 fatty acids, 15.3 mg
Vitamin B6, 0.3 mg
Vitamin B12, 0.6 mcg

*Grouper fillets are on average 8 oz.

HEALTH AND HEALING BENEFITS:

WEIGHT LOSS:

Grouper helps you feel fuller quicker and is low in calories and saturated fat. Magnesium is key to healthy metabolism.

BLOOD HEALTH:

Vitamin B12, vitamin B6, and iron maintain healthy red blood cells and improve their ability to carry oxygen to the body's cells. Growing children and adolescents, plus menstruating, pregnant, or lactating women have an increased need for iron. Low levels of B12 lead to anemia and potential damage to the spinal cord and brain. Vitamin B6 deficiency is found

Glycemic load: 0
Inflammatory index: Moderately anti-inflammatory

RECOMMENDED FOR HELP WITH:

- Weight loss
- Blood health
- Anemia deficiency
- Reduces risk of cardiovascular disease
- Strong bones
- Heart health
- Joint health
- Cancer protection

in people with heart disease, premenstrual syndrome, atherosclerosis, and carpal tunnel syndrome.

INTERNAL HEALTH:

Potassium keeps the organs and tissues in good condition. Protein and selenium are important for repairing new body tissue.

JOINT HEALTH:

Selenium and magnesium reduce joint inflammation.

CANCER PROTECTION:

Studies have shown a link between consumption of selenium and a reduction in the risk of cancer.

STRONG MUSCLES AND BONES:

Protein helps build and repair bones, tissues, hormones, and body chemicals. Phosphorus and magnesium assist healthy bone formation.

ENHANCED BRAIN FUNCTION:

Omega-3 improves brain function and is believed to aid memory.

Haddock

Like cod, haddock is a popular choice for those less keen on strong fishy flavors. Haddock is a mild white fish that is versatile in the kitchen, from the less-healthy breaded haddock to healthful baking or grilling. Containing essential amino acids, haddock is very low in saturated fat and an excellent source of protein. It is very high in cholesterol, and smoked haddock in particular is high in sodium and should be eaten in moderation. The high levels of vitamins and minerals in haddock help in the prevention of a number of chronic diseases, such as cancer, heart disease, and diabetes. In moderation, haddock is considered safe to eat while pregnant by the American Pregnancy Association, but smoked haddock should be avoided due to possible listeria contamination. Smoked haddock provides very similar nutrient levels, but it is very high in sodium.

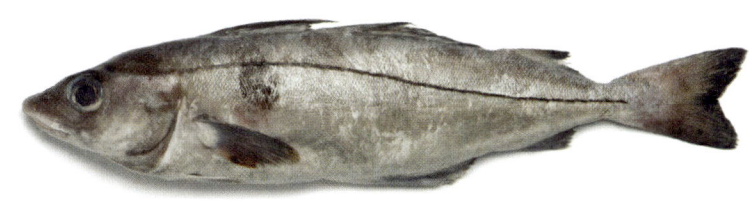

NUTRIENTS IN 3 OZ.* HADDOCK, COOKED:

Calories, 95
Calcium, 35.7 mg
Iron, 1.1 mg
Magnesium, 42.5 mg
Niacin, 3.9 g
Phosphorus, 205 mg
Potassium, 339 mg
Protein, 21 g
Selenium, 34.4 mcg
Total omega-3 fatty acids, 225 mg
Total omega-6 fatty acids, 10.2 mg
Vitamin B6, 0.3 mg
Vitamin B12, 1.2 mcg

*Haddock fillets are on average 6 oz.

HEALTH AND HEALING BENEFITS:

STRONG MUSCLES AND BONES:

Protein helps build and repair bones, tissues, hormones, and body chemicals. Amino acids help form muscle tissue and increase fat metabolism. This can help keep the body strong and increases athletic performance. Phosphorus and magnesium assist healthy bone formation.

GOOD INTERNAL HEALTH:

Amino acids work to keep organs healthy and functioning properly, including the heart, brain, and liver. Potassium keeps the organs and tissues in good condition. Protein and selenium are important for repairing new body tissue.

HEART AND BLOOD HEALTH:

Omega-3, omega-6, and potassium help protect against stroke, heart disease, and diabetes, and lower blood pressure. Vitamin B12, vitamin B6, and iron maintain healthy red blood cells and improve their ability to carry oxygen.

Glycemic load: 0
Inflammatory index: Moderately anti-inflammatory

CANCER PROTECTION:

Studies have shown a link between consumption of selenium and a reduction in the risk of cancer.

ENERGY:

Niacin plays a key role in energy production.

JOINT HEALTH:

Selenium and magnesium reduce joint inflammation.

RECOMMENDED FOR HELP WITH:

- Strong bones
- Blood health
- Reduces risk of cardiovascular disease
- Heart health
- Energy
- Joint health
- Cancer protection

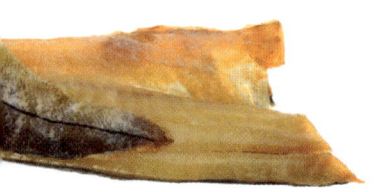

Halibut

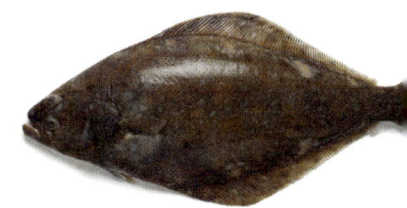

According to the USDA, halibut is one of the highest-protein fish available. Protein is important for muscle maintenance and energy, and halibut packs a punch with its high protein levels. Halibut also contains essential amino acids and is low in saturated fat and sodium. It is high in omega-3, selenium, and niacin, promoting heart health and boosting the immune system. In moderation, halibut is considered safe to eat while pregnant by the American Pregnancy Association.

NUTRIENTS IN 3 OZ.* HALIBUT, COOKED:

Calories, 119
Calcium, 51 mg
Iron, 0.9 mg
Magnesium, 90.9 mg
Niacin, 6.1 mg
Phosphorus, 242 mg
Potassium, 490 mg
Protein, 23 g
Riboflavin, 0.1 mg
Selenium, 39.8 mcg
Total omega-3 fatty acids, 569 mg
Total omega-6 fatty acids, 32.3 mg
Vitamin B6, 0.3 mg
Vitamin B12, 1.2 mcg

*Halibut fillets are on average 11 oz.

HEALTH AND HEALING BENEFITS:

STRONG MUSCLES AND BONES:

Protein helps build and repair bones, tissues, hormones, and body chemicals. Amino acids help form muscle tissue and increase fat metabolism. This can help keep the body strong and increases athletic performance. Calcium, as well as phosphorus and magnesium, assists healthy bone formation.

HEART AND BLOOD HEALTH:

Omega-3, omega-6, and potassium help protect against stroke, heart disease, and diabetes, and lower blood pressure. Vitamin B12, vitamin B6, and iron maintain healthy red blood cells and improve their ability to carry oxygen to the body's cells.

Glycemic load: 0
Inflammatory index: Moderately anti-inflammatory

RECOMMENDED FOR HELP WITH:

- Strong bones
- Heart health
- Reduces risk of cardiovascular disease
- Immunity
- Energy
- Joint health
- Cancer protection

INTERNAL HEALTH:

Amino acids work to keep organs healthy and functioning properly, including the heart, brain, and liver. Potassium keeps the organs and tissues in good condition. Protein and selenium are important for repairing new body tissue.

JOINT HEALTH:

Selenium and magnesium reduce joint inflammation.

CANCER PROTECTION:

Studies have shown a link between consumption of selenium and a reduction in the risk of cancer. It is thought that selenium promotes DNA repair in damaged cells and inhibits the increase of cancer cells.

IMMUNITY:

Selenium boosts immunity.

ENERGY:

Niacin and magnesium play a key role in energy production.

HERRING

Herring contains extremely high omega-3s and is high in protein, but also high in cholesterol. The fatty acids and protein promote healthy brain function and bone strength, and the potassium assists in nerve communication. Herring is rich in iron and vitamin B12, which keep red blood cells healthy. Herring is considered safe to eat during pregnancy due to its low mercury levels, but the American Pregnancy Association recommends avoiding kippered fish during pregnancy due to possible listeria contamination. If you suffer from gout, watch your consumption of this food. Grilling or poaching are the healthiest cooking options; kippered and pickled herring are high in sodium—eat these in moderation.

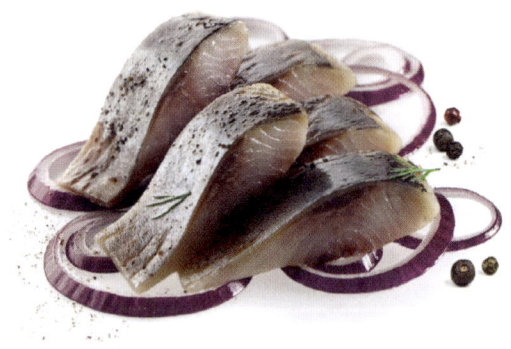

Herring (Atlantic)

NUTRIENTS IN 3 OZ.* ATLANTIC HERRING, COOKED:

Calories, 173
Calcium, 62.9 mg
Copper, 0.1 mg
Iron, 1.2 mg
Magnesium, 34.8 mg
Niacin, 3.5 mg
Pantothenic acid, 0.6 mg
Phosphorus, 258 mg
Potassium, 356 mg
Protein, 20 g
Selenium, 39.8 mcg
Riboflavin, 0.3 mg
Thiamin, 0.1 mg
Total omega-3 fatty acids, 1,885 mg
Total omega-6 fatty acids, 142 mg
Vitamin B6, 0.3 mg
Vitamin B12, 11.2 mcg
Vitamin E, 1.2 mg
Zinc, 1.1 mg

*Herring fillets are on average 6 oz.

Glycemic load: 0
Inflammatory index: Strongly anti-inflammatory

Herring (Pacific)

NUTRIENTS IN 3 OZ.* PACIFIC HERRING, COOKED:

Calories, 70
Niacin, 0.8 mg
Phosphorus, 81.8 mg
Potassium, 152 mg
Protein, 6 g
Riboflavin, 0.1 mg
Selenium, 13.1 mcg
Total omega-3 fatty acids, 677 mg
Total omega-6 fatty acids, 68.9 mg
Vitamin B6, 0.1 mg
Vitamin B12, 2.7 mcg

*Pacific herring fillets are on average 6 oz.

Glycemic load: 0
Inflammatory index: Strongly anti-inflammatory

HEALTH AND HEALING BENEFITS OF HERRING:

MUSCLES AND BONES:

Protein helps build and repair bones and tissues. Calcium, phosphorus, and magnesium assist healthy bone formation.

HEART AND BLOOD HEALTH:

Omega-3, omega-6, and potassium help protect against stroke, heart disease, and diabetes, and lower blood pressure. Vitamins B12 and B6, iron, and riboflavin maintain healthy red blood cells and improve their ability to carry oxygen to the body's cells. Growing children and adolescents, plus menstruating, pregnant, or lactating women, have an increased need for iron. Low levels of B12 lead to anemia and potential damage to the spinal cord and brain. Vitamin B6 deficiency is found in people with heart disease, premenstrual syndrome, atherosclerosis, and carpal tunnel syndrome.

ENHANCED BRAIN FUNCTION:

Omega fatty acids enhance brain function and are believed to aid memory.

IMMUNITY:

Selenium and omega-6 boost the immune system.

HEALTHY SKIN:

Riboflavin and zinc can prevent acne.

HEALTHY THYROID:

Riboflavin promotes healthy thyroid function.

EYE HEALTH:

Riboflavin and vitamin E promote eye health.

CANCER PROTECTION:

Studies have shown a link between consumption of selenium and a reduction in the risk of cancer.

Glycemic load: 1
Inflammatory index: Mildly anti-inflammatory

RECOMMENDED FOR HELP WITH:

- Anemia deficiency
- Cardiovascular disease
- Strong bones
- Brain function
- Healthy skin
- Immunity

Lobster

Lobster is a good source of vitamins and minerals. However, due to its high sodium and cholesterol content, it should be eaten in moderation. Lobster contains essential amino acids and is low in fat. The calcium and phosphorus build strong bones, vitamin B12 works toward brain function and nerve communication, and copper increases energy and assists in cell regeneration and skin health. Lobster has traditionally been considered an aphrodisiac. Because of higher mercury, lobster should be limited during pregnancy. Allergy to lobster and other shellfish is relatively common; if you suffer from any symptoms, get treatment immediately.

NUTRIENTS IN 3 OZ. LOBSTER (COOKED):

Calories, 83
Calcium, 51.8 mg
Copper, 1.6 mg
Magnesium, 29.8 mg
Niacin, 0.9 mg
Phosphorus, 157 mg
Potassium, 299 mg
Protein, 17 g
Selenium, 36.3 mcg
Sodium, 323 mg
Total omega-3 fatty acids, 73.1 mg
Total omega-6 fatty acids, 4.3 mg
Vitamin B12, 2.6 mcg
Vitamin E, 0.9 mg
Zinc, 2.5 mg

HEALTH AND HEALING BENEFITS:

BLOOD HEALTH:

Vitamin B12 maintains healthy red blood cells and improves their ability to carry oxygen to cells. Low levels of B12 lead to anemia and potential damage to the spinal cord and brain.

STRONG MUSCLES AND BONES:

Protein helps build and repair bones and tissues. Amino acids help form muscle tissue and increase fat metabolism. Phosphorus and copper assist healthy bone formation.

ENERGY:

Copper plays an important role in energy production.

INTERNAL HEALTH:

Amino acids keep organs healthy and functioning properly, including the heart, brain, and liver.

IMMUNITY:

Zinc has far-reaching effects on immune health, and selenium and omega-6 boost immunity.

CANCER PROTECTION:

Studies have shown a link between consumption of selenium and a reduction in the risk of cancer.

HEALTHY SKIN:

Copper and zinc keep skin strong and healthy.

Glycemic load: 1
Inflammatory index: Anti-inflammatory

RECOMMENDED FOR HELP WITH:

- Strong bones
- Anemia deficiency
- Blood health
- Energy
- Immunity
- Healthy skin
- Cancer protection

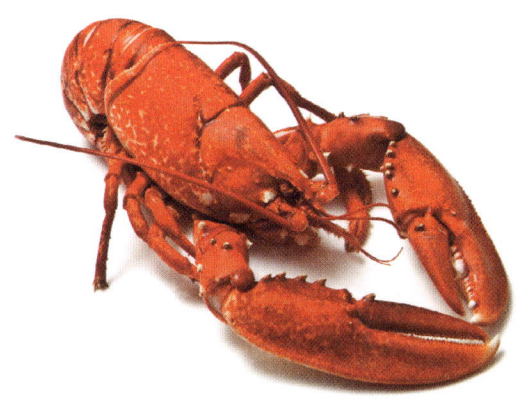

MACKEREL

Mackerel is an oily fish, and the name applies to several types. Mackerel provides high levels of omega-3—crucial for heart health—and jack mackerel is considered highest of all. Mackerel a good source of potassium, which, together with the high omega-3, works to control blood pressure, if eaten in moderation. The vitamin B12 strengthens red blood cells. The USDA. and American Pregnancy Association recommend avoiding king mackerel during pregnancy due to high mercury levels, but other types of mackerel can be eaten on occasion.

Mackerel (Atlantic)

The same amount of king mackerel has 114 calories, but lower fatty acids and trace vitamin B6.

NUTRIENTS IN 3 OZ.* ATLANTIC MACKEREL, COOKED:

Calories, 223
Iron, 1.3 mg
Magnesium, 82.5 mg
Niacin, 5.8 mg
Pantothenic acid, 0.8 mg
Phosphorus, 236 mg
Potassium, 341 mg
Protein, 20 g
Riboflavin, 0.4 mg
Selenium, 43.9 mcg
Thiamin, 0.1 mg
Total omega-3 fatty acids, 1,209 mg
Total omega-6 fatty acids, 125 mg
Vitamin B6, 0.4 mg
Vitamin B12, 16.1 mcg
Zinc, 0.8 mg

*Atlantic mackerel fillets are on average 3 oz.

Glycemic load: 0
Inflammatory index: Strongly anti-inflammatory

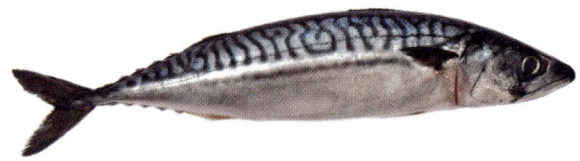

Mackerel (jack), canned

NUTRIENTS IN 3 OZ.* MACKEREL, CANNED:

Calories, 132
Calcium, 202.5 mg
Niacin, 5.1 mg
Phosphorus, 252.9 mg
Protein, 18 g
Selenium, 31.8 mcg
Sodium, 318 mg
Total omega-3 fatty acids, 1,155 mg
Total omega-6 fatty acids, 83.1 mg
Vitamin B12, 5.7 mcg
Vitamin D, 211.8 IU

*1 can of mackerel is roughly 12 oz.

HEALTH AND HEALING BENEFITS OF MACKEREL:

HEART AND BLOOD HEALTH:

Omega-3 and -6 and potassium protect against stroke, heart disease, and diabetes, and lower blood pressure. Vitamins B12 and B6, iron, and riboflavin maintain and oxygenate healthy red blood cells.

STRONG MUSCLES AND BONES:

Protein helps build and repair bones, tissues, hormones, and body chemicals. Calcium, phosphorus, and magnesium assist healthy bone formation.

ENHANCED BRAIN FUNCTION:

Omega fatty acids enhance brain function and memory.

IMMUNITY:

Selenium, zinc, and omega-6 boost the immune system.

CANCER PROTECTION:

Studies have shown a link between consumption of selenium and a reduction in the risk of cancer.

Glycemic load: 0
Inflammatory index: Strongly anti-inflammatory

Glycemic load: 1
Inflammatory index: Mildly anti-inflammatory

RECOMMENDED FOR HELP WITH:

- Heart health
- Reduces risk of cardiovascular disease
- Blood health
- Lowers blood pressure
- Enhanced brain function
- Strong bones
- Immunity
- Cancer protection

Monkfish

Monkfish is a type of anglerfish that, while not considered a thing of beauty, is a delicious and healthful fish. However, the sustainability of monkfish fishing has been brought into question in some parts of the world, so keep this under advisement when purchasing. Monkfish is a low-calorie, high-protein fish that contains essential amino acids and is low in sodium, as well as being high in selenium and phosphorus, great for energy and brain function. It is advised that monkfish consumption be limited during pregnancy due to mercury levels.

NUTRIENTS IN 3 OZ. MONKFISH, COOKED:

Calories, 82
Magnesium, 23 mg
Niacin, 2.2 mg
Phosphorus, 218 mg
Potassium, 436 mg
Protein, 16 g
Riboflavin, 0.1 mg
Selenium, 39.8 mcg
Vitamin B6, 0.2 mg
Vitamin B12, 0.9 mcg

HEALTH AND HEALING BENEFITS:

STRONG MUSCLES AND BONES:

Protein helps build and repair bones, tissues, hormones, and body chemicals. Phosphorus and magnesium assist healthy bone formation.

BLOOD HEALTH:

Vitamins B12 and B6 maintain healthy red blood cells and improve their ability to carry oxygen to the body's cells. Low levels of B12 lead to anemia and potential damage to the spinal cord and brain. Vitamin B6 deficiency is found in people with heart disease, premenstrual syndrome, atherosclerosis, and carpal tunnel syndrome.

IMMUNITY:

Selenium boosts the immune system. Selenium and potassium combat disease.

ENERGY:

Niacin plays a key role in energy production.

MOOD STABILIZER:

Vitamin B6 is crucial to brain function and is believed to help stabilize mood.

CANCER PROTECTION:

Studies have shown a link between consumption of selenium and a reduction in the risk of cancer. It is thought that selenium promotes DNA repair in damaged cells and inhibits the increase of cancer cells.

Glycemic load: 0
Inflammatory index: Neutral

RECOMMENDED FOR HELP WITH:

- Strong bones
- Blood health
- Anemia deficiency
- Immunity
- Energy
- Mood
- Cancer protection

Mullet

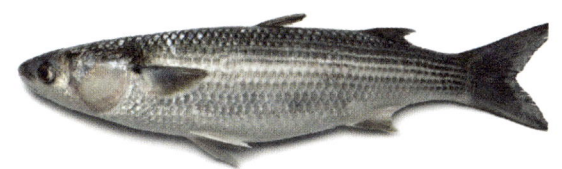

The striped mullet is found in various guises in the cuisines of the world, and the fish can be both farmed and wild. Mullet contains essential amino acids and is low in sodium, high in selenium, and provides a good source of iron and omega fatty acids. However, it is also high in cholesterol. Protein is important for strong bones, healthy blood, and tissue repair, and iron maintains healthy red blood cells and is particularly important for growing children, and women who are menstruating, pregnant, or lactating. Mullet is low in mercury and can be eaten in moderation during pregnancy.

NUTRIENTS IN 3 OZ.* MULLET, COOKED:

Calories, 128
Copper, 0.1 mg
Iron, 1.2 mg
Magnesium, 28.1 mg
Niacin, 5.4 mg
Pantothenic acid, 0.7 mg
Phosphorus, 207 mg
Potassium, 389 mg
Protein, 21 g
Riboflavin, 0.1 mg
Selenium, 39.8 mcg
Thiamin, 0.1 mg
Total omega-3 fatty acids, 357 mg
Total omega-6 fatty acids, 79.9 mg
Vitamin B6, 0.4 mg
Zinc, 0.7 mg

*Mullet fillets are on average 4 oz.

HEALTH AND HEALING BENEFITS:

MUSCLES AND BONES:

Protein helps build and repair bones and tissues. Amino acids help form muscle tissue and increase fat metabolism. Phosphorus and copper assist healthy bone formation.

INTERNAL HEALTH:

Amino acids work to keep organs healthy and functioning properly, including the heart, brain, and liver.

IMMUNITY:

Zinc affects immunity, and selenium and omega-6 boost the immune system.

ENERGY:

Niacin plays a key role in energy production.

BLOOD HEALTH:

Protein is a building block of blood, and vitamin B6 strengthens it. Iron improves oxygenation of the blood. Vitamin B6 deficiency is found in people with heart disease, premenstrual syndrome, atherosclerosis, and carpal tunnel syndrome.

Glycemic load: 0
Inflammatory index: Mildly anti-inflammatory

RECOMMENDED FOR HELP WITH:

- Strong bones
- Blood health
- Immunity
- Energy
- Cancer protection

Octopus

Octopus is an ocean mollusk related to squid and cuttlefish. It is believed there are over 300 species of octopus, but only a limited number of these are caught for human consumption. Octopus is a low-calorie seafood that contains essential amino acids and is low in saturated fat and high in protein, but also high in cholesterol and sodium. Both Atlantic and Pacific octopus provide high levels of copper, iron, zinc, and vitamin B12. Copper boosts energy and helps form connective tissue; it also metabolizes iron, itself important for healthy red blood cells. Together, copper and zinc strengthen the immune system.

NUTRIENTS IN 3 OZ. OCTOPUS (COOKED):

Calories, 139
Calcium, 90.1 mg
Copper, 0.6 mg
Folate, 20.4 mcg
Iron, 8.1 mg
Magnesium, 51 mg
Niacin, 3.2 mg
Pantothenic acid, 0.8 mg
Phosphorus, 237 mg
Potassium, 535 mg
Protein, 25 g
Selenium, 76.2 mcg
Sodium, 391 mg
Vitamin A (RAE), 76.5 mcg
Vitamin E, 1.0 mg
Total omega-3 fatty acids, 277 mg
Total omega-6 fatty acids, 15.3 mg
Vitamin B6, 0.6 mg
Vitamin B12, 30.6 mcg
Vitamin C, 6.8 mg
Zinc, 2.9 mg

HEALTH AND HEALING BENEFITS:

STRONG MUSCLES AND BONES:

Protein helps build and repair bones, tissues, hormones, and body chemicals. Amino acids help form muscle tissue and increase fat metabolism. This can help keep the body strong and increases athletic performance. Phosphorus and copper assist healthy bone formation.

INTERNAL HEALTH:

Amino acids keep organs healthy and functioning properly, including the heart, brain, and liver.

Glycemic load: 0
Inflammatory index: Moderately anti-inflammatory

RECOMMENDED FOR HELP WITH:

- Strong bones
- Blood health
- Immunity
- Energy
- Healthy skin
- Heart health
- Cancer protection

HEART AND BLOOD HEALTH:

Omega-3, omega-6, potassium, and vitamin E help protect against stroke, heart disease, and diabetes, and lower blood pressure. Vitamins B12 and B6, and iron maintain healthy red blood cells and improve their ability to carry oxygen to the body's cells. Growing children and adolescents, plus menstruating, pregnant, or lactating women, have an increased need for iron, and copper helps metabolize it. Vitamin B6 deficiency is found in people with heart disease, premenstrual syndrome, atherosclerosis, and carpal tunnel syndrome. Low levels of B12 lead to anemia and potential damage to the spinal cord and brain.

IMMUNITY:

Zinc, copper, and selenium boost the immune system, supported by vitamin C.

ENERGY:

Copper plays a key role in energy production.

HEALTHY SKIN:

Copper and zinc promote healthy skin.

CANCER PROTECTION:

Studies have shown a link between consumption of selenium and a reduction in the risk of cancer. It is thought that selenium promotes DNA repair in damaged cells and inhibits the increase of cancer cells.

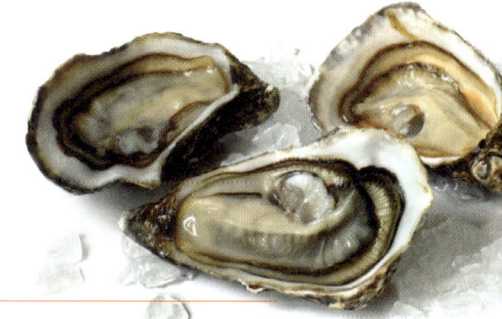

Oysters

Oysters are bivalve marine mollusks that live close to the shore and are served in coastal areas around the world. Oysters are low in fat and contain essential amino acids. They are also a good source of copper, iron, and zinc—which is especially high in canned oysters. Alongside copper, zinc boosts a healthy immune system, and iron promotes healthy red blood cells. However, oysters are very high in cholesterol and relatively low in protein; ensure your diet includes protein-rich food sources to complement your nutrient intake. Oysters are low in mercury and can be eaten in moderation during pregnancy.

NUTRIENTS IN 4 OZ.* OYSTERS, RAW:

Calories, 81
Copper, 1.6 mg
Iron, 5.1 mg
Manganese, 0.6 mg
Niacin, 2 mg
Phosphorus, 162 mg
Protein, 9 g
Riboflavin, 0.2 mg
Selenium, 77 mcg
Total omega-3 fatty acids, 740 mg
Total omega-6 fatty acids, 32.0 mg
Vitamin B12, 16 mcg
Vitamin C, 8 mg
Zinc, 16.6 mg

*1 medium oyster is roughly 2 oz.

HEALTH AND HEALING BENEFITS:

INTERNAL HEALTH:

Amino acids work to keep organs healthy and functioning properly, including the heart, brain, and liver.

STRONG MUSCLES AND BONES:

Protein helps build and repair bones, tissues, hormones, and body chemicals. Amino acids help form muscle tissue and increase fat metabolism. This can help keep the body strong and increases athletic performance. Phosphorus and copper assist healthy bone formation.

HEART AND BLOOD HEALTH:

Omega-3, omega-6, potassium, and vitamin E help protect against stroke, heart disease, and diabetes, and lower blood pressure. Vitamin B12 and iron maintain healthy red blood cells and improve their ability to carry oxygen to the body's cells. Growing children and adolescents, plus menstruating, pregnant, or lactating women, have an increased need for iron, and copper helps metabolize it. Low levels of B12 lead to anemia and potential damage to the spinal cord and brain.

IMMUNITY:

Zinc, copper, and selenium boost the immune system, supported by vitamin C.

ENERGY:

Copper and vitamin E play a key role in energy production.

Glycemic load: 4
Inflammatory index: Moderately inflammatory

RECOMMENDED FOR HELP WITH:

- Strong bones
- Blood health
- Immunity
- Energy
- Healthy skin
- Eye health
- Heart health
- Cancer protection

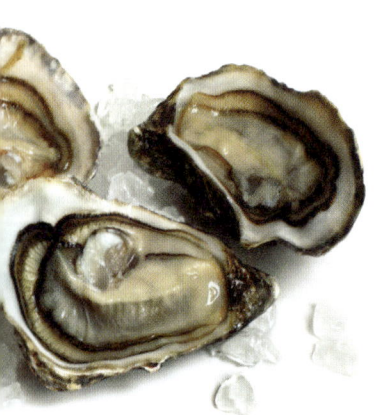

HEALTHY SKIN:

Copper, zinc, and vitamin A promote healthy skin, supported by manganese.

EYE HEALTH:

Zinc and vitamin E reduce the risk of cataracts and macular degeneration.

CANCER PROTECTION:

Studies have shown a link between consumption of selenium and a reduction in the risk of cancer. It is thought that selenium promotes DNA repair in damaged cells and inhibits the increase of cancer cells.

Perch (ocean)

Perch is low in saturated fat and rich in protein. It contains essential amino acids, selenium, phosphorus, vitamin B12, and calcium, but is high in cholesterol. Selenium promotes good metabolism and may reduce the risk of cancer, while phosphorus and calcium maintain healthy bones. Due to mercury l evels, the American Pregnancy Association recommends limiting perch consumption during pregnancy. The risk of mercury and other toxins in ocean perch can be reduced by careful preparation, especially by removing skin and fat and cooking to a high temperature.

NUTRIENTS IN 3 OZ.*
OCEAN PERCH, COOKED:

Calories, 103
Calcium, 112 mg
Iron, 1 mg
Magnesium, 33.2 mg
Niacin, 2.1 mg
Phosphorus, 235 mg
Potassium, 298 mg
Protein, 20 g
Riboflavin, 0.1 mg
Selenium, 47.2 mcg
Thiamin, 0.1 mg
Total omega-3 fatty acids, 405 mg
Total omega-6 fatty acids, 30.6 mg
Vitamin B6, 0.2 mg
Vitamin B12, 1 mg

*Ocean perch fillets are on average 2 oz.

HEALTH AND HEALING BENEFITS:

INTERNAL HEALTH:

Amino acids work to keep organs healthy and functioning properly, including the heart, brain, and liver.

STRONG MUSCLES AND BONES:

Protein helps build and repair bones, tissues, hormones, and body chemicals. Phosphorus and copper assist healthy bone formation, supported by calcium.

IMPROVED METABOLISM:

Amino acids form muscle tissue and increase fat metabolism. This can help keep the body strong and increases athletic performance.

HEART AND BLOOD HEALTH:

Omega-3, omega-6, potassium, and protein help protect against stroke, heart disease, and diabetes, and lower blood pressure. Vitamin B12 maintains healthy red blood cells and improves their ability to carry oxygen to the body's cells. Low levels of B12 lead to anemia and potential damage to the spinal cord and brain.

HEALTHY SKIN:

Manganese promotes healthy skin, supported by copper and zinc.

IMMUNITY:

Selenium, zinc, and copper boost the immune system.

ENERGY:

Niacin and copper play a key role in energy production.

CANCER PROTECTION:

Studies have shown a link between consumption of selenium and a reduction in the risk of cancer. It is thought that selenium promotes DNA repair in damaged cells and inhibits the increase of cancer cells.

Glycemic load: 0
Inflammatory index: Moderately anti-inflammatory

RECOMMENDED FOR HELP WITH:

- Strong bones
- Metabolism
- Blood health
- Healthy skin
- Immunity
- Energy
- Heart health
- Cancer protection

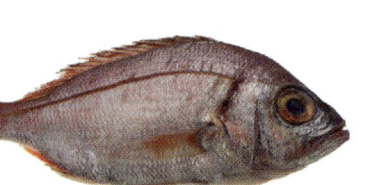

Pike

Pike is a freshwater fish with low sodium and high protein and vitamin B12. It is also very low in saturated fat and a good source of metabolism-boosting phosphorus, which makes pike a positive option for weight-loss programs. Pike comes in many types: Northern pike is common in the Northern Hemisphere; walleye pike (or simply "walleye" or "pikeperch") is native to North America and the official state fish of Minnesota. It is recommended that pike be avoided during pregnancy. Northern pike has lower potassium than walleye pike and lower omega-3.

NUTRIENTS IN 3 OZ.*
WALLEYE PIKE, COOKED:

Calories, 101
Calcium, 120 mg
Copper, 0.2 mg
Folate, 14.5 mcg
Iron, 1.4 mg
Magnesium, 32.3 mg
Manganese, 0.9 mg
Niacin, 2.4 mg
Pantothenic acid, 0.7 mg
Phosphorus, 229 mg
Potassium, 424 mg
Protein, 21 g
Riboflavin, 0.2 mg
Selenium, 13.8 mcg
Thiamin, 0.3 mg
Total omega-3 fatty acids, 395 mg
Total omega-6 fatty acids, 28.1 mg
Vitamin B6, 0.1 mg
Vitamin B12, 2 mcg
Zinc, 0.7 mg

*****Walleye pike fillets are on average 5 oz.**

HEALTH AND HEALING BENEFITS:

IMPROVED METABOLISM:

Phosphorus and magnesium are key to healthy metabolism.

STRONG MUSCLES AND BONES:

Protein helps build and repair bones, tissues, hormones, and body chemicals. Phosphorus and copper assist healthy bone formation, supported by calcium.

HEART AND BLOOD HEALTH:

Thiamin, fatty acids, and protein help protect against stroke, heart disease, and diabetes, and lower blood pressure. Vitamin B12 and iron maintain healthy red blood cells and improve their ability to carry oxygen to the body's cells. Growing children and adolescents, plus menstruating, pregnant, or lactating women, have an increased need for iron, and copper helps metabolize it. Low levels of B12 lead to anemia and potential damage to the spinal cord and brain.

Glycemic load: 0
Inflammatory index: Moderately anti-inflammatory

HEALTHY SKIN:

Manganese promotes healthy skin, supported by copper and zinc.

IMMUNITY:

Selenium, zinc, and copper boost the immune system.

FOR HELP WITH:

- Weight loss
- Strong bones
- Blood health
- Heart health
- Healthy skin
- Immunity

Pollock (Atlantic)

Pollock is a good source of protein and contains essential amino acids. It is low in saturated fat and is a source of vitamin B12, selenium, and phosphorus. However, it is quite high in cholesterol. Vitamin B12 is essential for a healthy nervous system, and phosphorus and selenium boost the immune system and strengthen bone and tissue. Due to low mercury, pollock is considered safe to eat in moderation while pregnant by the American Pregnancy Association.

NUTRIENTS IN 3 OZ.* ATLANTIC POLLOCK, COOKED:

Calories, 100
Calcium, 65.4 mg
Magnesium, 73.1 mg
Niacin, 3.4 mg
Pantothenic acid, 0.4 mg
Phosphorus, 241 mg
Potassium, 388 mg
Protein, 21 g
Riboflavin, 0.2 mg
Selenium, 80.8 mcg
Sodium, 93.5 mg
Total omega-3 fatty acids, 485 mg
Total omega-6 fatty acids, 10.2 mg
Vitamin B6, 0.3 mg
Vitamin B12, 3.1 mcg

*Atlantic pollock fillets are on average 12 oz.

HEALTH AND HEALING BENEFITS:

MUSCLES AND BONES:

Protein helps build and repair bones and tissues. Calcium, magnesium, and phosphorus aid healthy bone formation.

HEART AND BLOOD HEALTH:

Fatty acids and protein help protect the body against stroke, heart disease, and diabetes, and lower blood pressure. Vitamins B12 and B6 maintain healthy red blood cells and improve their ability to carry oxygen to the body's cells. Vitamin B6 deficiency is found in people with heart disease, premenstrual syndrome, atherosclerosis, and carpal tunnel syndrome. Low levels of B12 lead to anemia and potential damage to the spinal cord and brain.

ENHANCED BRAIN FUNCTION:

Omega-3 improves brain function and is believed to aid memory.

ENERGY:

Magnesium and niacin play a key role in energy production.

Glycemic load: 0
Inflammatory index: Strongly anti-inflammatory

RECOMMENDED FOR HELP WITH:

- Strong bones
- Blood health
- Enhanced brain function
- Energy
- Heart health
- Cancer protection

Red snapper

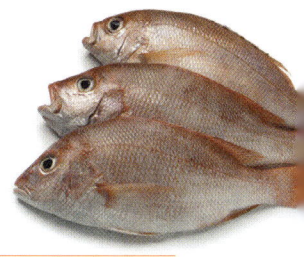

Red snapper is most prevalent along the southeastern Atlantic coast. Much of what is labeled as "red snapper" is actually snapper of a different type. Red snapper is low in calories, rich in protein, and contains all essential amino acids, as well as high levels of selenium and vitamin B12. It is also low in saturated fat and sodium. Due to higher levels of mercury, the American Pregnancy Association recommends limiting snapper during pregnancy. This fish may be in danger of overfishing and should be monitored prior to purchase.

NUTRIENTS IN 3 OZ.* RED SNAPPER, COOKED:

Calories, 109
Magnesium, 31.5 mg
Pantothenic acid, 0.7 mg
Phosphorus, 171 mg
Potassium, 444 mg
Protein, 22 g
Selenium, 41.6 mcg
Total omega-3 fatty acids, 485 mg
Total omega-6 fatty acids, 10.2 mg
Vitamin B6, 0.4 mg
Vitamin B12, 3.0 mcg

*Red snapper fillets are on average 7 oz.

HEALTH AND HEALING BENEFITS:

IMMUNITY:

Selenium boosts immunity.

HEART AND BLOOD HEALTH:

Fatty acids and protein help protect against stroke, heart disease, and diabetes, and lower blood pressure. Vitamins B12 and B6 maintain healthy red blood cells and improve their ability to carry oxygen to the body's cells. Vitamin B6 deficiency is found in people with heart disease, premenstrual syndrome, atherosclerosis, and carpal tunnel syndrome. Low levels of B12 lead to anemia and potential damage to the spinal cord and brain.

STRONG MUSCLES AND BONES:

Protein helps build and repair bones, tissues, hormones, and body chemicals. Phosphorus assists bone formation.

CANCER PROTECTION:

Studies have shown a link between consumption of selenium and a reduction in the risk of cancer. It is thought that selenium promotes DNA repair in damaged cells and inhibits the increase of cancer cells.

Glycemic load: 0
Inflammatory index: Strongly anti-inflammatory

RECOMMENDED FOR HELP WITH:

- Heart health
- Strong bones
- Blood health
- Immunity
- Cancer protection

Roe

Roe is the ripe ovaries or unfertilized eggs of fish, and cod and salmon are some of the more common types of roe. It is a delicacy in some countries, such as Norway, but less common in others, such as the United States. It comes as either "hard" or "soft" roe. The remarkably high omega-3 content makes this a very healthy food, despite the high cholesterol levels—although it should still be eaten in moderation. Roe is extremely high in vitamin B12, as well as being high in selenium, riboflavin, and phosphorus. Avoid eating uncooked fish eggs during pregnancy.

NUTRIENTS IN 3 OZ. ROE, COOKED:

Calories, 173
Copper, 0.1 mg
Folate, 78.2 mcg
Iron, 0.7 mg
Magnesium, 22.1 mg
Niacin, 1.0 mg
Pantothenic acid, 1 mg
Phosphorus, 438 mg
Potassium, 241 mg
Protein, 24 g
Riboflavin, 0.8 mg
Selenium, 43.9 mcg
Sodium, 99.5 mg
Thiamin, 0.2 mg
Total omega-3 fatty acids, 2,651 mg
Total omega-6 fatty acids, 31.5 mg
Vitamin A (RAE), 77.4 mcg
Vitamin B6, 0.2 mg
Vitamin B12, 9.8 mcg
Vitamin C, 13.9 mg
Zinc, 1.1 mg

HEALTH AND HEALING BENEFITS:

HEART AND BLOOD HEALTH:

Omega-3 helps protect against stroke, heart disease, and diabetes. Omega-6 regulates blood pressure, and the two together reduce high blood pressure. Vitamins B12 and B6, and iron maintain healthy red blood cells and improve their ability to carry oxygen to the body's cells. Growing children and adolescents, plus menstruating, pregnant, or lactating women, have an increased need for iron. Low levels of B12 lead to anemia and potential damage to the spinal cord and brain. Riboflavin helps create red blood cells.

Glycemic load: 2
Inflammatory index: Strongly anti-inflammatory

RECOMMENDED FOR HELP WITH:

- Reducing cardiovascular disease
- Blood health
- Enhanced brain function and memory
- Immunity
- Energy
- Cancer protection

STRONG MUSCLES AND BONES:

Protein helps build and repair bones, tissues, hormones, and body chemicals. Phosphorus assists healthy bone formation.

ENHANCED BRAIN FUNCTION:

Omega-3 improves brain function and is believed to aid memory. Folate is important for all aspects of brain function, and is especially important during pregnancy for reducing the risk of spinal and mental defects in the fetus. It may also help protect against Alzheimer's.

IMMUNITY:

Selenium, zinc, and omega-6 improve immune system function, supported by vitamin C. Riboflavin helps produce antibodies.

ENERGY:

Riboflavin plays a key role in energy production.

CANCER PROTECTION:

Studies have shown a link between consumption of selenium and a reduction in the risk of cancer. It is thought that selenium promotes DNA repair in damaged cells and inhibits the increase of cancer cells.

Roughy (orange)

Orange roughy, or deep-sea perch, is a widespread ocean fish with an incredible lifespan of over 100 years. They are vulnerable to overfishing, so it is important to monitor your region's advice on this fish prior to purchase. Orange roughy contains essential amino acids, is very low in saturated fat, and is high in omega-6, protein, and selenium—but this fish is very high in cholesterol. The American Pregnancy Association recommends avoiding orange roughy during pregnancy due to high mercury levels, and it is recommended that this fish be eaten in moderation by all others.

NUTRIENTS IN 3 OZ. ORANGE ROUGHY, COOKED:

Calories, 89
Iron, 1 mg
Magnesium, 15.3 mg
Niacin, 1.5 mg
Phosphorus, 86.7 mg
Potassium, 154 mg
Protein, 19 g
Selenium, 75 mcg
Total omega-3 fatty acids, 27.2 mg
Total omega-6 fatty acids, 107 mg
Vitamin B12, 0.4 mcg
Vitamin E, 1.6 mg

HEALTH AND HEALING BENEFITS:

HEART AND BLOOD HEALTH:

Iron maintains healthy red blood cells and improves their ability to carry oxygen to the body's cells. Growing children and adolescents, plus menstruating, pregnant, or lactating women, have an increased need for iron. Fatty acids and protein help protect against stroke, heart disease, and diabetes, and lower blood pressure. Vitamin E reduces the risk of heart disease and assists in cellular regeneration.

IMMUNITY:

Selenium and iron improve immune system function.

STRONG MUSCLES AND BONES:

Protein helps build and repair bones, tissues, hormones, and body chemicals. Amino acids help form muscle tissue and increase fat metabolism. This can help keep the body strong and increases athletic performance. Phosphorus assists healthy bone formation.

INTERNAL HEALTH:

Amino acids work to keep organs healthy and functioning properly, including the heart, brain, and liver.

CANCER PROTECTION:

Studies have shown a link between consumption of selenium and a reduction in the risk of cancer. It is thought that selenium promotes DNA repair in damaged cells and inhibits the increase of cancer cells. Vitamin E is believed to reduce the risk of cancer.

Glycemic load: 0
Inflammatory index: Mildly anti-inflammatory

RECOMMENDED FOR HELP WITH:

- Reducing cardiovascular disease
- Heart health
- Strong bones
- Immunity
- Cancer prevention
- Enhanced brain function and memory
- Immunity

SALMON

Salmon is believed to be among the top five most-consumed fish in the United States, and fresh salmon sales are on the rise in the UK. Salmon meat comes in many varieties, from salmon steaks to raw sushi, and lox/smoked to canned. Salmon is primarily found in the Atlantic and Pacific Oceans, with contention over the best farming and fishing practices. Salmon is full of essential vitamins and minerals: incredibly rich in omega-3 and omega-6, with essential amino acids, low sodium, and high selenium, vitamins B12 and B6, and folate. Salmon is lower in saturated fat than beef. Due to the low purine content, salmon is considered safe in moderation for those suffering from gout. The American Pregnancy Association recommends avoiding smoked fish during pregnancy due to possible listeria contamination, but fresh or canned salmon can be eaten in moderation.

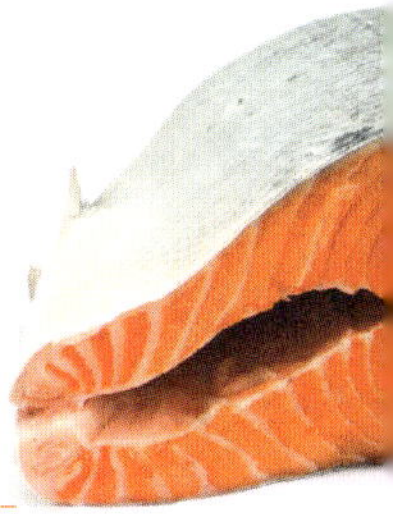

Salmon (farmed, Atlantic)

The same portion of wild salmon has 155 calories, 2,198 mg of omega-3, and 187 mg of omega-6.

NUTRIENTS IN 3 OZ.* FARMED ATLANTIC SALMON, COOKED:

Calories, 175
Folate, 28.9 mcg
Magnesium, 25.5 mg
Niacin, 6.8 mg
Pantothenic acid, 1.3 mg
Phosphorus, 214 mg
Potassium, 326 mg
Protein, 19 g
Riboflavin, 0.1 mg
Selenium, 35.2 mcg
Thiamin, 0.3 mg
Total omega-3 fatty acids, 1,921 mg
Total omega-6 fatty acids, 566 mg
Vitamin B6, 0.5 mg
Vitamin B12, 2.4 mcg
Vitamin C, 3.1 mg

*Farmed Atlantic salmon fillets are on average 14 oz.

Glycemic load: 0
Inflammatory index: Strongly anti-inflammatory

Salmon (chinook), smoked

NUTRIENTS IN 3 OZ. CHINOOK SALMON, SMOKED:

Calories, 99
Copper, 0.2 mg
Iron, 0.7 mg
Magnesium, 15.3 mg
Niacin, 4 mg
Pantothenic acid, 0.7 mg
Phosphorus, 139 mg
Potassium, 149 mg
Protein, 16 g
Riboflavin, 1 mg
Selenium, 27.5 mcg
Sodium, 666 mg
Total omega-3 fatty acids, 445 mg
Total omega-6 fatty acids, 401 mg
Vitamin B6, 0.2 mg
Vitamin B12, 2.8 mcg
Vitamin E, 1.1 mg

*Wild Atlantic salmon fillets are on average 12 oz.

Glycemic load: 0
Inflammatory index: Anti-inflammatory

Salmon (chum), cooked

NUTRIENTS IN 3 OZ.* CHUM SALMON, COOKED:

Calories, 131
Magnesium, 23.8 mg
Niacin, 7.2 mg
Pantothenic acid, 0.7 mg
Phosphorus, 309 mg
Potassium, 468 mg
Protein, 22 g
Riboflavin, 0.2 mg
Selenium, 39.8 mcg
Thiamin, 0.1 mg
Total omega-3 fatty acids, 807 mg
Total omega-6 fatty acids, 65.4 mg
Vitamin B6, 0.4 mg
Vitamin B12, 2.9 mcg

*Chum Atlantic salmon fillets are on average 12 oz.

Glycemic load: 0
Inflammatory index: Strongly anti-inflammatory

Salmon (pink), canned

Canned sockeye salmon provides roughly the same nutritional breakdown as pink salmon.

NUTRIENTS IN 3 OZ.* PINK SALMON, CANNED:

Calories, 117
Calcium, 178.8 mg
Niacin, 5.4 mg
Phosphorus, 276.3 mg
Potassium, 273.9 mg
Protein, 18 g
Riboflavin, 0.3 mg
Selenium, 27.9 mcg
Total omega-3 fatty acids, 1,476 mg
Total omega-6 fatty acids, 48.6 mg
Vitamin B6, 0.3 mg
Vitamin B12, 3.6 mcg

*1 can is roughly 5 oz.

Glycemic load: 0
Inflammatory index: Anti-inflammatory

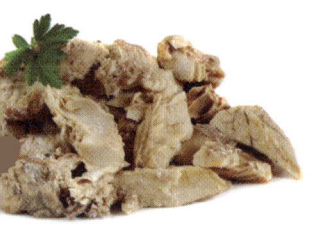

Salmon (red), smoked

NUTRIENTS IN 3 OZ. RED SALMON, SMOKED:

Calories, 174
Magnesium, 32.7 mg
Niacin, 11.1 mg
Phosphorus, 294 mg
Potassium, 396 mg
Protein, 30 g
Riboflavin, 0.3 mg
Selenium, 37.5 mcg
Sodium, 489 mg
Total omega-3 fatty acids, 1,545 mg
Total omega-6 fatty acids, 100.8 mg
Vitamin B6, 0.3 mg
Vitamin B12, 6.3 mcg

HEALTH AND HEALING BENEFITS OF SALMON:

HEART AND BLOOD HEALTH:

Omega-3 and -6 help protect against stroke, heart disease, and diabetes, as well as regulating blood pressure. Vitamins B12 and B6 maintain healthy red blood cells and improve their ability to carry oxygen to the body's cells. Growing children and adolescents, plus menstruating, pregnant, or lactating women have an increased need for iron. Low levels of B12 lead to anemia and potential damage to the spinal cord and brain. Folate assists in cholesterol metabolism.

ENHANCED BRAIN FUNCTION:

Omega-3 improves brain function and may aid memory. Folate is important for brain function, and is especially important during pregnancy for reducing the risk of spinal and mental defects in the fetus. It may also help protect against Alzheimer's.

STRONG MUSCLES AND BONES:

Protein helps build and repair bones, tissues, hormones, and body chemicals. Phosphorus assists healthy bone formation.

IMMUNITY:

Selenium and omega-6 improve immune system function.

Glycemic load: 0
Inflammatory index: Strongly anti-inflammatory

CANCER PROTECTION:

Studies have shown a link between consumption of selenium and a reduction in the risk of cancer. It is thought that selenium promotes DNA repair in damaged cells and inhibits the increase of cancer cells.

Glycemic load: 0
Inflammatory index: Mildly anti-inflammatory

RECOMMENDED FOR HELP WITH:

- Reducing cardiovascular disease
- Blood health
- Enhanced brain function and memory
- Strong bones
- Immunity
- Cancer protection

Sardines (Atlantic), canned

Sardines are small, oily saltwater fish known to promote heart health with high omega-6 and omega-3. It is recommended that you look for BPA-free canned sardines (or opt for fresh), as BPA is shown to increase cancer growth and diabetes. Sardines are also very high in cholesterol. They are a rich source of protein, vitamins, and minerals, and one of the few natural food sources of vitamin D. Sardines strengthen the cardiovascular and digestive systems and reduce the risk of disease. Sardines are low in mercury and can be eaten in moderation during pregnancy.

NUTRIENTS IN 1 OZ.* ATLANTIC SARDINES, CANNED:

Calories, 58
Calcium, 107 mg
Iron, 0.8 mg
Niacin, 1.5 mg
Phosphorus, 137 mg
Protein, 7 g
Riboflavin, 0.1 mg
Selenium, 14.8 mcg
Sodium, 141 mg
Total omega-3 fatty acids, 414 mg
Total omega-6 fatty acids, 992 mg
Vitamin B12, 2.5 mcg
Vitamin D, 76.2 IU

*1 can is roughly 4 oz.

HEALTH AND HEALING BENEFITS:

HEART AND BLOOD HEALTH:

Omega-3, omega-6, and protein protect against stroke, heart disease, and diabetes. Omega-6 regulates blood pressure. Vitamin B12 and iron maintain healthy red blood cells and improve their ability to carry oxygen to the body's cells. Growing children and adolescents, plus menstruating, pregnant, or lactating women have an increased need for iron. Low levels of B12 lead to anemia and potential damage to the spinal cord and brain.

MUSCLES AND BONES:

Protein helps build and repair bones, tissues, hormones, and body chemicals. Calcium and phosphorus assist healthy bone formation. Vitamin D promotes calcium absorption.

IMMUNITY:

Selenium and omega-6 improve immune system function.

Glycemic load: 0
Inflammatory index: Strongly anti-inflammatory

RECOMMENDED FOR HELP WITH:

- Regulating blood pressure
- Blood health
- Enhanced brain function and memory
- Strong bones
- Immunity

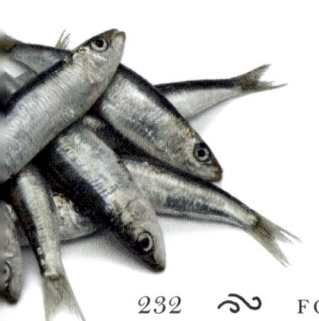

Scallops

Scallops are marine bivalve mollusks found in oceans all over the world. The name "scallop" applies to both the creature and the meat itself. Scallops are a lean source of protein that is low in calories and saturated fat, making them good for weight management. They are, however, high in cholesterol. They are high in vitamin B12 and super-rich in fatty acids—in particular, omega-6, which is integral to brain and immune system function, which, with omega-3, reduces the risk of heart disease and high blood pressure. If you suffer from gout, watch your consumption of this food. Scallops are low in mercury and can be eaten in moderation during pregnancy.

NUTRIENTS IN 3 OZ. SCALLOPS, STEAMED:

Calories, 93
Copper, 0.3 mg
Iron, 2.4 mg
Magnesium, 46.2 mg
Phosphorus, 283.8 mg
Potassium, 399 mg
Protein, 18 g
Selenium, 23.4 mcg
Total omega-3 fatty acids, 1,242 mg
Total omega-6 fatty acids, 2,976 mg
Vitamin B12, 1.2 mcg
Zinc, 2.4 mg

HEALTH AND HEALING BENEFITS:

WEIGHT LOSS:

Scallops are a lean source of protein, low in calories and saturated fat. Magnesium is key to healthy metabolism.

HEART AND BLOOD HEALTH:

Omega-3 and -6 help protect against stroke, heart disease, and diabetes, as well as regulating blood pressure. Iron maintains healthy red blood cells and improves their ability to carry oxygen. Growing children and adolescents, plus menstruating, pregnant, or lactating women have an increased need for iron.

ENHANCED BRAIN FUNCTION:

Omega-6 is integral to brain function. Omega-3 improves brain function and is believed to aid memory.

IMMUNITY:

Selenium and omega-6 improve immunity, as does zinc.

MUSCLES AND BONES:

Protein helps build and repair bones and tissues. Phosphorus and magnesium assist healthy bone formation.

Glycemic load: 0
Inflammatory index: Mildly anti-inflammatory

RECOMMENDED FOR HELP WITH:

- Weight loss
- Heart health
- Enhanced brain function
- Blood health
- Immunity
- Joint health

Shrimp

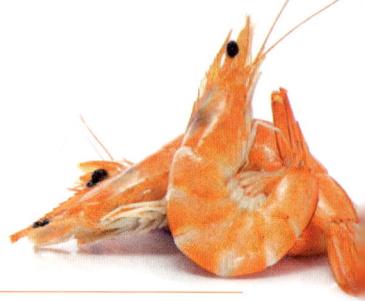

Shrimp are a widespread marine crustacean. The term "shrimp" is often used generally for a number of similarly shaped crustaceans and sometimes synonymously with "prawn." In North America, "shrimp" is the prevalent term, where they are the most popular seafood; however, in the UK, "prawn" is most often used, especially for larger shrimp. According to the American Heart Association, moderate consumption of shellfish (including shrimp) contributes to a heart-healthy diet. Shrimp contain essential amino acids, including tryptophan, which helps stabilize mood and sleep, as well as selenium, which boosts immunity. However, they are high in cholesterol. If you suffer from gout, watch your consumption. Shrimp are low in mercury and can be eaten in moderation during pregnancy. Allergy to shrimp and other shellfish is relatively common; if you show symptoms, get treatment immediately.

NUTRIENTS IN 3 OZ. SHRIMP, COOKED:

Calories, 101
Copper, 0.2 mg
Iron, 0.3 mg
Magnesium, 31.5 mg
Niacin, 2.3 mg
Phosphorus, 260.1 mg
Potassium, 144.5 mg
Protein, 19.4 g
Selenium, 42.1 mcg
Sodium, 804.9 mg
Total omega-3 fatty acids, 245 mg
Total omega-6 fatty acids, 179 mg
Vitamin A (RAE), 76.5 mcg
Vitamin B6, 0.2 mg
Vitamin B12, 1.4 mcg
Vitamin E, 1.9 mg
Zinc, 1.4 mg

HEALTH AND HEALING BENEFITS:

HEART AND BLOOD HEALTH:

Fatty acids and protein protect the body against stroke, heart disease, and diabetes, and lower blood pressure. Vitamin B12 and iron maintain healthy red blood cells and improve their ability to carry oxygen to the body's cells. Growing children and adolescents, plus menstruating, pregnant, or lactating women, have an increased need for iron. Low levels of B12 lead to anemia and potential damage to the spinal cord and brain. Copper contributes to blood vessel health.

STRONG MUSCLES AND BONES:

Protein helps build and repair bones, tissues, hormones, and body chemicals. Amino acids help form muscle tissue and increase fat metabolism. This can help keep the body strong and increases athletic performance. Phosphorus assists healthy bone formation.

GOOD INTERNAL HEALTH:

Amino acids work to keep organs healthy and functioning properly, including the heart, brain, and liver.

MOOD STABILIZER:

Vitamin B6 is crucial to brain function, and tryptophan and vitamin B6 are believed to help stabilize mood.

ENERGY:

Copper and niacin play a key role in energy production, and vitamin E boosts stamina.

IMMUNITY:

Selenium and zinc improve immune system function.

CANCER PROTECTION:

Studies have shown a link between consumption of selenium and a reduction in the risk of cancer. It is thought that selenium promotes DNA repair in damaged cells and inhibits the increase of cancer cells. Vitamin E is believed to reduce the risk of cancer.

Glycemic load: 0
Inflammatory index: Mildly anti-inflammatory

RECOMMENDED FOR HELP WITH:

- Heart health
- Strong bones
- Mood
- Blood health
- Energy
- Immunity
- Possible cancer protection

Sole (flatfish)

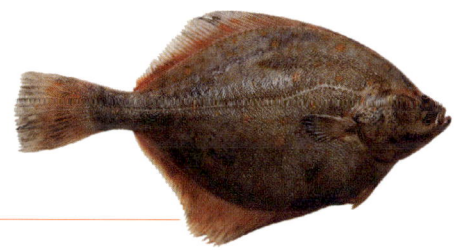

Sole is a flatfish, related to flounder, that dwells on the seabed. There are a number of types, from common or Dover sole to American sole. Like flounder, sole is a low-energy, dense fish, creating fullness on fewer calories. Sole is a good source of protein and low in saturated fat, but high in cholesterol. Due to the low purine content, sole is considered safe in moderation for gout sufferers, and due to low mercury is considered safe to eat in moderation during pregnancy. Common sole is at risk of unsustainable sourcing.

NUTRIENTS IN 3 OZ.* SOLE, COOKED:

Calories, 99
Magnesium, 49.3 mg
Niacin, 1.9 mg
Phosphorus, 246 mg
Potassium, 292 mg
Protein, 21 g
Selenium, 49.5 mcg
Sodium, 89.3 mg
Total omega-3 fatty acids, 61 mg
Total omega-6 fatty acids, 4.8 mg
Vitamin B6, 0.2 mg
Vitamin B12, 2.1 mcg

*Sole fillets are on average 5 oz.

HEALTH AND HEALING BENEFITS:

WEIGHT LOSS:

Sole helps you feel fuller quicker. Magnesium is key to healthy metabolism.

STRONG MUSCLES AND BONES:

Protein, phosphorus, and magnesium build and maintain strong bones, tissues, and body chemicals.

HEART AND BLOOD HEALTH:

Fatty acids and protein help protect against stroke, heart disease, and diabetes, and lower blood pressure. Vitamins B12 and B6 maintain healthy red blood cells and improve their ability to carry oxygen to the body's cells. Low levels of B12 lead to anemia and potential damage to the spinal cord and brain.

CANCER PROTECTION:

Studies have shown a link between consumption of selenium and a reduction in the risk of cancer.

JOINT HEALTH:

Magnesium and selenium reduce joint inflammation.

IMMUNITY:

Selenium and zinc boost immunity.

Glycemic load: 0
Inflammatory index: Strongly anti-inflammatory

RECOMMENDED FOR HELP WITH:

- Weight loss
- Heart health
- Strong bones
- Blood health
- Anemia deficiency
- Immunity
- Joint health
- Possible cancer protection

Sturgeon

Sturgeon is best known for its eggs, which produce caviar. However, sturgeon meat itself contains essential amino acids and is low in sodium, though high in cholesterol. It is a great source of vitamin A, pivotal to tissue regeneration, preventing acne, and reducing the chances of heart attack or stroke. Vitamin B12 maintains healthy red blood cells, and niacin is important for energy production.

NUTRIENTS IN 3 OZ. STURGEON, COOKED:

Calories, 115
Folate, 14.5 mcg
Iron, 0.8 mg
Magnesium, 38.2 mg
Niacin, 8.6 mg
Pantothenic acid, 0.7 mg
Potassium, 309 mg
Protein, 18 g
Selenium, 13.8 mcg
Total omega-3 fatty acids, 471 mg
Total omega-6 fatty acids, 73.9 mg
Vitamin A (RAE), 224 mcg
Vitamin B6, 0.2 mg
Vitamin B12, 2.1 mcg

HEALTH AND HEALING BENEFITS:

HEART AND BLOOD HEALTH:

Fatty acids and protein help protect against stroke, heart disease, and diabetes, and lower blood pressure. Vitamin A helps prevent cardiovascular disease. Folate reduces the risk of heart disease and hypertension. Vitamins B12 and B6, and iron maintain healthy red blood cells and improve their ability to carry oxygen. Growing children and adolescents, plus menstruating, pregnant, or lactating women have an increased need for iron. Low levels of B12 lead to anemia and potential damage to the spinal cord and brain.

STRONG BONES, MUSCLES, AND TISSUE:

Protein and magnesium build and maintain strong bones, tissues, and body chemicals. Vitamin A and fatty acids assist tissue repair.

ENHANCED BRAIN FUNCTION:

Fatty acids and folate are integral to brain function and are important during pregnancy for the developing fetus and may also protect against Alzheimer's.

TISSUE REGENERATION:

Vitamin A is central to tissue regeneration, and fatty acids and protein assist in cellular regeneration.

IMMUNITY:

Selenium and zinc boost immunity.

Glycemic load: 0
Inflammatory index: Moderately anti-inflammatory

RECOMMENDED FOR HELP WITH:

- Heart and blood health
- Strong bones and tissue
- Anemia deficiency
- Immunity
- Healthy skin
- Joint health
- Developing fetus during pregnancy

Swordfish

Swordfish is an excellent source of protein and omega-3, and one of the few natural food sources of vitamin D. The protein and fatty acids help build and protect bone and tissue, as well as protecting the body against stroke and heart disease. Vitamin D contributes to healthy bones. Selenium may help protect against cancer and, alongside vitamin D, boost immune system function. Swordfish is high in cholesterol and mercury. The USDA and American Pregnancy Association recommend avoiding swordfish during pregnancy, and swordfish should be limited in the diets of others.

NUTRIENTS IN 3 OZ. SWORDFISH, COOKED:

Calories, 132
Copper, 0.1 mg
Iron, 0.9 mg
Magnesium, 28.9 mg
Niacin, 10 mg
Phosphorus, 286 mg
Potassium, 314 mg
Protein, 22 g
Riboflavin, 0.1 mg
Selenium, 52.5 mcg
Sodium, 97.8 mg
Total omega-3 fatty
    acids, 898 mg
Total omega-6 fatty
    acids, 31.5 mg
Vitamin B6, 0.3 mg
Vitamin B12, 1.7 mcg
Vitamin D, 566 IU
Zinc, 1.2 mg

HEALTH AND HEALING BENEFITS:

ENERGY:

Niacin and copper aid energy production.

HEART AND BLOOD HEALTH:

Omega-3 and -6 protect against stroke, heart disease, and diabetes and regulate blood pressure. Vitamins B12 and B6 and iron maintain healthy red blood cells.

ENHANCED BRAIN FUNCTION:

Omega-3 and -6 improve brain function and memory.

HEALTHY SKIN:

Zinc, copper, and riboflavin promote healthy skin.

IMMUNITY:

Selenium and zinc boost immunity.

JOINT HEALTH:

Magnesium, omega-6, and selenium reduce joint inflammation.

STRONG MUSCLES AND BONES:

Protein helps maintain bones and tissues. Magnesium, phosphorus, and vitamin D aid healthy bone formation.

CANCER PROTECTION:

Studies have shown a link between consumption of selenium and a reduction in the risk of cancer.

Glycemic load: 0
Inflammatory index: Strongly anti-inflammatory

RECOMMENDED FOR HELP WITH:

- Heart health
- Enhanced brain function
- Strong bones
- Blood health
- Anemia deficiency
- Energy
- Healthy skin
- Immunity
- Joint health
- Possible cancer protection

Tilapia

Tilapia are believed to have originated in Africa but have since found their way to other warm climates and fish farms in colder climates, and are now one of the most commonly consumed fish in the United States. Tilapia are low in sodium and amino acids, but high in cholesterol. Protein is important for muscle maintenance and energy, and tilapia pack a punch with their high protein levels. Selenium improves immunity. Due to low mercury, tilapia are considered safe to eat in moderation while pregnant by the American Pregnancy Association. Serve tilapia grilled, baked, or steamed.

NUTRIENTS IN 3 OZ. TILAPIA, COOKED:

Calories, 110
Iron, 0.6 mg
Magnesium, 28.9 mg
Niacin, 4 mg
Phosphorus, 173.4 mg
Protein, 22 g
Riboflavin, 0.1 mg
Selenium, 46.2 mcg
Thiamin, 0.1 mg
Total omega-3 fatty acids, 240 mg
Total omega-6 fatty acids, 300 mg
Vitamin B6, 0.1 mg
Vitamin B12, 1.6 mcg

HEALTH AND HEALING BENEFITS:

HEART AND BLOOD HEALTH:

Omega-3 and -6 protect against stroke, heart disease, and diabetes, and lower blood pressure. Vitamins B12 and B6 and iron maintain and oxygenate blood.

INTERNAL HEALTH:

Amino acids work to keep organs healthy and functioning properly, including the heart, brain, and liver.

ENERGY:

Niacin, magnesium, and copper play a key role in energy production.

Glycemic load: 0
Inflammatory index: Mildly anti-inflammatory

RECOMMENDED FOR HELP WITH:

- Heart health
- Strong bones
- Blood health
- Energy
- Immunity
- Joint health
- Possible cancer protection

STRONG MUSCLES AND BONES:

Protein helps build and repair bones, tissues, hormones, and body chemicals. Amino acids help form muscle tissue and increase fat metabolism. This can help keep the body strong and increases athletic performance. Magnesium and phosphorus assist healthy bone formation.

JOINT HEALTH:

Magnesium, omega-6, and selenium reduce joint inflammation.

IMMUNITY:

Selenium and omega-6 improve immune system function.

CANCER PROTECTION:

Studies have shown a link between consumption of selenium and a reduction in the risk of cancer.

Trout

Trout refers to a large family of oily freshwater fish, although some do travel to the ocean. In the United States, there are a number of species, including lake trout and rainbow trout. Trout are rich in omega-3 and omega-6, as well as amino acids and protein, and low in sodium but high in cholesterol. Amino acids and protein work together to build and repair bones and tissue and maintain organ function. Omega fatty acids work together to decrease the risk of heart disease and high blood pressure, as well as helping with brain function. Vitamin B12 helps maintain healthy blood cells. Freshwater trout are low in mercury and can be eaten in moderation during pregnancy.

NUTRIENTS IN 3 OZ.* RAINBOW TROUT, COOKED:

Calories, 143
Calcium, 25.5 mg
Folate, 10.2 mcg
Magnesium, 25.5 mg
Niacin, 5.7 mg
Pantothenic acid, 1.7 mg
Phosphorus, 230 mg
Potassium, 382 mg
Protein, 20.2 g
Riboflavin, 0.1 mg
Selenium, 23.9 mcg
Thiamin, 0.1 mg
Total omega-3 fatty acids, 837 mg
Total omega-6 fatty acids, 547 mg
Vitamin A (RAE), 85 mcg
Vitamin B6, 0.3 mg
Vitamin B12, 3.5 mcg
Vitamin C, 2.5 mg

*Rainbow trout fillets are on average 3 oz.

Glycemic load: 0
Inflammatory index: Strongly anti-inflammatory

HEALTH AND HEALING BENEFITS:

GOOD INTERNAL HEALTH:

Amino acids work to keep organs healthy and functioning properly, including the heart, brain, and liver.

STRONG MUSCLES AND BONES:

Protein helps build and repair bones, tissues, hormones, and body chemicals. Amino acids help form muscle tissue and increase fat metabolism. This can help keep the body strong and increases athletic performance. Magnesium and phosphorus assist healthy bone formation.

CANCER PROTECTION:

Studies have shown a link between consumption of selenium and a reduction in the risk of cancer. It is thought that selenium promotes DNA repair in damaged cells and inhibits the increase of cancer cells.

ENHANCED BRAIN FUNCTION:

Omega-3 and -6 improve brain function and may improve memory.

IMMUNITY:

Selenium and omega-6 improve immune system function.

JOINT HEALTH:

Magnesium, omega-6, and selenium reduce joint inflammation.

ENERGY:

Niacin, magnesium, and copper play a key role in energy production.

HEART AND BLOOD HEALTH:

Omega-3 and -6 help protect against stroke, heart disease, and diabetes, as well as regulating blood pressure. Vitamins B12 and B6 maintain healthy red blood cells and improve their ability to carry oxygen to the body's cells. Low levels of B12 lead to anemia and potential damage to the spinal cord and brain.

Glycemic load: 0
Inflammatory index: Mildly anti-inflammatory

RECOMMENDED FOR HELP WITH:

- Heart health
- Strong bones
- Enhanced brain function
- Blood health
- Energy
- Immunity
- Joint health
- Possible cancer protection

TUNA

Tuna is a saltwater fish with widespread habitat and a number of species, including bluefin, yellowfin (ahi), bigeye, and albacore. Bluefin tuna is especially high in omega-3 and protein and low in sodium. It is also a good source of vitamins B12 and A. Yellowfin tuna is low in saturated fat

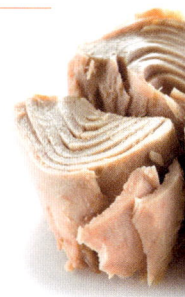

and sodium, but high in cholesterol. It is a good source of selenium, niacin, and vitamin B6. Both are protein-rich. Due to the low purine content, light canned tuna is considered safe in moderation for those suffering from gout. The American Pregnancy Association recommends avoiding ahi and bigeye tuna during pregnancy due to high mercury levels.

Tuna (bluefin)

NUTRIENTS IN 3 OZ. BLUEFIN TUNA, COOKED:

Calories, 156
Copper, 0.1 mg
Iron, 1.1 mg
Magnesium, 54.4 mg
Niacin, 9 mg
Pantothenic acid, 1.2 mg
Phosphorus, 277 mg
Potassium, 275 mg
Protein, 25 g
Riboflavin, 0.3 mg
Selenium, 39.8 mcg
Thiamin, 0.2 mg
Total omega-3 fatty acids, 1,414 mg
Total omega-6 fatty acids, 57.8 mg
Vitamin A (RAE), 643 mcg
Vitamin B6, 0.4 mg
Vitamin B12, 9.2 mcg
Zinc, 0.7 mg

Glycemic load: 0
Inflammatory index: Strongly anti-inflammatory

Tuna (yellowfin/ahi)

NUTRIENTS IN 3 OZ. YELLOWFIN TUNA, COOKED:

Calories, 118
Iron, 0.8 mg
Magnesium, 54.4 mg
Niacin, 10.1 mg
Pantothenic acid, 0.7 mg
Phosphorus, 208 mg
Potassium, 484 mg
Protein, 25 g
Selenium, 39.8 mcg
Thiamin, 0.4 mg
Total omega-3 fatty acids, 264 mg
Total omega-6 fatty acids, 8.5 mg
Vitamin B6, 0.9 mg
Vitamin B12, 0.5 mcg
Zinc, 0.6 mg

Glycemic load: 0
Inflammatory index: Mildly anti-inflammatory

Tuna (light), canned in oil

Light canned tuna in water has 32 calories for the same portion.

NUTRIENTS IN 3 OZ. TUNA, CANNED IN OIL

Calories, 165
Niacin, 10.5 mg
Phosphorus, 261.3 mg
Protein, 24 g
Selenium, 63.9 mcg
Total omega-3 fatty acids, 169.8 mg
Total omega-6 fatty acids, 2,253 mg
Vitamin B12, 1.8 mcg

*1 can is roughly 5 oz.

Glycemic load: 0
Inflammatory index: Moderately anti-inflammatory

HEALTH AND HEALING BENEFITS OF TUNA:

HEART AND BLOOD HEALTH:

Omega-3 and -6 help protect against stroke, heart disease, and diabetes, as well as regulating blood pressure. Vitamin A helps reduce cardiovascular disease. Vitamins B12 and B6, and iron maintain healthy red blood cells and improve their ability to carry oxygen to the body's cells. Growing children and adolescents, plus menstruating, pregnant, or lactating women have an increased need for iron. Low levels of B12 lead to anemia and potential damage to the spinal cord and brain. Vitamin B6 deficiency is found in people with heart disease, premenstrual syndrome, atherosclerosis, and carpal tunnel syndrome.

TISSUE REGENERATION:

Vitamin A is central to tissue regeneration, and fatty acids and protein assist in cellular regeneration.

ENERGY:

Niacin, magnesium, and copper play a key role in energy production.

ENHANCED BRAIN FUNCTION:

Omega-3 and -6 improve brain function and may aid memory.

JOINT HEALTH:

Magnesium, omega-6, and selenium reduce joint inflammation.

RECOMMENDED FOR HELP WITH:

- Heart health
- Strong bones
- Tissue regeneration
- Enhanced brain function
- Blood health
- Energy
- Immunity
- Joint health
- Possible cancer protection

IMMUNITY:

Selenium, zinc, and omega-6 boost immunity.

STRONG MUSCLES AND BONES:

Protein helps build and repair bones, tissues, hormones, and body chemicals. Magnesium and phosphorus assist healthy bone formation.

CANCER PROTECTION:

Studies have shown a link between consumption of selenium and a reduction in the risk of cancer. It is thought that selenium promotes DNA repair in damaged cells and inhibits the increase of cancer cells.

Whitefish

Whitefish is a large family of fish that are mainly of the freshwater variety. Outside of the United States, whitefish is not a common term found on menus or in stores; rather, the individual fish name is used. Whitefish are low in sodium, and whitefish meat is exceedingly high in omega-3, while the eggs are high in vitamin B12. However, whitefish are very high in cholesterol. These fish are low in mercury and can be eaten in moderation during pregnancy.

NUTRIENTS IN 3 OZ.*
WHITEFISH, COOKED:

Calories, 146
Copper, 0.1 mg
Folate, 14.5 mcg
Magnesium, 35.7 mg
Manganese, 0.1 mg
Niacin, 3.3 mg
Pantothenic acid, 0.7 mg
Phosphorus, 294 mg
Potassium, 345 mg
Protein, 21 g
Riboflavin, 0.1 mg
Selenium, 13.8 mcg
Thiamin, 0.1 mg
Total omega-3 fatty acids, 1,748 mg
Total omega-6 fatty acids, 297 mg
Vitamin B6, 0.3 mg
Vitamin B12, 0.8 mcg
Zinc, 1.1 mg

*Whitefish fillets are on average 6 oz.

HEALTH AND HEALING BENEFITS:

ENERGY:

Copper, niacin, and magnesium play a key role in energy production.

> **Glycemic load:** 0
> **Inflammatory index:** Strongly anti-inflammatory

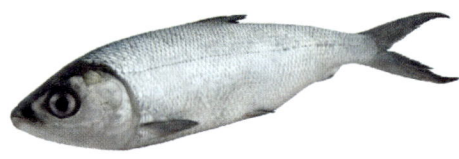

STRONG MUSCLES AND BONES:

Protein helps build and repair bones, tissues, hormones, and body chemicals. Calcium is integral to bone growth, and magnesium and phosphorus assist healthy bone formation.

IMMUNITY:

Selenium, zinc, and omega-6 improve immune system function.

HEART AND BLOOD HEALTH:

Omega-3 and -6 help protect against stroke, heart disease, and diabetes, as well as regulating blood pressure. Folate reduces the risk of heart disease and hypertension. Vitamins B12 and B6 maintain healthy red blood cells and improve their ability to carry oxygen to the body's cells. Low levels of B12 lead to anemia and potential damage to the spinal cord and brain. Vitamin B6 deficiency is found in people with heart disease, premenstrual syndrome, atherosclerosis, and carpal tunnel syndrome.

ENHANCED BRAIN FUNCTION:

Omega-3 improves brain function and is believed to aid memory. Folate is important for brain function, and is especially important during pregnancy for reducing the risk of spinal and mental defects in the fetus. It may also help protect against Alzheimer's.

JOINT HEALTH:

Magnesium, omega-6, and selenium reduce joint inflammation.

> **RECOMMENDED FOR HELP WITH:**
> - Heart health
> - Strong bones
> - Blood health
> - Enhanced brain function
> - Energy
> - Immunity
> - Joint health
> - Developing fetus during pregnancy

Whiting

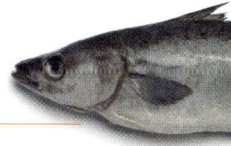

Whiting refers to a number of different species, including English, Japanese, and Pacific whiting, and can sometimes refer specifically to hake or pollock. Whiting contains essential amino acids and high protein, strengthening bones and protecting the heart. It is low in saturated fat but very high in cholesterol. Whiting is a good source of vitamin B12, selenium, phosphorus, and potassium. These nutrients maintain bone strength, blood health, and organ function, and strengthen the immune system. Whiting are low in mercury and can be eaten in moderation during pregnancy. Pacific whiting in particular is reported to be sustainably sourced.

Treats

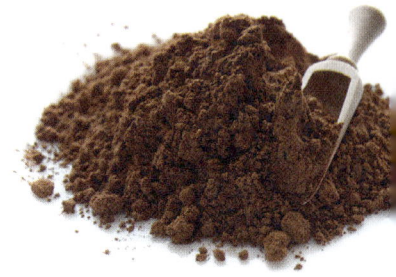

Treats rarely provide high-quality nutrition. The carbohydrates are generally sugar, and the fat varies but adds no value. Treats should only be consumed on occasion and balanced with a high intake of antioxidant foods.

Cocoa powder

For centuries, cocoa beans, the edible part of the cacao tree's seedpod, were prized as a medicine and aphrodisiac in South America. The Aztecs named it *yollotl eztli*, meaning "heart blood," and used it to make a health elixir drink called *xocoatl*. When the Europeans came to the New World, they added sugar, vanilla, and spices; chocolate became all the rage across Europe.

NUTRIENTS IN 1 TBSP. OF DRY, UNSWEETENED COCOA POWDER:

Calories, 12
Copper, 0.2 mg
Dietary fiber, 1.7 g
Iron, 0.7 mg
Magnesium, 26.2 mg
Manganese, 0.2 mg
Phosphorus, 38.5 mg
Potassium, 80.0 mg
Protein, 1.0 g
Zinc, 0.4 mg

HEALTH AND HEALING BENEFITS:

HEART AND BLOOD HEALTH:

Protein, calcium, carotene, thiamin, riboflavin, magnesium, sulfur, antioxidants, and fatty acids help lower LDL cholesterol and may reduce heart disease and cancer. Flavonols improve blood flow.

ANTIOXIDANT:

Antioxidants help decrease cell damage, protecting against disease.

Glycemic load: 4
Inflammatory index: Minimally inflammatory

RECOMMENDED FOR HELP WITH:

- Cholesterol
- Coronary heart disease
- Blood pressure

Dark chocolate (over 70%)

Good news: dark chocolate is rich in antioxidants, which help protect against cell damage. It also contains anandamide, a mood-enhancing neurotransmitter with a name that means "bliss" in Sanskrit. It's low in cholesterol and sodium, but high in saturated fat. The mineral benefits will outweigh this if eaten in moderate quantities—no more than one-third to two-thirds of an ounce per day. Milk chocolate does not offer the same health benefits, as it has a higher sugar content and the milk prevents compound absorption.

NUTRIENTS IN 1 BAR OF DARK CHOCOLATE, 70–85% COCOA SOLIDS*:

Calories, 604
Carbohydrate, 46.4 g
Calcium, 73.7 mg
Cholesterol, 3 mg
Copper, 1.8 mg
Dietary fiber, 11 g
Iron, 12 mg
Magnesium, 230 mg
Manganese, 2 mg
Potassium, 722 mg
Protein, 7.8 g
Saturated fat, 24.7 g
Selenium, 6.9 mcg
Sodium, 20.2 mg
Sugars, 24.2 g
Total fat, 43 g
Vitamin A (RAE), 2 mcg
Zinc, 3.3 mg

HEALTH AND HEALING BENEFITS:

HEART AND BLOOD HEALTH:

Potassium and sodium lower blood pressure, and magnesium maintains steady heart rhythm. Copper helps store iron, which oxygenates blood.

BONE HEALTH:

Potassium and magnesium maintain strong bones.

*1 bar is roughly 3.5 oz.

Glycemic load: 10
Inflammatory index: Moderately inflammatory

RECOMMENDED FOR HELP WITH:

- Maintaining blood pressure
- Bone formation
- Oxygenating blood

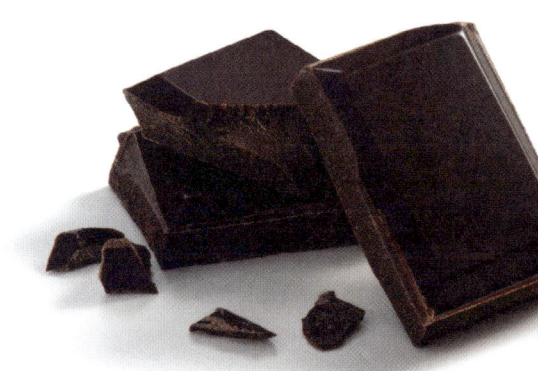

TREATS

Vegetables, non-starchy

Non-starchy vegetables contain lower amounts of carbohydrates and calories than starchy vegetables, and are packed with vitamins, antioxidants, and fiber.

Arugula (rocket), raw

This zesty salad leaf is an excellent source of nitric oxide, which improves heart health. It's loaded with health-boosting nutrients, from antioxidant vitamin A to immune-boosting zinc. A favorite in Italian cuisine, the younger, paler leaves have a more delicate flavor suited to salads and pesto, while the older, darker leaves pack a peppery punch, ideal for adding pizzazz to your pizza.

NUTRIENTS IN ½ CUP OF RAW ARUGULA:

Calories, 3
Calcium, 16 mg
Copper, 0 mg
Dietary fiber, 0.2 g
Folate, 9.7 mcg
Iron, 0.1 mg
Magnesium, 4.7 mg
Manganese, 0 mg
Pantothenic acid 0 mg
Phosphorus, 5.2 mg
Potassium, 36.9 mg
Protein, 0.3 g
Riboflavin, 0 mg
Thiamin, 0 mg
Vitamin A (RAE), 11.9 mcg
Vitamin B6, 0 mg
Vitamin C, 1.5 mg
Vitamin K, 10.9 mg
Zinc, 0 mg

Glycemic load: 1
Inflammatory index: Mildly anti-inflammatory

RECOMMENDED FOR HELP WITH:

- Cancer prevention
- Liver health
- Gastrointestinal ulcers

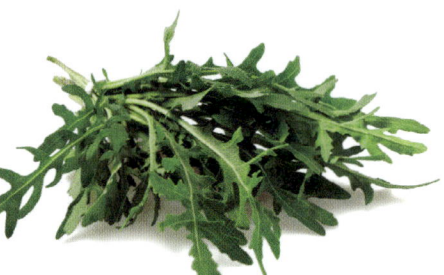

HEALTH AND HEALING BENEFITS:

CARDIOVASCULAR HEALTH:

Vitamin A helps prevent free radicals oxidizing cholesterol in the bloodstream—oxidized cholesterol can build up in blood vessel walls, initiating the development of atherosclerosis, which can result in heart attack or stroke.

ANTIOXIDANT:

Antioxidant vitamins A and C protect cells from free radical damage. Antioxidants are essential for optimal health. These compounds help decrease free radical molecules, which damage cells and lead to every known disease.

GASTROINTESTINAL HEALTH:

Studies have linked arugula with combating gastrointestinal ulcers due to its high antioxidant content.

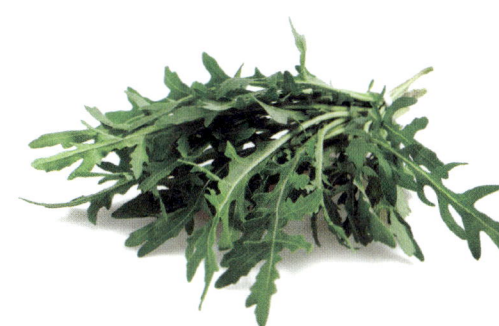

Artichoke

Artichokes contain more immune-boosting vitamin C than oranges. They're packed with vitamins and minerals, including vitamin K, essential for blood clotting, free-radical-zapping manganese, and cholesterol-regulating folate. They're also a very good source of fiber: just one ounce contains 10% of your recommended daily value, helping to maintain a healthy digestive system.

NUTRIENTS IN ½ CUP OF ARTICHOKE HEARTS, BOILED WITHOUT SALT:

Calories, 44
Copper, 0.1 mg
Dietary fiber, 4.8 g
Folate, 74.8 mcg
Magnesium, 35.3 mg
Manganese, 0.2 mg
Niacin, 0.9 mg
Phosphorus, 61.3 mg
Potassium, 240 mg
Vitamin C, 6.2 mg
Vitamin K, 12.4 mcg

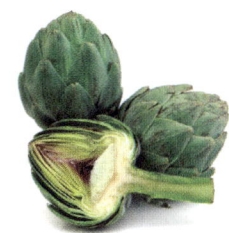

Glycemic load: 3
Inflammatory index: Mildly anti-inflammatory

RECOMMENDED FOR HELP WITH:

- Immunity
- Digestion

VEGETABLES, NON-STARCHY

HEALTH AND HEALING BENEFITS:

DIGESTION:

Fiber helps move food through your digestive system. Additionally, getting more fiber in your diet lowers blood cholesterol levels, prevents constipation, and helps you feel full faster.

IMMUNE HEALTH:

Nature's own powerful antioxidant vitamin C helps prevent cell damage from free radicals. Vitamin C is one of the most critical vitamins for supporting immune health.

MAINTAINING HEALTHY CHOLESTEROL:

A good source of folate, one of the most critical vitamins, especially during pregnancy, where deficiencies increase the risk of spinal defects and mental retardation in the fetus. In the general population, folate is particularly important in cholesterol metabolism and in all aspects of brain function.

Asparagus

Succulent asparagus spears have been considered a delicacy for many centuries. They're loaded with antioxidants, which help protect cells from free radicals, molecules which damage cells and lead to every known disease. Rich in phytonutrients known as saponins that have been shown to have anti-inflammatory and anti-cancer properties, asparagus packs a healthy, nutritious punch. Delicious in salads or on its own.

NUTRIENTS IN 4 SPEARS OF BOILED ASPARAGUS (HALF-INCH BASES):

Calories, 13
Calcium, 13.8 mg
Copper, 0.1 mg
Dietary fiber, 1.2 g
Folate, 89.4 mcg
Iron, 0.5 mg
Magnesium, 8.4 mg
Manganese, 0.1 mg
Niacin, 0.6 mg
Phosphorus, 32.4 mg
Potassium, 134 mg
Protein, 1.4 mg
Riboflavin, 0.1 mg
Selenium, 3.7 mcg
Thiamin, 0.1 mg
Vitamin A (RAE), 30 mcg
Vitamin C, 4.6 mg
Vitamin E, 0.9 mg
Vitamin K, 30.4 mg
Zinc, 0.4 mg

Glycemic load: 1
Inflammatory index: Mildly anti-inflammatory

RECOMMENDED FOR HELP WITH:

- Cancer prevention
- Regulating blood sugar levels and blood pressure

HEALTH AND HEALING BENEFITS:

ANTIOXIDANT:

Antioxidants are essential for optimal health. These compounds help decrease free radical molecules, which damage cells and lead to every known disease.

Asparagus is packed with antioxidant nutrients including vitamin C, beta-carotene, vitamin E, and the minerals zinc, manganese, and selenium.

ANTI-INFLAMMATORY:

Phytonutrients known as saponins have been shown to have anti-inflammatory and anti-cancer properties.

BLOOD REGULATION:

Intake of saponins has also been linked with improved blood pressure, improved blood sugar regulation, and better control of blood fat levels.

Beet greens

The leafy tops of the beetroot plant contain nitrates to help the body produce nitric oxide, which improves heart health. Beet greens are packed with even more health-boosting nutrients than the beetroot. They are very low in cholesterol, yet loaded with free-radical-zapping antioxidants, making them one of the healthiest greens. Just one ounce of beet greens contains in excess of your recommended daily value of vitamin K—raw greens provide about 140%, while cooked greens provide a huge 871%. Vitamin K helps blood to clot properly and promotes bone strength.

NUTRIENTS IN ½ CUP OF BEET GREENS, BOILED WITHOUT SALT:

Calories, 19
Calcium, 82.1 mg
Copper, 0.2 mg
Dietary fiber, 2.1 g
Folate, 10.1 mcg
Iron, 1.4 mg
Magnesium, 49 mg
Manganese, 0.4 mg
Pantothenic acid, 0.2 mg
Phosphorus, 29.5 mg
Potassium, 654 mg
Protein, 1.9 g
Riboflavin, 0.2 mg
Thiamin, 0.1 mg
Vitamin A (RAE), 276 mcg
Vitamin B6, 0.1 MG
Vitamin C, 17.9 mg
Vitamin E, 1.3 mg
Vitamin K, 348 mg
Zinc, 0.4 mg

Glycemic load: 4
Inflammatory index: Strongly anti-inflammatory

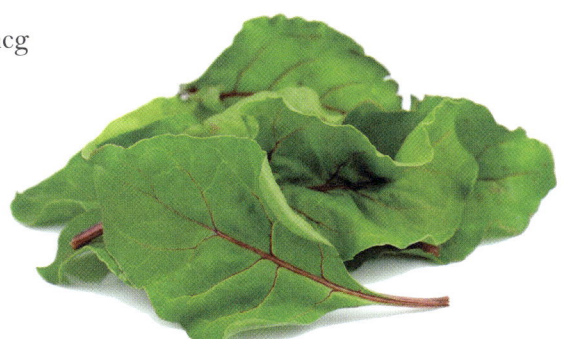

VEGETABLES, NON-STARCHY

HEALTH AND HEALING BENEFITS:

HEALTHY CIRCULATION:

Glycine betaine lowers homocysteine levels in the blood. Homocysteine can lead to atherosclerotic-plaque formation. Excess amounts of this compound in the blood can damage the blood vessels, resulting in the development of coronary heart disease, stroke, and peripheral vascular diseases.

ANTIOXIDANT:

Packed with free-radical-zapping antioxidants. Antioxidants are essential for optimal health. These compounds help decrease free radical molecules, which damage cells and lead to every known disease.

EYE HEALTH:

The carotenoid lutein plays an especially important role in eye health, including the health of the retina.

RECOMMENDED FOR HELP WITH:

- Weight loss
- Cardiovascular health
- Vision

BELL PEPPERS

Also known as sweet peppers or capsicums. Bell peppers are native to South America, but have spread to the rest of the world. They come in a variety of colors, red and green being the most common. Their crunchy, sweet, brightly colored skin makes them a favorite ingredient in a range of dishes from salads to sautées. Bell peppers are a great source of antioxidants, compounds that help decrease free radical molecules, which damage cells and lead to every known disease. Higher-heat cooking can damage some of the delicate phytonutrients in bell peppers, so use lower-heat methods for a short period of time to keep the nutrients intact.

NUTRIENTS IN 1 MEDIUM RAW GREEN BELL PEPPER:

Calories, 24
Copper, 0.1 mg
Dietary fiber, 2 g
Folate, 11.9 mcg
Magnesium, 11.9 mg
Manganese, 0.1
Niacin, 0.6 mg
Potassium, 208 mg
Thiamin, 0.1 mg
Vitamin A (RAE), 21.4 mcg
Vitamin B6, 0.3 mg
Vitamin C, 95.7 mg
Vitamin K, 8.8 mcg

Glycemic load: 2
Inflammatory index: Anti-inflammatory

Bell peppers (red)

One ounce of red bell pepper contains 16% of your recommended daily value of vision-boosting vitamin A and 80% of immune-boosting vitamin C, compared with 3% and 35% in the equivalent amount of green bell pepper.

HEALTH AND HEALING BENEFITS OF BELL PEPPERS:

ANTIOXIDANT:

Antioxidants are essential for optimal health. These compounds help decrease free radicals, which damage cells and lead to disease.

IMMUNE HEALTH:

Packed with vitamin C, which helps prevent damage from free radicals. Vitamin C is one of the most critical vitamins for supporting immunity.

RECOMMENDED FOR HELP WITH:
- Immunity
- Age-related macular degeneration

Broccoli

Broccoli is loaded with antioxidants to help protect cells against free radical damage, and sulforaphanes, molecules that may help to combat cancer. Nutrients in broccoli help the body to eliminate unwanted contaminants, resulting in a strong, positive detoxification impact. It's also rich in the flavanoid kaempferol, which lessens the impact of allergy-related substances on your body, providing broccoli with unique anti-inflammatory benefits. Its green or purple florets make a nutritious addition to a range of dishes from salads to stir fries.

NUTRIENTS IN ½ CUP OF CHOPPED OR DICED RAW BROCCOLI:

Calories, 15
Calcium, 20.7 mg
Dietary fiber, 1.1 g
Folate, 27.7 mcg
Iron, 0.3 mg
Magnesium, 9.2 mg
Pantothenic acid, 0.3 mg
Potassium, 139 mg
Protein, 1.2 g
Phosphorus, 29 mg
Riboflavin, 0.1 mg
Selenium, 1.1 mcg
Thiamin, 0 mg
Vitamin A (RAE), 13.6 mcg
Vitamin B6, 0.1 mg
Vitamin C, 39.2 mg
Vitamin E, 0.3 mg
Vitamin K, 44.9 mcg

Glycemic load: 1
Inflammatory index: Anti-inflammatory

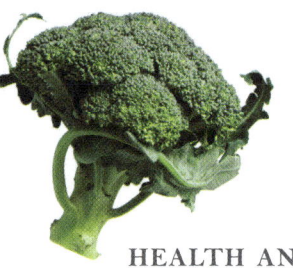

HEALTH AND HEALING BENEFITS:

DETOX SUPPORT:

Broccoli has a positive impact on your body's detoxification system. The phytonutrients glucoraphanin, gluconasturtiin, and glucobrassicin are found in a special combination in broccoli. Together they support the body's detox process, including activation, neutralization, and elimination of unwanted contaminants.

CANCER PREVENTION:

A storehouse of phytonutrients that have been linked with protecting against prostate, colon, pancreatic, and breast cancers.

IMMUNE HEALTH:

Packed with vitamin C, nature's own powerful antioxidant, which helps prevent cell damage from free radicals. Vitamin C is one of the most critical vitamins for supporting immune health.

RECOMMENDED FOR HELP WITH:

- Cancer prevention, especially prostate and colon
- Detoxing
- Immunity

Brussels sprouts

A great source of digestion-boosting fiber, immune-boosting vitamin C, and various phytochemical compounds, including glucosinolates which have been linked with protecting against cancer. Just one ounce of boiled Brussels sprouts contains nearly a third (29%) of your recommend daily value of vitamin C and almost half (49%) of vitamin K, which helps proper blood clotting and maintaining healthy bones.

NUTRIENTS IN ½ CUP OF BRUSSELS SPROUTS, BOILED WITHOUT SALT:

Calories, 28
Copper, 0.1 mg
Dietary fiber, 2 g
Folate, 46.8 mcg
Iron, 0.9 mg
Magnesium, 15.6 mg
Manganese, 0.2 mg
Phosphorus, 43.7 mg
Potassium, 247 mg
Riboflavin, 0.1 mg
Thiamin, 0.1 mg
Vitamin A (RAE), 30.4 mcg
Vitamin B6, 0.1 mg
Vitamin C, 48.4 mg
Vitamin K, 109 mcg

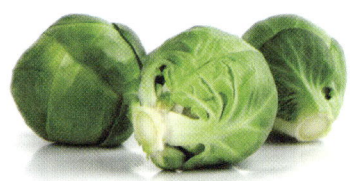

HEALTH AND HEALING BENEFITS:

CANCER PROTECTION:

Packed with important phytonutrients called glucosinolates, which have been linked with protecting against cancer.

IMMUNE HEALTH:

Packed with vitamin C, nature's own powerful antioxidant, which helps prevent cell damage from free radicals. Vitamin C is one of the most critical vitamins for supporting immune health.

DETOX SUPPORT:

Brussels sprouts are an outstanding source of glucosinolates, phytonutrients that help support your body's detoxification system.

Glycemic load: 1
Inflammatory index: Anti-inflammatory

RECOMMENDED FOR HELP WITH:

- Cancer prevention
- Immunity
- Detoxing

Burdock root

Burdock root is the tuber of the greater burdock plant. It is high in free-radical-zapping antioxidants, soothing mucilage, and carbohydrate- and fat-regulating insulin. Burdock root has long been used in traditional medicines to help purify the blood due to its diuretic properties. Its soothing, demulcent properties mean it has also traditionally been used to treat throat and chest problems.

NUTRIENTS IN 1 CUP OF BURDOCK ROOT (1-INCH PIECES), BOILED WITHOUT SALT:

Calories, 110
Magnesium, 48.8 mg
Manganese, 0.3 mg
Phosphorus, 26 mg
Potassium, 116 mg
Vitamin B6, 0.3 mg

HEALTH AND HEALING BENEFITS:

BLOOD SUGAR:

Insulin helps to reduce blood sugar levels and cholesterol.

CARDIOVASCULAR HEALTH:

Potassium helps to regulate heart rate and blood pressure.

BLOOD PURIFYING:

Burdock is a mild diuretic which helps expel toxins.

Glycemic load: 3
Inflammatory index: Mildly anti-inflammatory

RECOMMENDED FOR HELP WITH:

- Regulating blood sugar
- Mild laxative
- Cardiovascular health

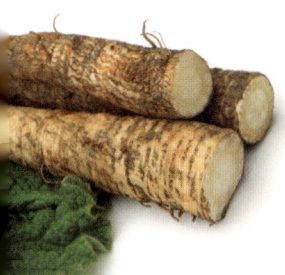

VEGETABLES, NON-STARCHY

CABBAGE

This leafy vegetable is packed with antioxidants and is high in fiber—one ounce contains 3% of your recommended daily value of dietary fiber. It's also packed with immune-boosting vitamin C and vitamin K, essential for blood clotting and bone nourishment. Steaming or sautéing cabbage can also provide special cholesterol-lowering benefits. The fiber-related components in cabbage do a better job of binding together with bile acids in your digestive tract when they've been steamed, making it easier for bile acids to be excreted. The result is a lowering of your cholesterol levels.

NUTRIENTS IN 1 CUP OF RAW CHOPPED CABBAGE:

Calories, 22
Calcium, 35.6 mg
Dietary fiber, 2.2 g
Folate, 38.3 mcg
Iron, 0.4 mg
Magnesium, 10.7 mg
Manganese, 0.1 mg
Phosphorus, 23.1 mg
Potassium, 151 mg
Thiamin, 0.1 mg
Vitamin B6, 0.1 mg
Vitamin C, 32.6 mg
Vitamin K, 67.6 mcg

Glycemic load: 1
Inflammatory index: Mildly anti-inflammatory

Cabbage, savoy

Savoy cabbage is a particularly good source of sinigrin, a glucosinolate which has been linked with unique cancer preventive properties, especially with respect to bladder cancer, colon cancer, and prostate cancer.

HEALTH AND HEALING BENEFITS OF CABBAGE:

DIGESTION:

Fiber helps move food through your digestive system. Additionally, getting more fiber in your diet lowers blood cholesterol levels, prevents constipation, and helps you feel full faster.

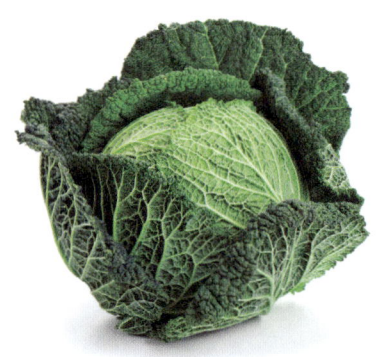

CANCER PREVENTION:

Studies have shown that sinigrin, one of the glucosinolates in cabbage, may be linked to cancer preventive properties, especially with respect to bladder cancer, colon cancer, and prostate cancer.

IMMUNE HEALTH:

Packed with vitamin C, nature's own powerful antioxidant, which helps prevent cell damage from free radicals. Vitamin C is one of the most critical vitamins for supporting immune health.

RECOMMENDED FOR HELP WITH:

- Digestion
- Cancer prevention, especially bladder, prostate, and colon
- Weight loss
- Lowering cholesterol

Celeriac

Also known as root celery, celeriac is loaded with antioxidants, which help prevent cell damage from free radicals. Research has shown that falcarinol, a polyacetylene antioxidant found in celeriac, may help to protect against colon cancer. It's also a good source of vitamin K, essential for blood clotting and bone nourishment. Enjoy celeriac in a range of dishes, from mash to soups and stews, for a healthy nutritional boost.

NUTRIENTS IN 1 CUP OF CELERIAC PIECES (BOILED WITHOUT SALT):

Calories, 42
Dietary fiber, 1.9 g
Magnesium, 18.6 g
Manganese, 0.1 mg
Phosphorus, 102 mg
Potassium, 268 mg
Vitamin B6, 0.2 mg
Vitamin C, 5.6 mg

HEALTH AND HEALING BENEFITS:

ANTIOXIDANT:

Antioxidants are essential for optimal health. These compounds help decrease free radical molecules, which damage cells and lead to every known disease.

CANCER PREVENTION:

Falcarinol, a polyacetylene antioxidant found in celeriac,

Glycemic load: 3
Inflammatory index: Anti-inflammatory

RECOMMENDED FOR HELP WITH:

- Cancer prevention, especially colon cancer
- Immunity

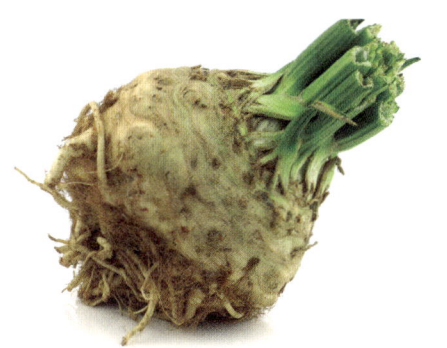

may help to protect against colon cancer.

BONE NOURISHMENT:

Rich in vitamin K, which provides bone nourishment and is essential to blood clotting. Vitamin K deficiency has been shown to result in a greater risk of bone fracture. For women who have passed through menopause and have started to experience unwanted bone loss, vitamin K has been shown to help prevent fractures.

Celery

Celery is one of the most alkaline foods you can eat. Since most people's bodies are far too acidic, celery is a welcome addition to any diet. Popular for its tasty leaves and shoots, and crunchy roots, celery is rich in immune-boosting, anticancerous antioxidants, which help protect cells against free radical damage; its leaves are a good source of vision-boosting vitamin A. Enjoy celery roots in salads for a healthy, nutritious crunch, or boiled in soups and stews.

NUTRIENTS IN 1 CUP OF RAW CHOPPED CELERY:

Calories, 14
Calcium, 40.4 mg
Dietary fiber, 1.6 g
Folate, 36.4 mcg
Magnesium, 11.1 mg
Manganese, 0.1 mg
Pantothenic acid, 0.2 mg
Phosphorus, 24.2 mg
Potassium, 263 mg
Riboflavin, 0.1 mg
Vitamin A (RAE), 22.2 mcg
Vitamin B6, 0.1 mg
Vitamin C, 3.1 mg
Vitamin K, 29.6 mcg

HEALTH AND HEALING BENEFITS:

ANTIOXIDANTS:

Anticancerous antioxidants are essential for optimal health. These compounds help decrease free radical molecules, which damage cells and lead to every known disease.

METABOLISM:

B vitamins, folate, riboflavin, and niacin are essential for optimum metabolism.

Glycemic load: 0
Inflammatory index: Mildly anti-inflammatory

HEART HEALTH:

Potassium, sodium, calcium, manganese, and magnesium help to regulate heart rate and blood pressure.

RECOMMENDED FOR HELP WITH:

- Lowering cholesterol
- Reducing anxiety levels
- Immunity

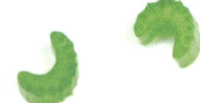

Chicory (curly endive)

Chicory is a woody plant native to Europe, North Africa, and Asia, which is now cultivated widely in the United States. Its long tap root is most commonly used as a caffeine-free coffee substitute, while its leaves are popular in salads. Chicory was prized by the ancient Egyptians for its healing benefits for the liver and gallbladder. It is loaded with free-radical-zapping antioxidants.

Chicory roots are a good source of inulin, which aids digestion and helps to regulate cholesterol. Chicory roots can also be roast, ground, and used as a caffeine-free coffee substitute.

Chicory greens, raw

Chicory greens are loaded with vitamin K, essential for blood clotting and bone nourishment—just one ounce is packed with 108% of your recommended daily value.

NUTRIENTS IN 1 CUP OF RAW CHOPPED CHICORY GREENS:

Calories, 7
Calcium, 29 mg
Copper, 0.1 mg
Dietary fiber, 1.2 g
Folate, 31.9 mcg
Iron, 0.3 mg
Magnesium, 8.7 mg
Manganese, 0.1 mg
Pantothenic acid, 0.3 mg
Phosphorus, 13.6 mg
Potassium, 122 mg
Riboflavin, 0 mg
Vitamin A, 82.9 mcg
Vitamin B6, 0 mg
Vitamin C, 7 mg
Vitamin E, 0.7 mg
Vitamin K, 86.4 mcg

HEALTH AND HEALING BENEFITS:

ANTIOXIDANTS:

Antioxidants are essential for optimal health. These compounds help decrease free radical molecules, which damage cells and lead to every known disease.

Glycemic load: 0
Inflammatory index: Mildly anti-inflammatory

RECOMMENDED FOR HELP WITH:

- Digestion
- Lowering cholesterol
- Liver detoxification

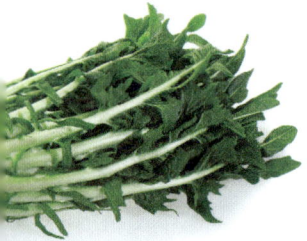

BONE NOURISHMENT:

Chicory leaves are rich in vitamin K, which provides bone nourishment and is essential to blood clotting. Vitamin K deficiency has been shown to result in a greater risk of bone fracture. For women who have passed through menopause and have started to experience unwanted bone loss, vitamin K has been shown to help prevent fractures.

DIGESTION:

Inulin in chicory roots, also known as "chicory root fiber," prevents constipation, helps maintain a healthy balance of "good" bacteria in the colon, and helps lower cholesterol levels.

Collards (collard greens)

Collards are a great source of phytonutrients—natural compounds that may help prevent disease and help to keep your body working properly. They're packed with vitamin K—just one ounce of raw collards contains a huge 179% of your recommended value of this bone-nourishing vitamin. Steamed collards may have the greatest cholesterol-lowering ability of all commonly eaten cruciferous vegetables, outshining steamed kale, broccoli, and mustard greens. The glucosinolates glucoraphanin, sinigrin, gluconasturtiian, and glucotropaeolin provide unique cancer protection, too, making collards a highly nutritious addition to any diet.

NUTRIENTS IN 1 CUP OF RAW CHOPPED COLLARDS:

Calories, 12
Calcium, 83.5 mg
Dietary fiber, 1.4 g
Folate, 46.4 mcg
Manganese, 0.2 mg
Niacin, 0.3 mg
Potassium, 76.7 mg
Protein, 1 g
Riboflavin, 0 mg
Thiamin, 0 mg
Vitamin A (RAE), 90.4 mcg
Vitamin B6, 0.1 mg
Vitamin C, 12.7 mg
Vitamin E, 0.8 mg
Vitamin K, 157 mcg

HEALTH AND HEALING BENEFITS:

CANCER PREVENTION:

The glucosinolates in collards, glucoraphanin, sinigrin, gluconasturtiian, and

Glycemic load: 1
Inflammatory index: Mildly anti-inflammatory

RECOMMENDED FOR HELP WITH:

- Cancer prevention
- Strong bones
- Immunity

glucotropaeolin, provide unique cancer protection, especially for prostate and colon cancer.

ANTIOXIDANTS:

Rich in nature's own powerful antioxidant, vitamin C, as well as other antioxidants, which help prevent cell damage from free radicals. Antioxidants are essential for optimal health. These compounds help decrease free radical molecules, which damage cells and lead to every known disease.

BONE NOURISHMENT:

Rich in vitamin K, which provides bone nourishment and is essential to blood clotting. Vitamin K deficiency has been shown to result in a greater risk of bone fracture. For women who have passed through menopause and have started to experience unwanted bone loss, vitamin K has been shown to help prevent fractures.

Cress, garden

Garden cress is packed with vitamins, essential minerals, and free-radical-zapping antioxidants. Just one ounce contains a huge 190% of your recommended daily value of bone-nourishing vitamin K. Cress is also loaded with vision-boosting vitamin A and immune-boosting vitamin C, as well as bone-building calcium, potassium, and phosphorus. The nutritional value of cress is often overlooked—it's so much more than just a garnish. Add cress to salads and sandwiches for a tasty, nutritious boost.

NUTRIENTS IN 1 CUP OF RAW GARDEN CRESS:

Calories, 16
Calcium, 40.5 mg
Copper, 0.1 mg
Dietary fiber, 0.6 g
Folate, 40 mcg
Iron, 0.7 mg
Magnesium, 19 mg
Manganese, 0.3 mg
Niacin, 0.5 mg
Phosphorus, 38 mg
Potassium, 303 mg
Riboflavin, 0.1 mg
Thiamin, 0 mg
Vitamin A (RAE), 173 mcg
Vitamin B6, 0.1 mg
Vitamin C, 34.5 mg
Vitamin E, 0.4 mg
Vitamin K, 271 mcg

Glycemic load: 1
Inflammatory index: Moderately anti-inflammatory

RECOMMENDED FOR HELP WITH:

- Iron-deficient anemia
- Diarrhea
- Immunity

HEALTH AND HEALING BENEFITS:

GASTROINTESTINAL HEALTH:

Garden cress helps purify blood and stimulate appetite. It is used during constipation as a laxative and a purgative. Paste made of the seeds can be taken internally with honey to treat amebic dysentery; the mucilage of the germinating seeds allays the irritation of the intestines in dysentery and diarrhea.

ANTIOXIDANTS:

Rich in nature's own powerful antioxidant, vitamin C, as well as other antioxidants, including vitamin E. Antioxidants are essential for optimal health. These compounds help decrease free radical molecules, which damage cells and lead to every known disease.

ANEMIA:

Rich in iron, which prevents anemia. Iron improves the ability of the red blood cells to carry oxygen from the lungs to the cells around the body in the form of hemoglobin. Iron is particularly important for menstruating women, who lose iron each month during menses. Growing children and adolescents have an increased need for iron, as do women who are pregnant or lactating.

Cucumber

Cool, refreshing cucumbers are low in calories and packed with nutritious vitamins and minerals. Because their rough outer skin can be difficult to chew and digest, cucumbers are often peeled. However, what many people don't know is that most of the beneficial nutritional value of cucumbers, including bone-nourishing vitamin K, comes from the peel. Leave the peel on to reap all of the nutritional benefits this vegetable has to offer.

NUTRIENTS IN 1 RAW CUCUMBER WITH PEEL:

Calories, 45
Magnesium, 39.1 mg
Manganese, 0.2 mg
Pantothenic acid, 0.8 mg
Phosphorus, 72.2 mg
Potassium, 442 mg
Vitamin A, 15 mcg
Vitamin C, 8.4 mg
Vitamin K, 49.4 mcg

Glycemic load: 0
Inflammatory index: Anti-inflammatory

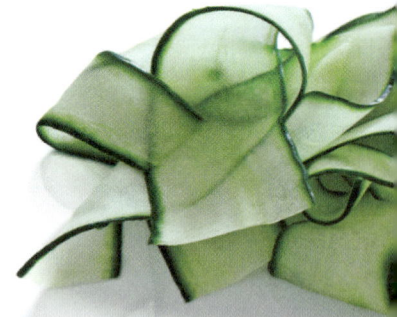

HEALTH AND HEALING BENEFITS:

DIGESTION:

Cucumbers are rich in fiber, which helps move food through your digestive system. Getting more fiber in your diet lowers blood cholesterol levels, prevents constipation, and helps you feel full faster.

BONE NOURISHMENT:

Rich in vitamin K, which provides bone nourishment and is essential to blood clotting. Vitamin K deficiency has been shown to result in a greater risk of bone fracture. For women who have passed through menopause and have started to experience unwanted bone loss, vitamin K has been shown to help prevent fractures.

VISION:

Cucumber peel is a good source of beta-carotene, a type of vitamin A, which contributes to healthy eyes and vision.

RECOMMENDED FOR HELP WITH:

- Digestion
- Strong bones
- Vision

Dandelion greens

Dandelions have long been revered for their healing properties. They are rich in free-radical-zapping antioxidants and other nutritious minerals and vitamins, including vitamin K, essential for blood clotting and bone nourishment. Just one ounce of raw dandelion greens contains a huge 272% of your recommended daily value of vitamin K. Dandelions are also a good source of vision-boosting vitamin A. Choose young, tender greens to add a tasty nutritional boost to salads.

NUTRIENTS IN 1 CUP OF RAW CHOPPED DANDELION GREENS:

Calories, 25
Calcium, 103 mg
Copper, 0.1 mg
Dietary fiber, 1.9 g
Folate, 14.8 mcg
Iron, 1.7 mg
Magnesium, 19.8 mg
Manganese, 0.2 mg
Phosphorus, 18.5 mg
Potassium, 36.3 mg
Riboflavin, 0.1 mg
Thiamin, 0.1 mg

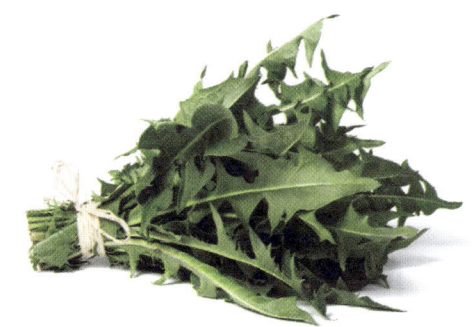

VEGETABLES, NON-STARCHY

HEALTH AND HEALING BENEFITS:

DIGESTION:

Fiber helps move food through your digestive system. Additionally, getting more fiber in your diet lowers blood cholesterol levels, prevents constipation, and helps you feel full faster.

BONE STRENGTH:

Rich in vitamin K, which provides bone nourishment and is essential to blood clotting. Vitamin K deficiency has been shown to result in a greater risk of bone fracture. For women who have passed through menopause and have started to experience unwanted bone loss, vitamin K has been shown to help prevent fractures.

VISION:

Vitamin A contributes to healthy eyes and vision.

NEUROLOGICAL HEALTH:

Vitamin K is used in the treatment of Alzheimer's disease patients; it's thought to limit neuronal damage in the brain.

Glycemic load: 1
Inflammatory index: Anti-inflammatory

RECOMMENDED FOR HELP WITH:

- Digestion
- Bone strength
- Vision
- Alzheimer's disease

Eggplant (aubergine)

Also known as aubergine and brinjal, eggplant is rich in free-radical-scavenging antioxidants, including nasunin, which has also been shown to contribute to healthy brain cells. Phytonutrients in eggplant help to lower cholesterol and have been linked with the prevention of cancer and rheumatoid arthritis. Many of the nutrients are contained in the glossy purple skin; be sure to include this to reap eggplant's full nutritional value in dishes from ratatouille to stews.

NUTRIENTS IN 1 CUP OF CUBED EGGPLANT (BOILED WITHOUT SALT):

Calories, 35
Copper, 0.1 mg
Dietary fiber, 2.5 g
Folate, 13.9 mcg
Magnesium, 10.9 mg
Manganese, 0.1 mg
Niacin, 0.6 mg
Pantothenic acid, 0.1 mg
Phosphorus, 14.8 mg
Potassium, 122 mg
Thiamin, 0.1 mg
Vitamin B6, 0.1 mg
Vitamin C, 1.3 mg
Vitamin K, 1 mcg

Glycemic load: 1
Inflammatory index: Anti-inflammatory

HEALTH AND HEALING BENEFITS:

AIDS DIGESTION:

Fiber helps move food through your digestive system. Additionally, getting more fiber in your diet lowers blood cholesterol levels, prevents constipation, and helps you feel full faster.

BRAIN HEALTH:

Studies have shown that nasunin protects the lipids (fats) in brain cell membranes. Cell membranes are almost entirely composed of lipids and are responsible for protecting the cell from free radicals, letting nutrients in and waste out, and receiving instructions from messenger molecules that tell the cell which activities it should perform.

CANCER PREVENTION

Phenolic antioxidant compounds in eggplant have been shown to have anticancerous properties.

RECOMMENDED FOR HELP WITH:

- Cancer prevention
- Digestion
- Lowering cholesterol

Endive, raw

This leafy green salad veg is rich in antioxidants, which protect cells in the body from free radical damage. It's bursting with bone-nourishing vitamin K, immune-boosting vitamin C, vision-boosting vitamin A, and energy-stoking B vitamins, as well as digestion-aiding dietary fiber. Include endives in salads for a tangy nutritional boost.

NUTRIENTS ½ CUP OF RAW CHOPPED ENDIVE:

Calories, 4
Calcium, 13 mg
Copper, 0 mg
Dietary fiber, 0.8 g
Folate, 35.5 mcg
Iron, 0.2 mg
Magnesium, 3.8 mg
Manganese, 0.1 mg
Pantothenic acid, 0.2 mg
Phosphorus, 7 mg
Potassium, 78.5 mg
Riboflavin, 0 mg
Thiamin, 0 mg
Vitamin A (RAE), 27 mcg
Vitamin C, 1.6 mg
Vitamin E, 0.1 mg
Vitamin K, 57.8 mcg
Zinc, 0.2 mg

Glycemic load: 0
Inflammatory index: Strongly anti-inflammatory

RECOMMENDED FOR HELP WITH:

- Lowering cholesterol
- Vision
- Immunity

HEALTH AND HEALING BENEFITS:

ANTIOXIDANTS:

A good source of various antioxidants, including vitamin C. Antioxidants are essential for optimal health. These compounds help decrease free radical molecules, which damage cells.

VISION:

Vitamin A and beta-carotene help to maintain healthy eyes and vision.

BONE STRENGTH:

Rich in vitamin K, which provides bone nourishment and is essential to blood clotting. Vitamin K deficiency has been shown to result in a greater risk of bone fracture. For women who have passed through menopause and have started to experience unwanted bone loss, vitamin K has been shown to help prevent fractures.

METABOLISM:

Energy-boosting B-complex vitamins, including niacin, thiamin, folate, and pantothenic acid, are essential for the metabolism of fat, protein, and carbohydrate.

Fennel bulb

Succulent fennel bulb is loaded with free-radical-zapping antioxidants and dietary fiber. Its anise-like flavor makes it a favorite in Mediterranean dishes. Anethole, the essential oil that gives fennel its distinctive flavor, has been shown to have antifungal and antibacterial properties, while heart-friendly potassium contributes to a healthy cardiovascular system, helping to regulate heart rate and blood pressure. Fennel is a tasty, healthy addition to many dishes, from roast chicken to seared salmon.

NUTRIENTS IN 1 CUP OF RAW SLICED FENNEL BULB:

Calories, 27
Calcium, 42.6 mg
Copper, 0.1 mg
Dietary fiber, 2.7 g
Folate, 23.5 mcg
Iron, 0.6 mg
Magnesium, 14.8 mg
Manganese, 0.2 mg
Niacin, 0.6 mg
Phosphorus, 43.5 mg
Potassium, 360 mg
Vitamin C, 10.4 mg

Glycemic load: 1
Inflammatory index: Anti-inflammatory

RECOMMENDED FOR HELP WITH:

- Lowering blood pressure
- Digestion

HEALTH AND HEALING BENEFITS:

AIDS DIGESTION:

Fiber helps move food through your digestive system. Additionally, getting more fiber in your diet lowers blood cholesterol levels, prevents constipation, and helps you feel full faster.

ANTIFUNGAL/ANTIBACTERIAL:

The essential oil anethole, which gives fennel its distinctive anise-like flavor, has been shown to have antifungal and antibacterial properties.

HEART HEALTH:

Heart-friendly potassium helps to regulate blood pressure and heart rate.

Garlic

Garlic has long been celebrated as a king of healing plants in cultures around the world, used in traditional remedies for a wide range of ailments, from heart problems to premature aging. It also has a reputation as a natural antibiotic. Add garlic to soups, stews, fish, and meat dishes for a delicious, healthy boost, or chop it raw into salads. Not only does it pack a tasty punch, it's loaded with health-boosting nutrients. Allowing garlic to sit after you've chopped or crushed it, before heating or adding to other ingredients, increases the health benefits.

NUTRIENTS IN 1 CLOVE OF RAW GARLIC:

Calories, 4
Calcium, 5.4 mg
Manganese, 0.1 mg
Phosphorus, 4.6 mg
Selenium, 0.4 mcg
Vitamin B6, 0 mg
Vitamin C, 0.9 mg

HEALTH AND HEALING BENEFITS:

CHOLESTEROL AND HEART HEALTH:

Allicin, a substance found in garlic, has been shown to reduce cholesterol by inhibiting enzymes in the liver. Allacin also facilitates nitric oxide release, which improves heart health, reduces blood pressure, and lowers the risk of coronary artery disease and stroke.

Glycemic load: 5
Inflammatory index: Strongly anti-inflammatory

RECOMMENDED FOR HELP WITH:

- Cancer prevention
- Lowering cholesterol
- Immunity

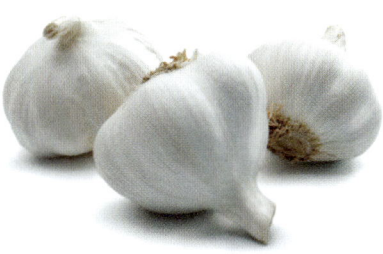

VEGETABLES, NON-STARCHY

Kale

Green leafy kale is rich in antioxidants and high in calcium. It's also a good source of immune-boosting vitamin C, vision-boosting vitamin A, and vitamin K, essential for blood clotting and bone nourishment. Flavonoids in kale have been shown to have strong antioxidant and anti-cancer properties.

NUTRIENTS IN 1 CUP OF RAW KALE

Calories, 7
Calcium, 53.3 mg
Copper, 0 mg
Dietary fiber, 0.9 g
Folate, 13 mcg
Iron, 0.3 mg
Magnesium, 6.9 mg
Manganese, 0.2 mg
Potassium, 73.1 mg
Protein, 0.6 g
Riboflavin, 0.1 mg
Thiamin, 0 mg
Vitamin A (RAE), 50.6 mcg
Vitamin B6, 0 mg
Vitamin C, 19.6 mg
Vitamin E, 0.1 mg
Vitamin K, 81.9 mcg

HEALTH AND HEALING BENEFITS:

CANCER PREVENTION:

Consumption of kale may help to lower the risk of cancer, including cancer of the bladder, breast, colon, ovary, and prostate.

ANTIOXIDANT/ ANTI-INFLAMMATORY:

Flavonoids in kale, including kaempferol and quercetin, combine antioxidant and anti-inflammatory benefits. Antioxidants are essential for optimal health. These compounds help decrease free radical molecules, which damage cells and lead to every known disease.

DETOX:

Kale helps to regulate the body's detoxification system.

Glycemic load: 1
Inflammatory index: Strongly anti inflammatory

RECOMMENDED FOR HELP WITH:

- Cancer prevention, especially prostate and colon
- Detoxing
- Macular degeneration

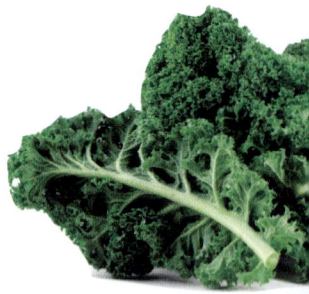

Leek

Delicate-flavored leeks are rich in antioxidants, protecting cells against damage from free radicals. They're also a good source of immune-boosting vitamin C, vision-boosting vitamin A, and vitamin K, essential for blood clotting and bone nourishment. For a healthy cooking option, slice thinly and briefly sauté. As with garlic and onions, allowing leeks to sit after chopping, before heating or adding to other ingredients, enhances their nutritional benefits.

NUTRIENTS IN 1 CUP OF RAW LEEK:

Calories, 54
Dietary fiber, 1.6 g
Folate, 57 mcg
Iron, 1.9 mg
Magnesium, 24.9 mg
Manganese, 0.4 mg
Vitamin A (RAE), 73.9 mcg
Vitamin B6, 0.2 mg
Vitamin C, 10.7 mg
Vitamin K, 41.8 mcg

HEALTH AND HEALING BENEFITS:

CHOLESTEROL AND HEART HEALTH:

Allicin, a substance found in leeks, has been shown to reduce cholesterol by inhibiting enzymes in the liver. Allacin also facilitates nitric oxide release, which improves heart health, reduces blood pressure, and lowers the risk of coronary artery disease and stroke.

ANTIOXIDANT:

Antioxidants are essential for optimal health. These compounds help decrease free radical molecules, which damage cells and lead to every known disease.

METABOLISM:

Energy-boosting B-complex vitamins are essential for the metabolism of fat, protein, and carbohydrate.

Glycemic load: 2
Inflammatory index: Mildly anti-inflammatory

RECOMMENDED FOR HELP WITH:

- Lowering cholesterol
- Heart health
- Immune health

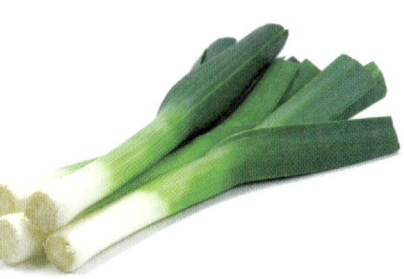

LETTUCE

Lettuce is a very low-calorie food loaded with vision-boosting vitamin A and vitamin K, essential for blood clotting and bone nourishment, as well as dietary fiber, iron, and energy-enhancing B vitamins. A good rule of thumb is that the nutritional value becomes greater the darker green the leaves, with iceberg at the lower end and green leaf lettuce at the higher end of the spectrum. However, all varieties are low in calories and provide fiber, vitamins, and minerals, making lettuce a healthy addition to any diet.

Lettuce, green leaf

This loose-headed variety is growing in popularity in the United States, and is among the most nutritious of the lettuces. One ounce provides 41% of your recommended daily value of vision-boosting vitamin A, and 61% of vitamin K, essential for blood clotting and bone nourishment.

NUTRIENTS IN 1 CUP OF SHREDDED GREEN LEAF LETTUCE:

Calories, 5
Calcium, 13 mg
Dietary fiber, 0.5 g
Folate, 13.7 mcg
Iron, 0.3 mg
Magnesium, 4.7 mg
Manganese, 0.1 mg
Phosphorus, 10.4 mg
Potassium, 69.8 mg
Protein, 0.5 g
Thiamin, 0 mg
Vitamin A (RAE), 133 mcg
Vitamin B6, 0 mg
Vitamin C, 3.3 mg
Vitamin K, 45.4 mcg

Glycemic load: 0
Inflammatory index: Anti-inflammatory

Lettuce, iceberg

Also known as crisphead lettuce, this type of lettuce has a tight, dense head, resembling a cabbage. One ounce provides 3% of your recommended daily value of vision-boosting vitamin A, and 8% of vitamin K.

Lettuce, red leaf

Red lettuce is a loose-headed variety, with leaves tinged shades of red to dark reddish purple. One ounce provides 42% of your recommended daily value of vision-boosting vitamin A, and 49% of vitamin K, essential for blood clotting and bone nourishment.

NUTRIENTS IN 1 CUP OF SHREDDED RED LEAF LETTUCE:

Calories, 4
Calcium, 9.2 mg
Dietary fiber, 0.3 g
Folate, 10.1 mcg
Iron, 0.3 mg
Magnesium, 3.4 mg
Manganese, 0.1 mg
Phosphorus, 7.8 mg
Potassium, 52.4 mg
Riboflavin, 0 mg
Selenium, 0.4 mcg
Thiamin, 0 mg
Vitamin A (RAE), 105 mcg
Vitamin B6, 0 mg
Vitamin C, 1 mg
Vitamin K, 39.2 mcg

HEALTH AND HEALING BENEFITS OF LETTUCE:

VISION:

Vitamin A is a powerful antioxidant that protects cells from free radical damage. It is also important for maintaining healthy vision.

BONE NOURISHMENT:

Rich in vitamin K, which provides bone nourishment and is essential to blood clotting. Vitamin K deficiency has been shown to result in a greater risk of bone fracture. For women who have passed through menopause and have started to experience unwanted bone loss, vitamin K has been shown to help prevent fractures.

Glycemic load: 0
Inflammatory index: Anti-inflammatory

DIGESTION:

Fiber helps move food through your digestive system. Additionally, getting more fiber in your diet lowers blood cholesterol levels, prevents constipation, and helps you feel full faster.

RECOMMENDED FOR HELP WITH:

- Digestion
- Vision
- Immunity

Okra

Also known as "lady finger," okra is high in fiber, which is beneficial for digestion, as well as being a good source of vision-boosting vitamin A, immune-boosting vitamin C, brain-boosting folate, and vitamin K, essential for blood clotting and bone nourishment. Okra is popular pickled, fried, or grilled and in dishes such as gumbo. It is sometimes known as "gumbo pod."

NUTRIENTS IN 8 PODS OF RAW OKRA:

Calories, 31
Calcium, 77.9 mg
Copper, 0.1 mg
Dietary fiber, 3 g
Folate, 57 mcg
Iron, 0.6 mg
Magnesium, 54.2 mg
Manganese, 0.7 mg
Niacin, 1 mg
Phosphorus, 58 mg
Potassium, 284 mg
Protein, 1.8 g
Riboflavin, 0.1 mg
Thiamin, 0.2 mg
Vitamin A (RAE), 34.2 mcg
Vitamin B6, 0.2 mg
Vitamin C, 21.8 mg
Vitamin K, 29.7 mcg
Zinc, 0.6 mg

HEALTH AND HEALING BENEFITS:

BRAIN FUNCTION:

A good source of folate, one of the most critical vitamins, especially during pregnancy, where deficiencies increase the risk of spinal defects and mental retardation in the fetus. In the general population, folate is particularly important in all aspects of brain function and in cholesterol metabolism.

VISION:

Vitamin A is a powerful antioxidant that protects cells from free radical damage. It is also important for maintaining healthy vision.

Glycemic load: 1
Inflammatory index: Anti-inflammatory

DIGESTION:

Fiber helps move food through your digestive system. Additionally, getting more fiber in your diet lowers blood cholesterol levels, prevents constipation, and helps you feel full faster.

RECOMMENDED FOR HELP WITH:

- Digestion
- Vision
- Immunity

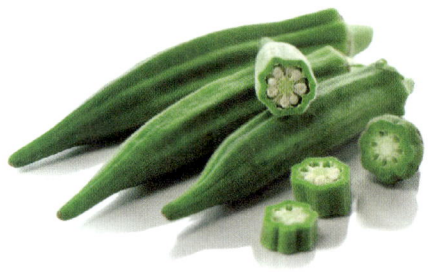

ONION

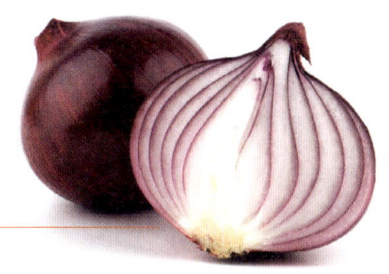

Onions are with antioxidants, which help prevent cell damage from free radicals. Many of the nutrients in onions are concentrated in the outer layers of the flesh. To reap maximum health benefits from the outer layers, avoid over-peeling onions. Onion is a wonderfully versatile ingredient, adding a healthy boost to a huge range of dishes, from salads to soups, to sauces and curries. As with garlic and leeks, allowing onions to sit after chopping, before heating or adding to other ingredients, enhances their nutritional benefits.

Onion, red

Red onions are distinct from other onions because of their dark purplish color. They have a milder flavor than white onions, making them a popular choice raw in burgers or salads.

NUTRIENTS IN 1 RED ONION:

Calories, 87
Calcium, 33.5 mg
Dietary fiber, 4.3 g
Magnesium, 22.5 mg
Manganese, 0.2 mg
Potassium, 388 mg
Vitamin C, 16 mg

Glycemic load: 0
Inflammatory index: Anti-inflammatory

Onion, white

Sharper and more pungent than red onions, white onions add a crisp bite to burgers and salad dishes, or provide a pungent, robust base for a wide range of savory dishes.

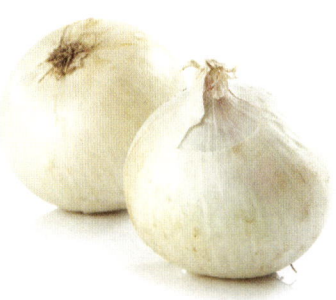

NUTRIENTS IN 1 WHITE ONION:

Calories, 36
Dietary fiber, 1.2 g
Manganese, 0.1 mg
Potassium, 141 mg

HEALTH AND HEALING BENEFITS OF ONIONS:

CHOLESTEROL AND HEART HEALTH:

Allicin, a substance found in onions, has been shown to reduce cholesterol by inhibiting enzymes in the liver, as well as facilitating nitric oxide release, which improves heart health, reduces blood pressure, and lowers the risk of coronary artery disease and stroke.

CANCER PREVENTION:

Onions contain antioxidant flavonoids, including quercetin, which protect cells from free radical damage, and have been linked with protecting cells from cancer.

BLOOD SUGAR:

Rich in the trace mineral chromium, which helps tissues respond appropriately to glucose levels in the blood, assisting in the regulation of insulin levels in diabetics. Allicin has also been shown to help lower blood sugar levels in diabetics.

Glycemic load: 1
Inflammatory index: Strongly anti-inflammatory

RECOMMENDED FOR HELP WITH:

- Cancer prevention
- Diabetes
- Heart health

Pepper, jalapeño

Native to Mexico, these hot, fiery green peppers contain the natural plant compound capsaicin, which has anti-inflammatory properties. These little peppers pack a nutritious punch—one jalapeño contains in excess of your recommended daily value of immune-boosting vitamin C, as well as providing bone-nourishing vitamin K, vision-boosting vitamin A, and health-boosting minerals. Add jalapeños to salsa, guacamole, or eggs for a spicy, nutritious kick.

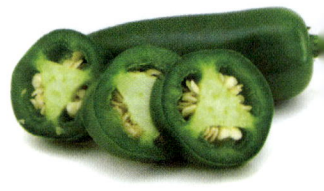

NUTRIENTS IN 1 CUP OF SLICED JALAPEÑO PEPPERS:

Calories, 26
Dietary fiber, 2.5 g
Folate, 24.3 mcg
Iron, 0.2 mg
Magnesium, 13.5 mg
Manganese, 0.1 mg
Niacin, 1.2 mg
Phosphorus, 23.4 mg
Potassium, 223 mg
Riboflavin, 0.1 mg
Thiamin, 0 mg
Vitamin A (RAE), 48.6 mcg
Vitamin B6, 0.4 mg
Vitamin C, 107 mg
Vitamin K, 16.6 mcg

HEALTH AND HEALING BENEFITS:

CHOLESTEROL:

Capsaicin, which gives jalapeño peppers their strong spicy characteristics, has been shown to reduce cholesterol levels in obese individuals.

ANTIOXIDANTS:

Antioxidants are essential for optimal health. These compounds help decrease free radical molecules, which damage cells and lead to every known disease.

IMMUNITY:

A good source of nature's own powerful antioxidant vitamin C, which helps prevent cell damage from free radicals. Vitamin C is one of the most critical vitamins for supporting immune health.

Glycemic load: 2
Inflammatory index: Strongly anti-inflammatory

RECOMMENDED FOR HELP WITH:

- Lowering cholesterol
- Immunity

Radicchio (red chicory)

This Mediterranean, cabbage-like vegetable is rich in antioxidants It's also loaded with the flavonoids zeaxanthin and lutein, which help to protect your eyes from harmful ultraviolet rays, as well as bone-nourishing vitamin K and energy-enhancing B vitamins. Its wine-red, bitter-flavored leaves have long been a popular ingredient in Italian salads.

NUTRIENTS IN 1 CUP OF SHREDDED RAW RADICCHIO:

Calories, 9
Copper, 0.1 mg
Folate, 24 mcg
Manganese, 0.1 mg
Potassium, 121 mg
Vitamin C, 3.2 mg
Vitamin E, 0.9 mg
Vitamin K, 102 mcg

HEALTH AND HEALING BENEFITS:

EYE HEALTH:

The flavonoids zeaxanthin and lutein contribute to healthy

eyes, helping to protect against age-related macular disease by filtering harmful ultraviolet rays.

ANTIOXIDANTS:

Antioxidants are essential for optimal health. These compounds help decrease free radical molecules, which damage cells and lead to every known disease.

BONE NOURISHMENT:

Rich in vitamin K, which provides bone nourishment and is essential to blood clotting. Vitamin K deficiency has been shown to result in a greater risk of bone fracture. For women who have passed through menopause and have started to experience unwanted bone loss, vitamin K has been shown to help prevent fractures.

Glycemic load: 1
Inflammatory index: Anti-inflammatory

RECOMMENDED FOR HELP WITH:

- Macular degeneration
- Strong bones
- Immunity

Scallion (spring onion)

These small, slender bulbs have a milder, more delicate flavor than onions. On a weight to weight basis, scallions are richer in minerals, vitamins, and antioxidants than other types of onions, making them a welcome addition to any diet. Scallions are rich in antioxidants, which help cells combat free radicals, and are a good source of vision-boosting vitamin A. As with onions, allowing scallions to sit after chopping enhances their nutritional benefits.

NUTRIENTS IN 1 TBSP. OF RAW CHOPPED SCALLIONS:

Calories, 7
Folate, 3.4 mcg
Manganese, 0 mg
Potassium, 33.4 mg
Vitamin A, 0 mcg
Vitamin B6, 0 mg
Vitamin C, 0.8 mg

Glycemic load: 2
Inflammatory index: Anti-inflammatory

RECOMMENDED FOR HELP WITH:

- Cancer prevention
- Lowering cholesterol

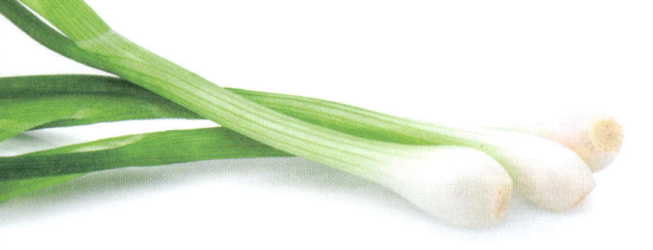

HEALTH AND HEALING BENEFITS:

CHOLESTEROL AND HEART HEALTH:

Allicin, a substance found in onions, has been shown to reduce cholesterol by inhibiting enzymes in the liver, as well as facilitating nitric oxide release, which improves heart health, reduces blood pressure, and lowers the risk of coronary artery disease and stroke.

BRAIN FUNCTION:

A good source of folate, one of the most critical vitamins, especially during pregnancy, where deficiencies increase the risk of spinal defects and mental retardation in the fetus. In the general population, folate is particularly important in all aspects of brain function and in cholesterol metabolism.

PREVENTING CANCER:

Studies have shown that diets rich in allium vegetables have been linked with a reduced rate of cancer, especially stomach and colorectal cancers.

Spinach

Spinach is one of the most alkaline foods you can eat. Since most people's bodies are far too acidic, spinach is a welcome addition to any diet. Spinach is a storehouse of vitamins and minerals—one ounce of raw spinach contains 169% of your recommended daily value of vitamin K, essential for blood clotting and bone nourishment, over half (53%) of your recommended daily value of vision-boosting vitamin A, and 4% of iron.

NUTRIENTS IN 1 CUP OF RAW SPINACH:

Calories, 7
Calcium, 29.7 mg
Copper, 0 mg
Dietary fiber, 0.7 g
Folate, 58.2 mcg
Iron, 0.8 mg
Magnesium, 23.7 mg
Manganese, 0.3 mg
Niacin, 0.2 mg
Phosphorus, 14.7 mg
Potassium, 167 mg
Protein, 0.9 g
Riboflavin, 0.1 mg
Thiamin, 0 mg
Vitamin A (RAE), 141 mcg
Vitamin B6, 0.1 mg
Vitamin C, 8.4 mg
Vitamin E, 0.6 mg
Vitamin K, 145 mcg
Zinc, 0.2 mg

Glycemic load: 0
Inflammatory index: Anti-inflammatory

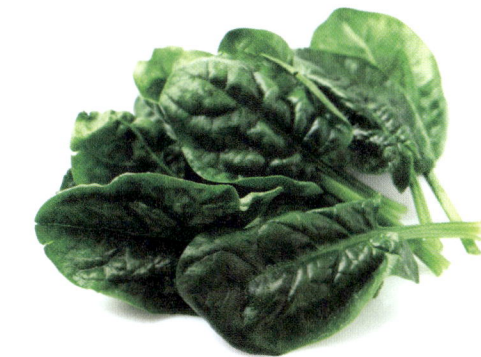

VEGETABLES, NON-STARCHY

HEALTH AND HEALING BENEFITS:

OXYGENATION OF THE BLOOD:

Spinach is rich in iron, which improves the ability of red blood cells to transport oxygen from the lungs to cells around the body in the form of hemoglobin. Iron is particularly important for menstruating women, who lose iron each month during menses. Growing children and adolescents have an increased need for iron, as do women who are pregnant or lactating.

CANCER PREVENTION:

Spinach contains more than a dozen flavonoid compounds. Studies have shown that these work together as cancer-fighting antioxidants, neutralizing free radicals in the body, thus helping to prevent cancer.

CARDIOVASCULAR HEALTH:

The antioxidant properties of spinach work together to promote cardiovascular health by preventing harmful oxidization of cholesterol, which can lead to artery and heart problems, while magnesium helps to lower blood pressure.

Glycemic load: 0
Inflammatory index: Anti-inflammatory

RECOMMENDED FOR HELP WITH:

- Anemia
- Cancer prevention
- Lowering blood pressure

Swiss chard

Also known as silverbeet or spinach chard, this leafy green vegetable is a storehouse of nutrients. It's rich in antioxidants and loaded with immune-boosting vitamin C, bone-nourishing vitamin K, and vision-boosting vitamin A, as well as health-boosting flavonoids.

NUTRIENTS IN 1 CUP OF RAW SWISS CHARD:

Calories, 7
Calcium, 18.4 mg
Copper, 0.1 mg
Dietary fiber, 0.6 g
Folate, 5 mcg
Iron, 0.6 mg
Magnesium, 29.2 mg
Manganese, 0.1 mg
Phosphorus, 16.6 mg
Potassium, 136 mg
Riboflavin, 0 mg
Thiamin, 0 mg
Vitamin A (RAE), 110 mcg
Vitamin B6, 0 mg
Vitamin C, 10.8 mg
Vitamin E, 0.7 mg
Vitamin K, 299 mcg
Zinc, 0.1 mg

HEALTH AND HEALING BENEFITS:

IMMUNE HEALTH:

Rich in nature's own powerful antioxidant vitamin C, which helps prevent cell damage from free radicals. Vitamin C is one of the most critical vitamins for supporting immune health.

BONE NOURISHMENT:

Rich in vitamin K, which provides bone nourishment and is essential to blood clotting. Vitamin K deficiency has been shown to result in a greater risk of bone fracture. For women who have passed through menopause and have started to experience unwanted bone loss, vitamin K has been shown to help prevent fractures.

BLOOD SUGAR:

The flavonoid syringic acid helps regulate blood sugar levels by inhibiting activity of the enzyme called alpha-glucosidase. This results in fewer carbs being broken down into simple sugars, meaning blood sugar is able to stay more steady.

Glycemic load: 1
Inflammatory index: Anti-inflammatory

RECOMMENDED FOR HELP WITH:

- Immunity
- Bone strength
- Regulating blood sugar levels

TOMATO

Tomatoes are a nutritional powerhouse. Tomatoes and tomato products, including tomato sauce and tomato juice, are rich in vitamins and antioxidants, including lycopene. Research has shown that diets rich in lycopene may help decrease the risk of heart disease, age-related macular degeneration, stroke, high cholesterol, and certain types of cancer. Cooked tomatoes and tomato products in the form of tomato paste or sauce contain significantly more lycopene than raw tomatoes. However, whether eaten raw or cooked, freshly picked or canned, tomatoes provide a healthy addition to most diets, though high acidic levels may aggravate reflux or heartburn in those prone to these conditions. Include a mixture of cooked and raw tomatoes in your weekly meal plan to reap the most health benefits from tomatoes.

Tomato, red

Raw red tomatoes are rich in dietary fiber, vision-boosting vitamin A, immune-boosting vitamin C, and bone-nourishing vitamin K.

NUTRIENTS IN 1 MEDIUM RAW RED TOMATO:

Calories, 22
Copper, 0.1 mg
Dietary fiber, 1.5 g
Folate, 18.4 mcg
Magnesium, 13.5 mg
Manganese, 0.1 mg
Niacin, 0.7 mg
Phosphorus, 29.5 mg
Potassium, 292 mg
Thiamin, 0 mg
Vitamin A (RAE), 51.7 mcg
Vitamin B6, 0.1 mg
Vitamin C, 16.9 mg
Vitamin E, 0.7 mg
Vitamin K, 9.7 mcg

Glycemic load: 0
Inflammatory index: Anti-inflammatory

Tomato, orange

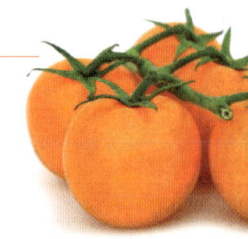

Lycopene is the antioxidant that gives tomatoes their rich red color. However, tomatoes do not necessarily have to be deep red to be an outstanding source of lycopene. Research suggests that lycopene from orange tomatoes may actually be better absorbed by the body.

Tomato juice, canned without salt

Like other tomato products, canned tomato juice contains the antioxidant lycopene. The lycopene content in all-natural or homemade tomato juice is similar to that found in fresh raw tomatoes. Look for products with no added salts, sugars, or chemicals.

Tomato sauce, no salt

Cooking tomatoes increases the lutein content, which helps prevent prostate cancer. Cooking also increases the content of the antioxidant lycopene. Eating cooked tomatoes with a healthy source of fat or oil enhances the absorption of lycopene, so try tomato sauce made with olive oil to maximize lycopene uptake.

Tomatoes, sun-dried

Due to their moisture content, tomatoes deteriorate rapidly after being picked. Sun-drying removes the water to preserve the tomato, while retaining the flavor and many of the nutrients. Sun-dried tomatoes are low in fat, and high in fiber and immune-boosting vitamin C.

HEALTH AND HEALING BENEFITS OF TOMATOES:

CANCER PREVENTION:

Lycopene, the carotenoid found in tomatoes, is a potent antioxidant, protecting cells against damage from free radicals. Research has shown it may prevent the development of certain cancers, including prostate, rectal, colon, and some stomach cancers.

MAINTAINING OPTIMAL HEALTH:

Research has shown that diets rich in lycopene may help decrease the risk of various diseases and conditions, including heart disease, age-related macular degeneration, stroke, and high cholesterol.

IMMUNITY:

Rich in nature's own powerful antioxidant vitamin C, which helps prevent cell damage from free radicals. Vitamin C is one of the most critical vitamins for supporting immune health.

RECOMMENDED FOR HELP WITH:

- Cancer prevention
- Heart disease
- Age-related macular degeneration
- Stroke
- Lowering cholesterol

Wakame seaweed

Wakame seaweed has a delicate briny flavor and is popular in Japanese cuisine in dishes such as miso soup. It is traditionally cultivated in Japan on ropes tied to offshore rafts. Wakame seaweed is one of the few foods containing iodine, which improves thyroid function, and has been linked to the prevention of breast cancer. It can be eaten raw or cooked. Enjoy in salads or soups for a healthy umami flavor boost. However, it is high in sodium, so should be consumed in moderation.

NUTRIENTS IN 2 TBSP. OF RAW WAKAME SEAWEED:

Calories, 5
Calcium, 15 mg
Copper, 0 mg
Folate, 19.6 mcg
Iron, 0.2 mg
Magnesium, 10.7 mg
Manganese, 0.1 mg
Niacin, 0.2 mg
Pantothenic acid, 0.1 mg
Phosphorus, 8 mg
Riboflavin, 0 mg
Vitamin A (RAE), 1.8 mcg
Vitamin C, 0.3 mg
Vitamin E, 0.1 mg
Vitamin K, 0.5 mcg

HEALTH AND HEALING BENEFITS:

THYROID FUNCTION:

Rich in iodine, which contributes to healthy thyroid function. Thyroid hormones regulate metabolism in every cell of the body and play a role in virtually all physiological functions. Iodine deficiency can have a negative impact on your health and well-being.

CANCER PREVENTION:

Studies suggest that the iodine content of wakame seaweed may be linked to the prevention of breast cancer.

HEART HEALTH:

Fucoxanthin, a compound found in wakame, has been shown to stimulate the liver to produce more DHA, an omega-3 acid that helps lower the "bad" cholesterol linked to obesity and heart disease.

Glycemic load: 1
Inflammatory index: Anti-inflammatory

RECOMMENDED FOR HELP WITH:

- Thyroid function
- Lowering cholesterol
- Cancer prevention, especially breast cancer

Watercress

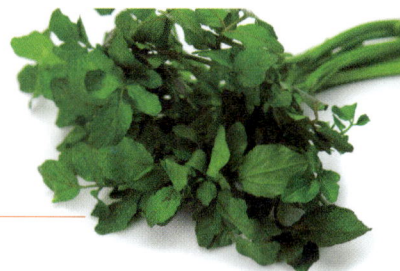

This aquatic leafy green plant is found near springs and slow-moving streams. It's a close cousin to arugula (rocket) and cabbage, yet it is often overlooked as a nutritional food source. Watercress is packed with vitamins and contains more vitamin C than oranges—one ounce of raw watercress provides 20% of your recommended daily value of this immune-boosting vitamin, as well as 18% of vision-boosting vitamin A, and a huge 87% of bone-nourishing vitamin K. It's also rich in iron. Add raw to salads or steam as a side vegetable for a subtle, peppery health boost.

NUTRIENTS IN 1 CUP OF RAW CHOPPED WATERCRESS:

Calories, 4
Folate, 3.1 mcg
Pantothenic acid, 0.1 mg
Potassium, 112 mg
Protein, 0.8 g
Riboflavin, 0 mg
Thiamin, 0 mg
Vitamin A (RAE), 54.4 mcg
Vitamin B6, 0 mg
Vitamin C, 14.6 mg
Vitamin E, 0.3 mg
Vitamin K, 85 mg

HEALTH AND HEALING BENEFITS:

IMMUNE HEALTH:

Rich in nature's own powerful antioxidant vitamin C, which helps prevent cell damage from free radicals. Vitamin C is one of the most critical vitamins for supporting immune health.

BONE NOURISHMENT:

Rich in vitamin K, which provides bone nourishment and is essential to blood clotting. Vitamin K deficiency has been shown to result in a greater risk of bone fracture. For women who have passed through menopause and have started to experience unwanted bone loss, vitamin K has been shown to help prevent fractures.

OXYGENATION OF THE BLOOD:

Rich in iron, which improves the ability of the red blood cells to carry oxygen from the lungs to the cells around the body in the form of hemoglobin. Iron is particularly important for menstruating women, who lose iron each month during menses. Growing children and adolescents have an increased need for iron, as do women who are pregnant or lactating.

Glycemic load: 0
Inflammatory index: Anti-inflammatory

RECOMMENDED FOR HELP WITH:

- Immunity
- Anemia
- Bone strength

Zucchini (courgette)

Zucchini is one of the most popular summer squashes in the Americas. Zucchinis are low in calories, and high in vision-boosting vitamin A and heart-friendly potassium. The skin is particularly rich in nutrients, so leave it on to reap the full nutritional benefits of zucchini.

NUTRIENTS IN 1 MEDIUM RAW ZUCCHINI:

Calories, 33
Copper, 0.1 mg
Dietary fiber, 2 g
Folate, 47 mcg
Magnesium, 35.3 mg
Manganese, 0.3 mg
Niacin, 0.9 mg
Phosphorus, 74.5 mg
Potassium, 512 mg
Riboflavin, 0.2 mg
Thiamin, 0.1 mg
Vitamin A (RAE), 19.6 mcg
Vitamin B6, 0.3 mg
Vitamin C, 35.1 mg
Vitamin K, 8.4 mcg

HEALTH AND HEALING BENEFITS:

HEART HEALTH:

Heart-friendly potassium helps to reduce blood pressure and regulate heart rate by countering the effects of sodium.

VISION:

Rich in vitamin A, a powerful antioxidant that protects cells from free radical damage and plays an important role in maintaining healthy eyesight. The carotenoids lutein and zeaxanthin also contribute to healthy eyes and vision, protecting against age-related macular degeneration.

ANTIOXIDANTS:

Loaded with antioxidants, including the carotenoids lutein and zeaxanthin, and vitamin C, one of the most critical vitamins for supporting immune health. Antioxidants are essential for optimal health. These compounds help decrease free radical molecules, which damage cells and lead to every known disease.

Glycemic load: 2
Inflammatory index: Anti-inflammatory

RECOMMENDED FOR HELP WITH:

- Immunity
- Macular degeneration
- Regulating blood pressure

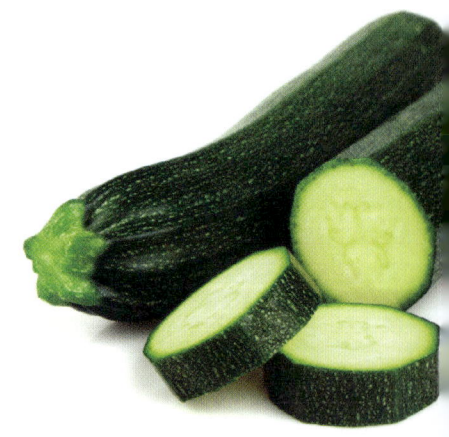

Vegetables, starchy

Starchy vegetables are higher in calories than non-starchy vegetables, but their health benefits are enormous as they are rich in vitamins, minerals, and fiber. They are also high-quality carbohydrates, so those with diabetes need to be wary of their intake.

BEET

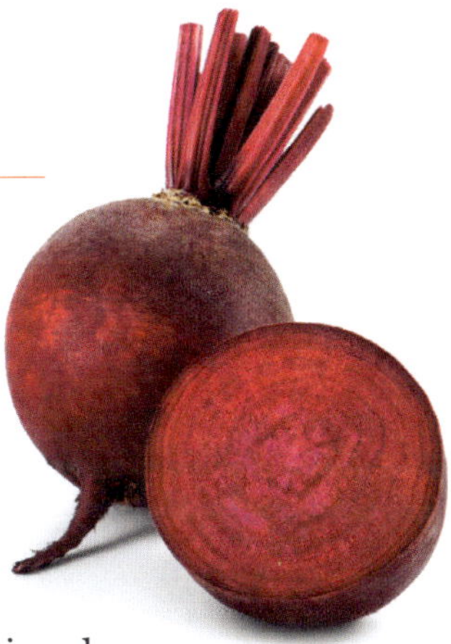

Beets are commonly found sliced in Greek salads, boiled down in Russian borscht, and can be delicious roasted or served in a salad. The most commonly found beets are reddish-purple, but beets also come in white, orange, and yellow. Beets are a good source of many nutrients, including vitamin C, iron, magnesium, potassium, folate, manganese, and dietary fiber. The nitrates in beets help the body to produce nitric oxide, which improves heart health. The traditional red beets are a gorgeous color, but do be careful when preparing, as they easily stain surfaces and skin. Avoid eating beets if you suffer from kidney stones.

NUTRIENTS IN 1 CUP OF RAW BEET:

Calories, 58
Dietary fiber, 4 g
Folate, 148 mcg
Iron, 1.1 mg
Magnesium, 31.3 mg
Manganese, 0.4 mg
Potassium, 442 mg
Protein, 2 g
Vitamin C, 6.7 mg

Glycemic load: 2
Inflammatory index: Neutral

Beet, pickled

NUTRIENTS IN 1 CUP OF PICKLED BEET:

Calories, 148
Copper, 0.3 mg
Dietary fiber, 6 g
Folate, 61.3 mcg
Iron, 0.9 mg
Manganese, 0.5 mg
Protein, 2 g
Sodium, 599 mg
Vitamin C, 5.2 mg

HEALTH AND HEALING BENEFITS OF BEETS:

INTESTINAL HEALTH:

Dietary fiber helps food move through your digestive system and prevents constipation and diarrhea.

HEALTHY BONES:

Magnesium plays a role in maintaining healthy bones and controlling inflammation. Magnesium deficiency can lead to a significant amount of bone loss.

CARDIOVASCULAR HEALTH:

Fiber helps to lower blood cholesterol levels. Folate assists in cholesterol metabolism. Iron maintains healthy red blood cells and improves their ability to carry oxygen to cells around the body. Growing children and adolescents, as well as menstruating, pregnant, or lactating women, have an increased need for iron.

INCREASES BRAIN FUNCTION:

Folate is important in all aspects of brain function. It is helpful for pregnant women in particular, as it decreases the risk of spinal defects and brain delay in the fetus.

ANTIOXIDANTS:

Vitamin C is nature's own powerful antioxidant, helping to prevent cell damage. It is one of the most critical vitamins for supporting immune health. Manganese is a strong antioxidant that protects cells against damage and contributes to healthy skin.

Glycemic load: 5
Inflammatory index: Neutral

RECOMMENDED FOR HELP WITH:

- Constipation and diarrhea
- Lowering cholesterol levels
- Improves heart health
- Increasing brain function
- Immune health
- Healthy bones
- Healthy skin
- Good for pregnant women
- Iron-deficient anemia

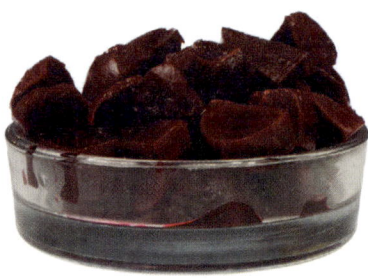

Carrot

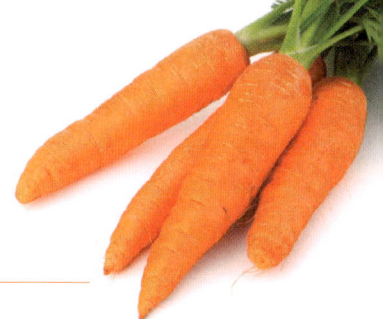

With the nickname of rabbit food, carrots are anything but basic animal feed. Raw carrots are a delicious, crunchy snack, but carrots also make tasty soups, nutritious sides, and are a delightful and colorful addition to stir-fries, casseroles, and stews. Carrots can now be found in white, purple, or red due to inventive breeding programs. Carrots are one of the richest sources of beta-carotene, which the body converts into vitamin A. Carrots also have no fat and no cholesterol, which makes them a great snack for anyone watching their weight.

Carrot, raw

NUTRIENTS IN 1 MEDIUM RAW CARROT:

Calories, 25
Dietary fiber, 1.7 g
Folate, 11.6 mcg
Manganese, 0.1 mg
Potassium, 195 mg
Vitamin A (RAE), 509 mcg
Vitamin K, 8.1 mcg

HEALTH AND HEALING BENEFITS:

INTESTINAL HEALTH:

Dietary fiber helps food move through your digestive system and prevents constipation and diarrhea.

LOWERS CHOLESTEROL:

Vitamin A lowers cholesterol in the bloodstream, reducing the risk of heart attack and stroke.

HEART AND BLOOD HEALTH:

Vitamin A reduces the risk of heart disease. Vitamin K is known as the "clotting" nutrient, as it helps blood to clot.

STRONG MUSCLES:

Potassium helps to build muscle and maintain body growth.

IMMUNE HEALTH:

Vitamin A is a powerful antioxidant that helps prevent cells from damage and promotes good immune health.

Glycemic load: 3
Inflammatory index: Mildly anti-inflammatory

RECOMMENDED FOR HELP WITH:

- Weight loss
- Good intestinal health
- Stroke and heart attack prevention
- Lowering cholesterol
- Improves heart health
- Immunity
- Promotes eye health

IMPROVED VISION AND EYE HEALTH:

Vitamin A works with other nutrients to improve vision, and night vision in particular, as well as promoting eye health.

Cauliflower

Most vegetables that are highly rated for their nutritional value are deep greens or bright reds—but in spite of its pale color, cauliflower is just as jam-packed with nutrients as its vivid cousins. It is very low in saturated fat and cholesterol, and a good source of both protein and dietary fiber. Delicious raw on its own or in dips, excellent in stir-fries and casseroles, cauliflower is a real powerhouse for its immune system and anti-cancer benefits.

NUTRIENTS IN 1 CUP OF CHOPPED CAULIFLOWER:

Calories, 27
Dietary fiber, 2.1 g
Folate, 61 mcg
Potassium, 320 mg
Protein, 2.1 g
Vitamin C, 51.6 mg
Vitamin K, 16.6 mcg

HEALTH AND HEALING BENEFITS:

GOOD IMMUNE HEALTH:

Vitamin C and folate strengthen the immune system, helpful for fighting colds and other illnesses.

STRONG MUSCLES:

Potassium helps to build muscle and maintain body growth.

CANCER PROTECTION:

An excellent source of phytonutrients that prevent cancer by reducing levels of hormones that stimulate tumor growth.

STRONG MUSCLES AND BONES:

A great source of complete protein, a building block of bones, muscles, blood, skin, nails, and hair. Protein helps build bones and repair tissues, hormones, and body chemicals.

HEART AND BLOOD HEALTH:

Vitamin K is known as the "clotting" nutrient, as it helps blood to clot. Folate reduces the risk of cardiovascular disease.

Glycemic load: 1
Inflammatory index: Mildly anti-inflammatory

RECOMMENDED FOR HELP WITH:

- Weight loss
- Good intestinal health
- Immunity
- Cancer protection
- Reducing risk of cardiovascular disease

INTESTINAL HEALTH:

Dietary fiber helps food move through your digestive system and prevents constipation and diarrhea.

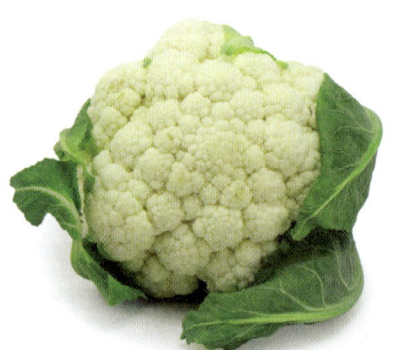

Corn

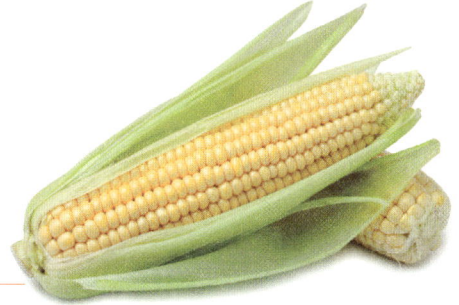

Corn is considered a nutritional powerhouse: it is a healthy, alkalizing food that is rich in antioxidants, low in saturated fat, cholesterol, and sodium, and is a good source of dietary fiber. Corn can be eaten as corn on the cob, boiled from frozen, or as baby corn in stir-fries or as a side dish. Corn also comes in a variety of colors, although yellow corn is the most common. This is often referred to as "sweetcorn" in the UK, but just simply "corn" in the United States. Corn is good for your heart, eyes, and digestion. If you suffer from kidney trouble, discuss potassium intake with your doctor.

NUTRIENTS IN 1 MEDIUM EAR OF YELLOW CORN (BOILED WITHOUT SALT):

Calories, 99
Dietary fiber, 2.5 g
Folate, 23.7 mcg
Potassium, 225 mg
Protein, 3.5 g
Thiamin, 0.1 mg
Vitamin C, 5.7 mg

HEALTH AND HEALING BENEFITS:

IMMUNE HEALTH:

Vitamin C and folate strengthen the immune system, helpful for fighting colds and other illnesses.

STRONG MUSCLES AND BONES:

A great source of complete protein, a building block of bones, muscles, blood, skin, nails, and hair. Protein helps build bones and repair tissues, hormones, and body chemicals.

INTESTINAL HEALTH:

Dietary fiber helps food move through your digestive system and prevents constipation and diarrhea.

HEART HEALTH AND CIRCULATION:

Corn is rich in antioxidants, which can reduce the risk of heart disease, as can folate. Potassium can improve blood pressure.

STRONG MUSCLES:

Potassium helps to build muscle and maintain body growth.

PROMOTES EYE HEALTH:

Corn contains lutein and zeaxanthin, which promote eye health and may protect against macular degeneration and cataracts.

Glycemic load: 3
Inflammatory index: Mildly anti-inflammatory

RECOMMENDED FOR HELP WITH:

- Immunity
- Good intestinal health, alleviating constipation and diarrhea
- Heart health and circulation
- Eye health, protecting against macular degeneration and cataracts
- Reducing risk of cardiovascular disease

Ginger root

Long used for its medicinal properties, fresh ginger root has a very high level of antioxidants. It can be used fresh or dried and is popular in Asian cooking, as well as in some desserts and teas, and has a fresh and distinctive flavor. Ginger has traditional uses as a nausea suppressant, and has been recommended to stave off feelings of nausea from chemotherapy, morning sickness, and travel sickness. If you experience heartburn or gallstones, consult your doctor before incorporating too much ginger into your diet.

NUTRIENTS: IN 1 TSP. FRESH CHOPPED GINGER:

Calories, 2
Calcium, 0.3 mg
Folate, 0.2 mcg
Magnesium, 0.9 mg
Phosphorus, 0.7 mg
Potassium, 9.3 mg
Vitamin C, 0.1 mg

HEALTH AND HEALING BENEFITS:

NAUSEA SUPPRESSANT:

Ginger is effective at reducing nausea, vomiting, and travel sickness.

IMMUNE HEALTH:

Magnesium supports a healthy immune system.

IMPROVED CIRCULATION AND HEART HEALTH:

The stimulatory effects of ginger can increase circulation. Potassium helps to keep the heart in good condition and maintains blood pressure.

REDUCES INFLAMMATION:

Ginger can help to reduce joint inflammation and reduces osteoarthritic pain.

STRONG BONES AND TEETH:

The mineral phosphorus plays an important role in bones and teeth. It helps in healthy bone formation, hormonal balance, and cellular repair.

Glycemic load: 0
Inflammatory index: Moderately anti-inflammatory

RECOMMENDED FOR HELP WITH:

- Nausea and upset stomach
- Nausea due to chemotherapy, travel sickness, pregnancy, and menstruation
- Improves immune health
- Improved circulation
- Reduces inflammation and osteoarthritic pain

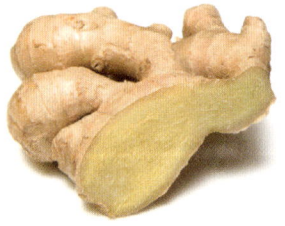

Parsnip

Parsnips are related to carrots, celeriac, and fennel. Parsnips are not a widely used root vegetable in the United States, but they are popular as a roasted side dish in Europe, and can also be made into a delicious spiced or curried soup. Parsnips are rich in antioxidants and a very good source of potassium, dietary fiber, vitamin C, folate, and manganese. They are also very low in saturated fat, cholesterol, and sodium.

NUTRIENTS IN 1 PARSNIP (BOILED WITHOUT SALT):

Calories, 114
Dietary fiber, 5.8 g
Folate, 92.6 mcg
Magnesium, 46.4 mg
Manganese, 0.5 mg
Phosphorus, 110 mg
Potassium, 587 mg
Vitamin C, 20.8 mg

HEALTH AND HEALING BENEFITS:

ENHANCED BRAIN FUNCTION:

Folate is important in all aspects of brain function, and is particularly important during pregnancy, for decreasing the risk of spinal defects and brain deficiencies in the fetus.

DIGESTIVE HEALTH:

Fiber can help ease constipation and promotes digestive health.

IMPROVED BLOOD AND HEART HEALTH:

Potassium helps to keep the heart in good condition and maintains blood pressure. Fiber can help lower high cholesterol and risk of heart disease. Vitamin K assists in healthy blood clotting.

Glycemic load: 2
Inflammatory index: Mildly anti-inflammatory

STRONG BONES AND TEETH:

The mineral phosphorus plays an important role in bones and teeth. It helps in healthy bone formation, hormonal balance, and cellular repair. Vitamin C also strengthens bone and teeth. Magnesium helps in bone formation.

RECOMMENDED FOR HELP WITH:

- Digestive health
- Maintaining blood pressure and cholesterol
- Enhanced brain function
- Strong bones and teeth

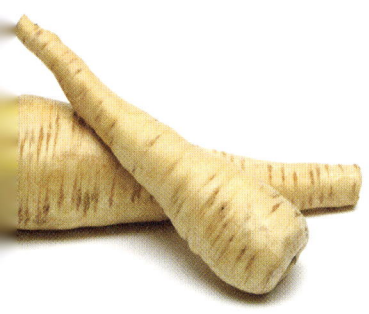

VEGETABLES, STARCHY

PUMPKIN

Not just a fun Halloween tradition, pumpkin is also a delicious and nutritious food. Beautiful in color and versatile to cook with, pumpkin is equally delicious in curries and casseroles as it is in desserts (but, of course, the sugars in most pies will outweigh the nutritional benefits, so keep this in moderation). While fresh whole pumpkin is best, canned pumpkin does still maintain a good amount of vitamins and minerals for a healthy diet. Pumpkin is a low-calorie, appetite-satisfying, alkalizing food that is rich in antioxidants.

Pumpkin, boiled without salt

NUTRIENTS IN 1 CUP OF MASHED PUMPKIN (BOILED WITHOUT SALT):

Calories, 44
Calcium, 36.8 mg
Folate, 22 mcg
Iron, 1.4 mg
Magnesium, 22 mg
Phosphorus, 73.5 mg
Potassium, 564 mg
Vitamin A (RAE), 706 mcg
Vitamin C, 11.5 mg

Glycemic load: 0
Inflammatory index: Moderately anti-inflammatory

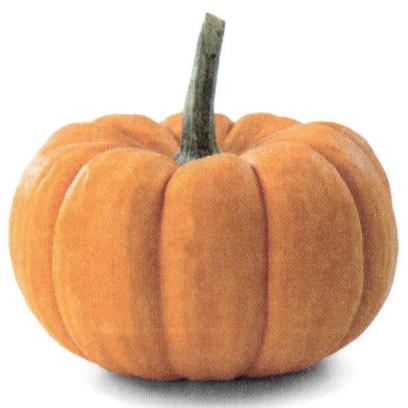

Pumpkin, canned without salt

NUTRIENTS IN 1 CUP OF PUMPKIN (CANNED WITHOUT SALT):

Calories, 83
Calcium, 63.7 mg
Dietary fiber, 7.1 g
Folate, 29.4 mcg
Magnesium, 56.4 mg
Phosphorus, 85.8 mg
Potassium, 505 mg
Vitamin A (RAE), 1,910 mcg
Vitamin C, 10.3 mg
Vitamin K, 39.2 mcg

HEALTH AND HEALING BENEFITS OF PUMPKINS:

ANTIOXIDANTS:

Vitamin A is a powerful antioxidant that helps strengthen and protect cells.

WEIGHT LOSS

Pumpkin is incredibly low in calories, which makes it a recommended food for controlling weight and cholesterol.

STRONG BONES AND TEETH:

The mineral phosphorus plays an important role in bones and teeth. It helps in healthy bone formation, hormonal balance, and cellular repair. Vitamin C also strengthens bones and teeth. Magnesium helps in bone formation.

EYE HEALTH AND VISION:

Pumpkin provides lutein and zeaxanthin, which promote eye health and protect against macular degeneration and cataracts.

ENHANCED BRAIN FUNCTION:

Folate is important in all aspects of brain function, and is particularly important during pregnancy, for decreasing the risk of spinal defects and brain deficiencies in the fetus.

PROMOTES DIGESTIVE HEALTH:

Fiber can help ease constipation and promotes digestive health.

Glycemic load: 1
Inflammatory index: Strongly anti-inflammatory

IMPROVED BLOOD AND HEART HEALTH:

Potassium helps to keep the heart in good condition and maintains blood pressure. Fiber can help lower high cholesterol and risk of heart disease. Vitamin K assists in healthy blood clotting. Vitamin A lowers cholesterol in the blood and reduces the risk of heart attack or stroke.

RECOMMENDED FOR HELP WITH:

- Digestive health
- Maintaining blood pressure and cholesterol
- Reducing risk of stroke and heart attack
- Eye health
- Enhanced brain function
- Strong bones and teeth
- Weight loss

Radish

A healthy, alkalizing food, radishes are often overlooked as a foodstuff and relegated to the place of a pretty garnish on the side of a plate. But think again. Radishes can be a tasty snack or crunchy salad addition, as well as great in soups or casseroles, and are packed with vitamin C, potassium, and fiber. As a low-calorie food, they are excellent for anyone watching their weight. White icicle radishes provide slightly more vitamin C.

NUTRIENTS IN 1 MEDIUM RAW RADISH:

Calories, 1
Calcium, 1.1 mg
Folate, 1.1 mcg
Magnesium, 0.5 mg
Phosphorus, 0.9 mg
Potassium, 10.5 mg
Vitamin C, 0.7 mg

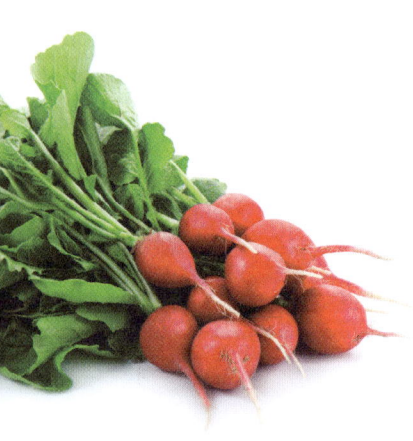

HEALTH AND HEALING BENEFITS:

WEIGHT LOSS

Radishes are incredibly low in calories, which makes them a recommended food for controlling weight and cholesterol.

CANCER PREVENTION:

Vitamin C helps to fight cellular damage that can lead to cancer.

STRONG BONES AND TEETH:

Vitamin C strengthens bones and teeth and helps rebuild tissues. The mineral phosphorus plays an important role in bones and teeth. It helps in healthy bone formation, hormonal balance, and cellular repair. Magnesium helps in bone formation.

ENHANCED BRAIN FUNCTION:

Folate is important in all aspects of brain function, and is particularly important during pregnancy, for decreasing the risk of spinal defects and brain deficiencies in the fetus.

IMPROVED BLOOD AND HEART HEALTH:

Potassium helps to keep the heart in good condition and maintains blood pressure. Vitamin C rebuilds blood vessels.

Glycemic load: 0
Inflammatory index: Anti-inflammatory

RECOMMENDED FOR HELP WITH:

- Enhanced brain function
- Blood pressure and cholesterol
- Strong bones and teeth
- Possible cancer prevention
- Weight loss

Rutabaga (swede)

A rutabaga (also called the swede or Swedish turnip) is a cruciferous root vegetable that is closely related to the turnip. Both the purple-yellow vegetable itself and the green leaves can be eaten. Rutabaga is most commonly either roasted or mashed. It is high in antioxidants and a good source of both fiber and vitamin C.

NUTRIENTS IN 1 MEDIUM RAW RUTABAGA:

Calories, 143
Calcium, 166 mg
Dietary fiber, 8.9 g
Folate, 81.1 mcg
Magnesium, 77.2 mg
Phosphorus, 205 mg
Potassium, 1,180 mg
Vitamin C, 96.5 mg

HEALTH AND HEALING BENEFITS:

ENHANCED BRAIN FUNCTION:

Folate is important in all aspects of brain function, and is particularly important during pregnancy, for decreasing the risk of spinal defects and brain deficiencies in the fetus.

IMMUNE HEALTH:

Vitamin C supports immune health.

DIGESTIVE HEALTH:

Potassium keeps the digestive tract moving and promotes digestive health.

IMPROVED BLOOD AND HEART HEALTH:

Potassium helps to keep the heart in good condition and maintains blood pressure. Vitamin C rebuilds blood vessels.

STRONG BONES AND TEETH:

Vitamin C strengthens bones and teeth and helps rebuild tissues. Calcium and the mineral phosphorus play an important role in bones and teeth, helping in healthy bone formation, hormonal balance, and cellular repair. Magnesium helps in bone formation.

HEALTHY SKIN:

Vitamin C keeps skin healthy by making collagen.

CANCER PREVENTION:

Vitamin C helps to fight cellular damage that can lead to cancer.

Glycemic load: 1
Inflammatory index: Anti-inflammatory

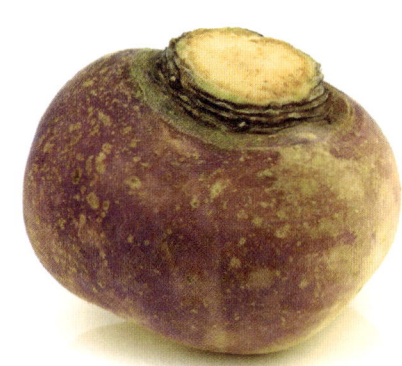

RECOMMENDED FOR HELP WITH:

- Immune health
- Digestive health
- Strong bones and teeth
- Healthy skin
- Cancer prevention, especially prostate and colon

SWEET POTATO

One of the healthiest of all vegetables, and certainly the healthiest of all starchy vegetables, sweet potatoes are delicious and versatile. Why not try them in place of a baked potato, mashed, or in casseroles for a healthy and filling meal? As mashed potatoes, they require very little butter and milk, making them a healthful alternative. Sweet potatoes are loaded with antioxidants and are a good source of dietary fiber (especially if you leave the skin on), potassium, and a huge array of vitamins, as well as being low in sodium, saturated fat, and cholesterol.

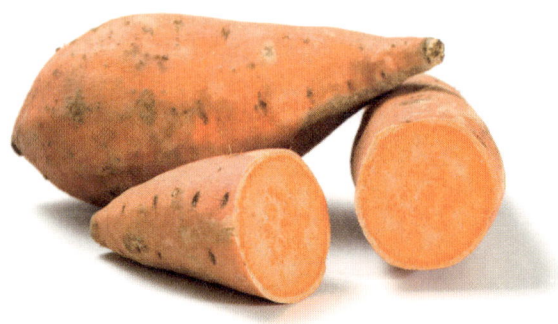

Sweet potato, baked in skin without salt

NUTRIENTS IN 1 MEDIUM SWEET POTATO (BAKED IN SKIN WITHOUT SALT):

Calories, 103
Calcium, 43.3 mg
Dietary fiber, 4 g
Folate, 6.8 mcg
Magnesium, 30.8 mg
Manganese, 0.6 mg
Niacin, 1.7 mg
Phosphorus, 61.6 mg
Potassium, 542 mg
Protein, 2 g
Riboflavin, 0.1 mg
Sodium, 41 mg
Thiamin, 0.1 mg
Vitamin A (RAE), 1,100 mcg
Vitamin B6, 0.3 mg
Vitamin C, 22.3 mg

Glycemic load: 10
Inflammatory index: Strongly anti-inflammatory

HEALTH AND HEALING BENEFITS:

IMMUNE HEALTH:

Vitamin A is a powerhouse for promoting immune health, supported by vitamin C. Vitamin A and copper are among the antioxidants in sweet potatoes, helping to boost the body's defenses.

DIGESTIVE HEALTH:

Dietary fiber promotes digestive regularity. Potassium keeps the digestive tract moving and promotes digestive health. Sweet potatoes are a huge source of dietary fiber, which encourages digestive efficiency.

MAINTAINS GOOD HEART AND BLOOD HEALTH:

Dietary fiber and vitamin A maintain good cholesterol levels in the blood and reduce the risk of stroke and heart attack. Copper promotes blood vessel health. Potassium helps to keep the heart in good condition and maintains blood pressure. Vitamin C rebuilds blood vessels.

EYE HEALTH:

Vitamin A promotes eye health and vision.

INCREASED ENERGY:

Copper is a good energy booster.

HEALTHY SKIN:

Vitamin C keeps skin healthy by making collagen. Manganese is a strong antioxidant that protects cells against damage and contributes to healthy skin.

STRONG BONES:

Protein helps build bones and repair tissues, hormones, and body chemicals. Phosphorus and calcium assist healthy bone formation.

ENHANCED BRAIN FUNCTION:

Folate is important in all aspects of brain function, and is particularly important during pregnancy, for decreasing the risk of spinal defects and brain deficiencies in the fetus.

CANCER PREVENTION:

Vitamin C helps to fight cellular damage that can lead to cancer.

RECOMMENDED FOR HELP WITH:

- Weight loss
- Immune health
- Digestive health and regularity
- Strong bones
- Healthy skin
- Eye health
- Increased energy
- Lowering cholesterol
- Reducing risk of stroke and heart attack
- Possible cancer prevention

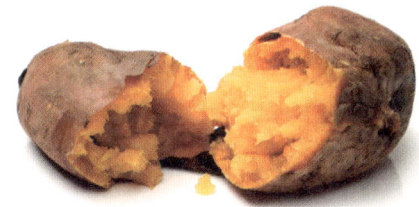

Turnip

Turnips are an incredibly nutritious root vegetable that are high in antioxidants. They are also a good source of dietary fiber, vitamins A, C, and K, as well as a range of other minerals. They are low in saturated fat, sodium, and cholesterol. Turnips are underused in everyday cooking, but they are delicious roasted on their own or alongside carrots and paired with meats and in casseroles. Turnips have a central role in Scottish tradition, being served in the Burns Night dish of haggis, neeps (turnips), and tatties (potatoes). Turnip greens provide fiber, folate, and very high vitamin K.

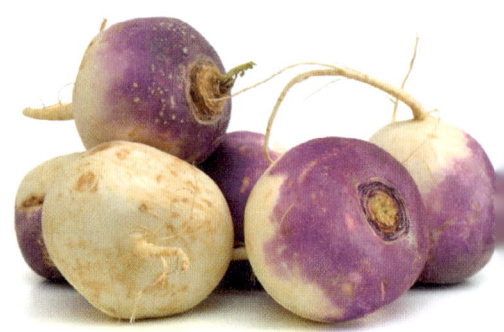

NUTRIENTS IN 1 CUP OF MASHED TURNIPS (BOILED WITHOUT SALT):

Calories, 51
Calcium, 75.9 mg
Dietary fiber, 4.6 g
Folate, 20.7 mcg
Magnesium, 20.7 mg
Phosphorus, 59.8 mg
Potassium, 407 mg
Vitamin C, 26.7 mg

HEALTH AND HEALING BENEFITS:

DIGESTIVE HEALTH:

Dietary fiber promotes digestive regularity and encourages digestive efficiency. Potassium keeps the digestive tract moving and promotes digestive health.

IMMUNE HEALTH:

Vitamin A is a powerhouse for promoting immune health, supported by vitamin C. Vitamin A helps to boost the energy's defenses.

MAINTAINS GOOD HEART AND BLOOD HEALTH:

Dietary fiber and vitamin A maintain good cholesterol levels in the blood and reduce the risk

Glycemic load: 0
Inflammatory index: Strongly anti-inflammatory

of stroke and heart attack. Potassium helps to keep the heart in good condition and maintains blood pressure. Vitamin C rebuilds blood vessels. Vitamin K promotes healthy blood clotting.

EYE HEALTH:

Vitamin A promotes eye health and vision.

GOOD METABOLISM:

Magnesium is a key mineral in healthy metabolism and energy production.

HEALTHY SKIN:

Vitamin C keeps skin healthy by making collagen.

STRONG BONES:

Protein helps build bones and repair tissues, hormones, and body chemicals. Phosphorus and calcium assist healthy bone formation, and magnesium helps to maintain healthy bones.

CANCER PREVENTION:

Vitamin C helps to fight cellular damage that can lead to cancer.

RECOMMENDED FOR HELP WITH:

- Immune health
- Digestive health and regularity
- Strong bones
- Healthy skin
- Eye health
- Lowering cholesterol
- Reducing risk of stroke and heart attack
- Possible cancer prevention, especially prostate and colon
- Weight loss

WINTER SQUASH

Winter squash comes in several varieties, including acorn, butternut, spaghetti, and more. Winter squash is a healthy, alkalizing food that is versatile and delectable—bake it whole, add it to a casserole, or make a warming winter soup. Winter squash is full of vitamin A, which improves lung health, and is a good source of folate, a beneficial vitamin during pregnancy.

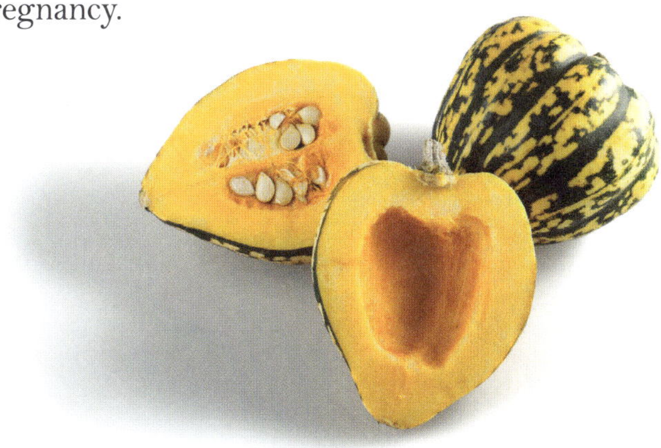

VEGETABLES, STARCHY

Winter squash, acorn

NUTRIENTS IN 1 CUP OF CUBED WINTER ACORN SQUASH (BAKED WITHOUT SALT):

Calories, 115
Calcium, 90.2 mg
Dietary fiber, 9 g
Folate, 39 mcg
Magnesium, 88.2 mg
Manganese, 0.5 mg
Phosphorus, 92.2 mg
Potassium, 896 mg
Vitamin B6, 0.4 mg
Vitamin C, 22.1 mg

Glycemic load: 0
Inflammatory index: Mildly anti-inflammatory

Winter squash, butternut, baked without salt

NUTRIENTS IN 1 CUP OF CUBED WINTER BUTTERNUT SQUASH (BAKED WITHOUT SALT):

Calories, 82
Calcium, 84 mg
Folate, 39 mcg
Iron, 1.2 mg
Magnesium, 59.4 mg
Phosphorus, 55.4 mg
Potassium, 582 mg
Vitamin A (RAE), 1,140 mcg
Vitamin C, 31 mg
Vitamin E, 2.6 mg

HEALTH AND HEALING BENEFITS OF WINTER SQUASH:

LUNG HEALTH:

Vitamin A is believed to promote lung health and may help to protect against emphysema.

PREGNANCY:

Folate is important in all aspects of brain function, and is particularly important during pregnancy, for decreasing the risk of spinal defects and brain deficiencies in the fetus.

Glycemic load: 0
Inflammatory index: Moderately anti-inflammatory

DIGESTIVE HEALTH:

Potassium keeps the digestive tract moving and promotes digestive health.

IMMUNE HEALTH:

Vitamin A is a powerhouse for promoting immune health, supported by vitamin C. Vitamin A and C help to boost the energy's defenses.

MAINTAINS GOOD HEART AND BLOOD HEALTH:

Vitamin A maintains good cholesterol levels in the blood and reduces the risk of stroke and heart attack. Potassium helps to keep the heart in good condition and maintains blood pressure. Vitamin C rebuilds blood vessels.

EYE HEALTH:

Vitamin A promotes eye health and vision.

GOOD METABOLISM:

Magnesium is a key mineral in healthy metabolism and energy production.

HEALTHY SKIN:

Vitamin C keeps skin healthy by making collagen.

STRONG BONES:

Phosphorus and calcium assist healthy bone formation, and magnesium helps to maintain healthy bones.

CANCER PREVENTION:

Vitamin C helps to fight cellular damage that can lead to cancer.

RECOMMENDED FOR HELP WITH:

- Lung health
- Pregnancy and health of fetus
- Immune health
- Digestive health
- Healthy skin
- Eye health
- Lowering cholesterol
- Reduce risk of stroke and heart attack

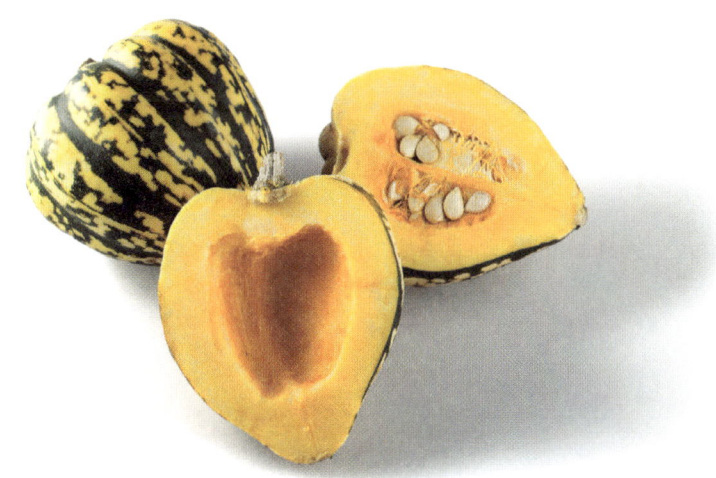

INDEX

abalone 188–189
acai 43–44
acerola 45
acid/basic balance 25
additives, artificial
   and processed 25
alfalfa seeds 130–131
allspice 112
almonds 161
   butter 161
   milk 33
   oil 162
amino acids:
   conditionally
     essential 16–19
   essential 13–16
   non-essential 19–21
anchovy 190
   canned in oil 190
   raw 190–191
antioxidants 6
apple 46
   juice 47
apricot 47–48
artichoke 249–250
arugula (rocket)
   248–249
asparagus 250–251
aubergine (eggplant)
   238–239
avocado 48–49

bacon:
   Canadian 146
   cured 146
banana 50
basil 113
bass 191
   freshwater 191
   sea 192–193
beef 138
   kidney 139
   liver 140
   raw, grass-fed 139
   round steak 140

tongue 141
beet 255
   greens 251–252
   pickled 256
bell peppers 252
   green 252
   red 253
beverages 25–26
blackberries 51
blueberries 52–53
bran flakes 103–104
Brazil nuts 162–163
bream (sea) 193–194
broccoli 253–254
Brussels sprouts
   254–255
burdock root 255

cabbage 256
   savoy 256–257
cantaloupe 53–54
carbohydrates 10–11
carp 195
carrot 287
   raw 287
cashew:
   butter 163
   nuts 164
catfish 196–197
cauliflower 288
caviar 197–198
celeriac 257–258
celery 258
cheese 27–28
cherries 54
   sour 55
   sweet 55
   tart juice 55–56
chestnuts 164–165
chia seeds 165–166
chicken 178
   breast meat 178
   dark meat (and
     thigh) 179
   drumstick 179

giblets 179
   liver 180
chickpeas (garbanzo
   beans) 131–132
chicory (curly endive)
   259
   greens 259–260
cinnamon 114
clams 198–199
cloves 115
cocoa powder 246
coconut:
   milk 34
   oil 58
   raw 57
cod 199
   Atlantic 200
   Pacific 200–201
collard greens
   261–262
corn 289
courgette (zucchini)
   258
crab (Alaska King),
   cooked 201–202
cranberries:
   juice, unsweetened
     59
   raw 58–59
crappie (wild) 203
cress, garden
   262–262
cucumber 262–263
cumin 116
curly endive (chicory)
   259
currants 59
   black 60

dairy 27–38
dandelion greens
   263–264
dark chocolate 247
dates 60–61
dill 117

duck 181

eel 203–204
eggplant (aubergine)
   238–239
eggs 39
   boiled 40
   chicken 39
   duck 42
   poached 40
   scrambled 41
   whole fried 41
elderberries, black
   62–63
endive, raw 265–266

fats 11–13
fennel 118
   bulb 266–267
figs 63–64
flaxseeds 167
   oil 167–168
flounder 204–205
French beans (green
   beans) 136
fruits and fruits
   juices 43–102

garbanzo beans
   (chickpeas)
   131–132
garlic 267–268
ginger root 290
ginkgo nuts 168–169
goat's milk 35
goose 182
grains 103–109
granola 104–103
grapefruit 64
   juice (pink) 65
   pink and red 64
   white 65
grapes 65
   green 66
   juice 67–68

   red 66–67
   white 66
green beans (French
   beans) 136
grouper 206–207
guava 68
   common 69
   nectar 70

haddock 207–208
halibut 209–210
ham:
   rump 148
   whole leg 148
haricot beans
   106–107
hazelnuts 169–170
herbs, spices, and
   seasonings
   110–129
herring 210
   Atlantic 111
   Pacific 111–112
honeydew 70–71

jalapeño, pepper
   274–275

kale 268
kefir 29
kidney beans
   133–134
kiwifruit 71–72

lamb 142
   chops 143
   leg of 143
   liver 144
   loin, cooked 142
leek 269
legumes 130–137
lemon 72–73
lemongrass 73–74
lettuce 270
   green leaf 270

iceberg 270
red leaf 271
lime 74–75
lobster 212–213
lychee 75–76

macadamia nuts 170
mackerel 214
   Atlantic 214
   jack 215
mandarin (satsuma) 76–77
mango:
   dried 79
   nectar, canned 79
   raw 77–78
meats 138–155
milk 30
   almond 33
   coconut 34
   goat's 35
   low-fat 31
   skim 32
   soy 36
   whole 30
minerals:
   toxic 24
   trace 21–24
mixed meats 145–150
monkfish 216
muesli 105–106
mullet 217
mushrooms 156–160
   morel 156
   Portobello 157
   shiitake 158
   shiitake, dried 159
   shiitake, raw 158
   white, button 160

nectarine 79–80
nuts and seeds 161–177

oats 106
   cereal 106–107
   whole (rolled) 107
   groats, whole 107
octopus 218–219
oils, culinary 26
okra 272
olives 80–81
onion 273
   red 273
   white 273–274
orange 81–82
   juice 83–84
oregano 119
oyster 219–221

Paleo diet 4
papaya 84–85
parsley 120
parsnip 291
passion fruit 85–86
peach 87
   canned 87–88
   fresh 87
   nectar (canned) 88
peanut butter 135
peanuts 134
pear 89
   dried 90
pecan nut 171
pepper
   bell 252-253
   jalapeño 274–275
peppermint 121
perch (ocean) 221–222
pheasant 183
pike 222–223
pine nuts 171–172
pineapple 90–91
   juice (unsweetened) 91
pistachio nuts 172–173
plum 92
   fresh 92–93
   prune (dried plum) 93–94
pollock (Atlantic) 224
pomegranate 94
   fresh 95–95
   juice 96
pork 145–149
   bacon, Canadian 146
   bacon, cured 146
   chops, center loin 147
   ground 147
   ham, rump 148
   ham, whole leg 148
   liver cheese, pork 149
   tenderloin 149–150
poultry 178–187
prune (dried plum) 93–94
pumpkin 292
   boiled without salt 292
   canned without salt 293
   seeds 173–174

quail 184

radicchio (red chicory) 275–276
radish 294
raspberries 96–97
red chicory (radicchio) 275–276
red snapper 225
rhubarb 98
rice:
   black 108
   brown 109
rocket (arugula) 248–249
roe 226–227
rose hips 99
rosemary 122
roughy (orange) 227–228
rutabaga (swede) 295

saffron 123
sage 124
salmon 228
   chinook, smoked 229
   chum, cooked 230
   farmed, Atlantic 229
   pink, canned 230
   red, smoked 231
sardines (Atlantic) 232
satsuma (mandarin) 76–77
scallion (spring onion) 276–277
scallops 233
sea bream 193–194
seafood and fish 188–245
sesame seeds 174–175
shrimp 234–235
snow peas 137
sole (flatfish) 235–236
sorghum bran 9125
soy milk 36
soy sauce 126
spinach 277–278
spring onion (scallion) 276-277
strawberries 100
sturgeon 236–237
sugar snap peas 137
sunflower seeds 175–176
sweet potato 296
   baked in skin without salt 296–297
Swiss chard 278–279
swede (rutabaga) 295
swordfish 237–238

tangerine 101
tarragon 127
thyme 128
tilapia 239–240
tomato 279
   juice, canned without salt 280
   orange 280
   red 280
   sauce, no salt 281
   sun-dried 281
treats 246–247
trout 240–241
tuna 241–242
   bluefin 242
   light, canned in oil 243–244
   yellowfin/ahi 242
turkey 185
   bacon 185
   breast 185
   dark meat (and thigh) 186
   drumstick 186
   giblets 186
   ground 186
   liver 187
turmeric 129
turnip 298–299

veal 150
   breast 151
   chops, sirloin 151
   liver 151
   loin 152
   rump 152
   shoulder 153
vegetables:
   non-starchy 248–284
   starchy 285–301
venison 154
   ground 154
   loin 155
vitamins, essential 7–10

wakame seaweed 282
walnuts 176
   black 177
   English 177
watercress 283
watermelon 101–102
whitefish 244–245
whiting 245
winter squash 299
   acorn 300
   butternut, baked without salt 300–301

yogurt:
   Greek 38
   plain 37

zucchini (courgette) 258

SELECT BIBLIOGRAPHY

American Heart Association website: www.heart.org

American Pregnancy Association website: www.americanpregnancy.org

Calorie Count website: http://www.caloriescount.com

Davis, W. (2012) *Wheat Belly*. New York, NY: Harper Collins

Duffy, W. (1976) *Sugar Blues*. New York, NY: Warner Books.

Eat This Much diet website: http://www.eatthismuch.com/

Fazekas, I. (2005) *The Alkalizing Diet*. Virginia Beach, VA: A.R.E. Press.

Filippo, D. (2012) *Practical Paleo*. Riverside, NJ: Victory Belt Publishing.

Heal with Food website: http://www.healwithfood.org

Livestrong Nutrition website: http://www.livestrong.com/food/

McKeith, G. (2006) *You Are What You Eat: The Plan That Will Change Your Life*. New York, NY: Penguin Adult.

Nutrition and You website: http://www.nutrition-and-you.com

Perlmutter, D. (2013) *Grain Brain*. New York, NY: Little Brown & Company

Price, W.A. (2004) *Nutrition and Physical Degeneration*, 6th Edition. Loveland, CO: Price-Pottenger Nutrition Foundation.

Schlosser, E. (2001) *Fast Food Nation*. Boston, MA: Houghton Mifflin Co.

U.S. Department of Agriculture Food and Nutrition website: http://www.usda.gov/wps/portal/usda/usdahome?navid=food-nutrition

U.S. Department of Agriculture FoodData Central website: https://fdc.nal.usda.gov

White, E.G. (1976) *A Study Guide: Counsels on Diet and Foods*. Hagerstown, MD: Review and Harold Publishing Association.

Every care has been taken to trace copyright holders. However, if there have been unintentional omissions or failure to trace copyright holders, we apologize and will, if informed, endeavor to make corrections in any future edition.